DSM-5-TR™
CLINICAL CASES

DSM-5-TR™ CLINICAL CASES

EDITED BY

John W. Barnhill, M.D.

Professor of Clinical Psychiatry
DeWitt Wallace Senior Scholar
Vice Chair for Psychosomatic Medicine
Department of Psychiatry
Weill Cornell Medical College

Chief, Consultation-Liaison Service
New York-Presbyterian Hospital/
Weill Cornell Medical Center

Faculty, Columbia University Center
for Psychoanalytic Training & Research
New York, New York

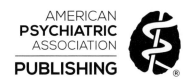

AMERICAN
PSYCHIATRIC
ASSOCIATION
PUBLISHING

If you wish to buy 50 or more copies of the same title, please go to www.appi.org/specialdiscounts for more information.

Copyright © 2023 American Psychiatric Association Publishing

ALL RIGHTS RESERVED

First Edition

Manufactured in the United States of America on acid-free paper
27 26 25 24 23   5 4 3 2 1
ISBN 978-1-61537-361-1 (print), 978-1-61537-362-8 (ebook)

American Psychiatric Association Publishing
800 Maine Avenue SW, Suite 900
Washington, DC 20024-2812
www.appi.org

Library of Congress Cataloging-in-Publication Data
Names: Barnhill, John W. (John Warren), 1959– editor. | American
    Psychiatric Association Publishing, issuing body.
Title: DSM-5-TR clinical cases / edited by John W. Barnhill.
Description: First edition. | Washington : American Psychiatric Association
    Publishing, [2023] | Includes bibliographical references and index.
Identifiers: LCCN 2022049312 (print) | LCCN 2022049313 (ebook) | ISBN
    9781615373611 (paperback) | ISBN 9781615373628 (ebook)
Subjects: MESH: Diagnostic and statistical manual of mental disorders. ‡s
    5th ed | Mental Disorders–diagnosis | Case Reports
Classification: LCC RC473.D54 (print) | LCC RC473.D54 (ebook) | NLM WM 40
    | DDC 616.89/075–dc23/eng/20230113
LC record available at https://lccn.loc.gov/2022049312
LC ebook record available at https://lccn.loc.gov/2022049313

British Library Cataloguing in Publication Data
A CIP record is available from the British Library.

Contents

19 Paraphilic Disorders. 345

Contributors

Jamie Miller Abelson, M.S.W.
Program Manager, Curtis Center for Health Equity Research and Training, University of Michigan (Ann Arbor, MI)

Stewart Adelson, M.D.
Clinical Associate Professor of Psychiatry, Weill Cornell Medicine (New York City)

Anthony O. Ahmed, Ph.D.
Associate Professor of Psychology in Clinical Psychiatry, Weill Cornell Medicine (White Plains, NY)

Salman Akhtar, M.D.
Professor of Psychiatry, Thomas Jefferson Medical College (Philadelphia, PA)

George S. Alexopoulos, M.D.
Professor Emeritus of Psychiatry, Weill Cornell Medicine (White Plains, NY)

Margaret Altemus, M.D.
Associate Professor of Psychiatry, Yale University School of Medicine (New Haven, CT)

Paul S. Appelbaum, M.D.
Elizabeth K. Dollard Professor of Psychiatry, Medicine, and Law, Vagelos College of Physicians and Surgeons, Columbia University (New York City)

Evelyn Attia, M.D.
Professor of Psychiatry, Vagelos College of Physicians and Surgeons, Columbia University and Professor of Clinical Psychiatry, Weill Cornell Medicine (New York City)

Elizabeth L. Auchincloss, M.D.
Clinical Professor of Psychiatry, Weill Cornell Medicine (New York City)

Jonathan Avery, M.D.
Stephen P. Tobin and Dr. Arnold M. Cooper Associate Professor in Consultation-Liaison Psychiatry, Weill Cornell Medicine (New York City)

Richard Balon, M.D.
Professor of Clinical Psychiatry and Anesthesiology, Wayne State University School of Medicine (Detroit, MI)

John W. Barnhill, M.D.
Professor of Clinical Psychiatry and DeWitt Wallace Senior Scholar, Weill Cornell Medicine, and Adjunct Clinical Professor of Psychiatry, Vagelos College of Physicians and Surgeons, Columbia University (New York City)

Anne E. Becker, M.D., Ph.D.
Maude and Lillian Presley Professor of Global Health and Social Medicine, Harvard Medical School (Boston, MA)

Eugene Beresin, M.D.
Professor of Psychiatry, Harvard Medical School (Boston, MA)

Silvia Bernardi, M.D.
Assistant Professor of Clinical Psychiatry, Vagelos College of Physicians and Surgeons, Columbia University (New York City)

Carlos Blanco, M.D., Ph.D.
Director, Division of Epidemiology, Services, and Prevention Research, National Institute on Drug Abuse, National Institutes of Health (Bethesda, MD)

Susan Bögels, Ph.D.
Professor in Psychology, University of Amsterdam (Amsterdam, Netherlands)

Robert Boland, M.D.
Brown Foundation Endowed Chair and Professor of Psychiatry, Baylor College of Medicine (Houston, TX)

James A. Bourgeois, O.D., M.D.
Professor of Psychiatry, University of California Davis School of Medicine (Sacramento, CA)

Benjamin Brody, M.D.
Associate Professor of Clinical Psychiatry, Weill Cornell Medicine (New York City)

Deborah L. Cabaniss, M.D.
Professor of Clinical Psychiatry, Vagelos College of Physicians and Surgeons, Columbia University (New York City)

Kristin Cadenhead, M.D.
Professor of Psychiatry, University of California San Diego School of Medicine (La Jolla, CA)

Jason P. Caplan, M.D.
Chair of Psychiatry, St. Joseph's Hospital and Medical Center (Phoenix, AZ)

Emil F. Coccaro, M.D.
George T. Harding III, M.D., Endowed Chair in Psychiatry and Professor, Department of Psychiatry and Behavioral Health, Wexner Medical Center, Ohio State University (Columbus, OH)

Victoria E. Cosgrove, Ph.D.
Clinical Associate Professor of Psychiatry, Stanford University School of Medicine (Stanford, CA)

Catherine Crone, M.D.
Associate Professor of Psychiatry, George Washington University School of Medicine (Washington, DC)

Jessica Daniels, M.D.
Psychiatrist, Edward P. Boland Department of Veterans Affairs Medical Center (Leeds, MA)

Lori L. Davis, M.D.
Clinical Professor of Psychiatry, University of Alabama Health System (Birmingham, AL)

Anna Dickerman, M.D.
Associate Professor of Clinical Psychiatry, Weill Cornell Medicine (New York City)

Andrea DiMartini, M.D.
Professor of Psychiatry, Surgery, and Clinical and Translational Science, University of Pittsburgh School of Medicine (Pittsburgh, PA)

Arden D. Dingle, M.D.
Professor of Psychiatry & Behavioral Sciences, School of Medicine, University of Nevada (Reno, NV)

Coreen Domingo, D.P.H., M.P.H.
Assistant Professor of Psychiatry and Behavioral Sciences, Baylor College of Medicine (Houston, TX)

Carlo Faravelli, M.D.
Professor of Psychiatry, University of Florence (Florence, Italy)

J. Paul Fedoroff, M.D.
Professor of Psychiatry, University of Ottawa (Ottawa, Ontario, Canada)

Lorena Fernández de la Cruz, Ph.D.
Associate Professor, Centre for Psychiatry Research, Department of Clinical Neuroscience, Karolinska Institutet (Stockholm, Sweden)

Stephen J. Ferrando, M.D.
Har Esh Professor and Chair, Department of Psychiatry and Behavioral Sciences, New York Medical College (Valhalla, NY)

Robert L. Findling, M.D., M.B.A.
Professor and Chair, Department of Psychiatry, Virginia Commonwealth University (Richmond, VA)

Eve K. Freidl, M.D.
Associate Professor of Psychiatry, Icahn School of Medicine at Mount Sinai (New York City)

Matthew J. Friedman, M.D., Ph.D.
Professor of Psychiatry, Geisel School of Medicine, Dartmouth College (Hanover, NH)

Richard A. Friedman, M.D.
Professor of Clinical Psychiatry, Weill Cornell Medicine (New York City)

James E. Galvin, M.D., M.P.H.
Professor of Neurology and of Psychiatry & Behavioral Sciences, Miller School of Medicine, University of Miami (Miami, FL)

Michael Gitlin, M.D.
Professor of Clinical Psychiatry, Geffen School of Medicine at UCLA (Los Angeles, CA)

Joseph F. Goldberg, M.D.
Clinical Professor of Psychiatry, Icahn School of Medicine at Mount Sinai (New York City)

Janna Gordon-Elliott, M.D.
Associate Professor of Clinical Psychiatry, Weill Cornell Medicine (New York City)

Cynthia A. Graham, Ph.D.
Professor in Sexual and Reproductive Health, Department of Psychology, University of Southampton (Southampton, England)

Robert E. Hales, M.D., M.B.A.
Professor of Psychiatry and Behavioral Sciences, University of California Davis School of Medicine (Sacramento, CA)

Robert Haskell, M.D.
Psychiatrist, Department of Mental Health, Los Angeles County Department of Children and Family Services (Los Angeles, CA)

Donald M. Hilty, M.D.
Professor of Psychiatry and Behavioral Sciences, University of California Davis School of Medicine (Sacramento, CA)

Heather B. Howell, M.S.W.
Clinical Social Worker, Yale University School of Medicine (New Haven, CT)

Ian Jones, M.R.C.Psych., Ph.D.
Professor of Psychiatry, Division of Psychological Medicine and Clinical Neurosciences, Cardiff University School of Medicine (Cardiff, Wales)

Loes Jongerden, M.A.
Psychologist, GGZ Ingeest (Amstelveen, Netherlands)

Vishesh K. Kapur, M.D., M.P.H.
Professor of Medicine, University of Washington School of Medicine (Seattle, WA)

Otto Kernberg, M.D.
Professor Emeritus of Psychiatry, Weill Cornell Medicine (New York City)

Barbara J. Kocsis, M.D.
Psychiatrist, Sacramento, California

Thomas R. Kosten, M.D.
Jay H. Waggoner Endowed Chair and Professor of Psychiatry, Baylor College of Medicine (Houston, TX)

Peter D. Kramer, M.D.
Clinical Professor Emeritus of Psychiatry and Human Behavior, Alpert Medical School, Brown University (Providence, RI)

Britney Lambert, M.D.
Fellow, Department of Psychiatry and Behavioral Sciences, Baylor College of Medicine (Houston, TX)

Ryan E. Lawrence, M.D.
Associate Professor of Psychiatry, Vagelos College of Physicians and Surgeons, Columbia University (New York City)

Christopher M. Layne, Ph.D.
Associate Professor of Psychology, Nova Southeastern University (Colorado Springs, CO)

James L. Levenson, M.D.
Rhona Arenstein Professor of Psychiatry, Virginia Commonwealth University School of Medicine (Richmond, VA)

Petros Levounis, M.D., M.A.
Professor and Chair of Psychiatry, Rutgers New Jersey Medical School (Newark, NJ)

Roberto Lewis-Fernández, M.D.
Professor of Clinical Psychiatry, Vagelos College of Physicians and Surgeons, Columbia University (New York City)

Russell F. Lim, M.D.
Clinical Professor of Psychiatry and Behavioral Sciences, University of California Davis School of Medicine (Sacramento, CA)

Richard J. Loewenstein, M.D.
Clinical Professor of Psychiatry, School of Medicine, University of Maryland (Baltimore, MD)

Catherine Lord, Ph.D.
George Tarjan Distinguished Professor of Psychiatry, Geffen School of Medicine at UCLA (Los Angeles, CA)

Dolores Malaspina, M.D., M.P.H.
Professor of Psychiatry, Neuroscience, and Genetics and Genomic Science, Icahn School of Medicine at Mount Sinai (New York City)

José R. Maldonado, M.D.
Professor of Psychiatry and John and Terry Levin Family Professor of Medicine, Stanford University School of Medicine (Stanford, CA)

David Mataix-Cols, Ph.D.
Honorary Senior Research Fellow, Institute of Psychiatry, King's College London (London, England)

Sofia E. Matta, M.D.
Psychiatrist, Salem Hospital, Mass General Brigham (Salem, MA)

Christopher McDougle, M.D.
Nancy Lurie Marks Professor of Psychiatry, Harvard Medical School (Boston, MA)

Susan L. McElroy, M.D.
Professor of Psychiatry, University of Cincinnati College of Medicine (Cincinnati, OH)

Thomas W. Meeks, M.D.
Associate Professor of Psychiatry, Oregon Health & Science University (Portland, OR)

Katharina Meyerbröker, Ph.D.
Assistant Professor of Clinical Psychology, University of Utrecht (Utrecht, Netherlands)

Robert Michels, M.D.
Walsh McDermott University Professor of Medicine and University Professor of Psychiatry, Weill Cornell Medicine (New York City)

Barbara L. Milrod, M.D.
Professor of Psychiatry and Behavioral Sciences. Albert Einstein College of Medicine (New York City)

James E. Mitchell, M.D.
Chester Fritz University Professor of Psychiatry, School of Medicine, University of North Dakota (Fargo, ND)

Lianne K. Morris Smith, M.D.
Psychiatrist, New York, New York

Megan Mroczkowski, M.D.
Assistant Professor of Psychiatry, Vagelos College of Physicians and Surgeons, Columbia University (New York City)

Cheryl C. Munday, Ph.D.
Retired Professor of Psychology, College of Liberal Arts and Education, University of Detroit Mercy (Detroit, MI)

Joseph F. Murray, M.D.
Associate Professor of Clinical Psychiatry, Weill Cornell Medicine (New York City)

Melissa Nau, M.D.
Psychiatrist, Park City, Utah

Nancy J. Needell, M.D.
Assistant Professor of Clinical Psychiatry, Weill Cornell Medicine (New York City)

Jeffrey H. Newcorn, M.D.
Professor of Psychiatry and Pediatrics, Icahn School of Medicine at Mount Sinai (New York City)

Edward V. Nunes, M.D.
Professor of Psychiatry, Vagelos College of Physicians and Surgeons, Columbia University (New York City)

Maurice M. Ohayon, M.D., D.Sc., Ph.D.
Professor of Psychiatry and Behavioral Sciences, Stanford University School of Medicine (Stanford, CA)

Mayumi Okuda, M.D.
Assistant Professor of Psychiatry, Vagelos College of Physicians and Surgeons, Columbia University (New York City)

Maria A. Oquendo, M.D.
Ruth Meltzer Professor and Chair of Psychiatry, Perelman School of Medicine, University of Pennsylvania (Philadelphia, PA)

Brian Palen, M.D.
Associate Professor of Medicine, University of Washington School of Medicine (Seattle, WA)

Kathy P. Parker, Ph.D., R.N.
Psychiatric Nurse Practitioner, Rochester, New York

Juan D. Pedraza, M.D.
Assistant Professor of Psychiatry, Icahn School of Medicine at Mount Sinai (New York City)

Julie B. Penzner, M.D.
Associate Professor of Psychiatry and Behavioral Sciences, Duke University School of Medicine (Durham, NC)

J. Christopher Perry, M.P.H., M.D.
Professor of Psychiatry, Faculty of Medicine and Health Sciences, McGill University (Montreal, Quebec, Canada)

Cynthia R. Pfeffer, M.D.
Professor of Psychiatry, Weill Cornell Medicine (New York City)

Katharine A. Phillips, M.D.
Professor of Psychiatry and DeWitt Wallace Senior Scholar, Weill Cornell Medicine (New York City)

Robert S. Pynoos, M.D., M.P.H.
Professor of Psychiatry and Biobehavioral Sciences, Geffen School of Medicine at UCLA (Los Angeles, CA)

Raymond Raad, M.D., M.P.H.
Psychiatrist, New York, New York

Peter V. Rabins, M.D., M.P.H.
Richman Family Professor of Alzheimer's and Related Diseases, Johns Hopkins University School of Medicine (Baltimore, MD)

Charles F. Reynolds III, M.D.
UPMC Endowed Professor in Geriatric Psychiatry, University of Pittsburgh School of Medicine (Pittsburgh, PA)

Stephen Ross, M.D.
Associate Professor of Psychiatry, Grossman School of Medicine, New York University (New York City)

Anthony J. Rothschild, M.D.
Irving S. and Betty Brudnick Endowed Chair and Professor of Psychiatry, T.H. Chan School of Medicine, University of Massachusetts (Worcester, MA)

David H. Rubin, M.D.
Assistant Professor of Psychiatry, Harvard Medical School (Boston, MA)

Lauren Z. Rynar, Ph.D.
Assistant Professor, Department of Psychiatry and Behavioral Sciences, Rush University Medical College (Chicago, IL)

Susan Samuels, M.D.
Assistant Professor of Clinical Psychiatry, Weill Cornell Medicine (New York City)

Daniel S. Schechter, M.D.
Associate Professor of Psychiatry, Lausanne University (Vaud, Switzerland)

Lorin M. Scher, M.D.
Roy T. Brophy Endowed Chair and Professor of Psychiatry and Behavioral Sciences, University of California Davis School of Medicine (Sacramento, CA)

Marc A. Schuckit, M.D.
Professor of Psychiatry, University of California San Diego School of Medicine (La Jolla, CA)

Charles L. Scott, M.D.
Professor of Psychiatry and Behavioral Sciences, University of California Davis School of Medicine (Sacramento, CA)

Daryl Shorter, M.D.
Associate Professor of Psychiatry, Baylor College of Medicine (Houston, TX)

Collin Shumate, M.D.
Fellow, Department of Psychiatry and Behavioral Sciences, University of California Davis School of Medicine (Sacramento, CA)

Larry J. Siever, M.D.‡
Formerly Director, Mood and Personality Disorders Program, Icahn School of Medicine at Mount Sinai (New York City)

Charles H. Silberstein, M.D.
Psychiatrist, Martha's Vineyard, Massachusetts

Daphne Simeon, M.D.
Associate Clinical Professor of Psychiatry, Icahn School of Medicine at Mount Sinai (New York City)

Helen Blair Simpson, M.D., Ph.D.
Professor of Psychiatry, Vagelos College of Physicians and Surgeons, Columbia University (New York City)

Dan J. Stein, M.D., Ph.D.
Professor and Chair of the Department of Psychiatry, Faculty of Health Sciences, University of Cape Town (Cape Town, South Africa)

Alan M. Steinberg, Ph.D.
Chief Science Officer, Behavioral Health Innovations (Los Angeles, CA)

Theodore A. Stern, M.D.
Ned H. Cassem Professor of Psychiatry, Harvard Medical School (Boston, MA)

William S. Stone, Ph.D.
Associate Professor of Psychology, Department of Psychiatry, Harvard Medical School (Boston, MA)

Trisha Suppes, M.D., Ph.D.
Professor of Psychiatry and Behavioral Sciences, Stanford University School of Medicine (Stanford, CA)

Holly A. Swartz, M.D.
Professor of Psychiatry, University of Pittsburgh School of Medicine (Pittsburgh, PA)

Carol A. Tamminga, M.D.
Lou and Ellen McGinley Distinguished Chair and McKenzie Chair in Psychiatry, University of Texas Southwestern Medical School (Dallas, TX)

Rajiv Tandon, M.D.
Professor Emeritus of Psychiatry, Homer Stryker M.D. School of Medicine, Western Michigan University (Kalamazoo, MI)

---

‡ Deceased.

Rosemary Tannock, Ph.D.
Canada Research Chair, University of Toronto (Toronto, Ontario, Canada)

Robyn Thom, M.D.
Instructor of Psychiatry, Harvard Medical School (Boston, MA)

Jennifer J. Thomas, Ph.D.
Associate Professor of Psychology in the Department of Psychiatry, Harvard Medical School (Boston, MA)

Ming T. Tsuang, M.D., Ph.D., D.Sc.
Behavioral Genomics Endowed Chair and University Professor, University of California, and Distinguished Professor of Psychiatry, University of California San Diego School of Medicine (La Jolla, CA)

John T. Walkup, M.D.
Margaret C. Osterman Professor and Chair of Psychiatry, Ann and Robert H. Lurie Children's Hospital of Chicago; Professor of Psychiatry, Feinberg School of Medicine, Northwestern University (Chicago, IL)

Michael F. Walton, M.D.
Associate Professor, Department of Psychiatry and Behavioral Sciences, University of Washington School of Medicine, Seattle; Medical Director, St. Luke's Behavioral Health (Boise and McCall, ID)

Heather Warm, M.D.
Psychiatrist, San Francisco, California

Roger D. Weiss, M.D.
Professor of Psychiatry, Harvard Medical School (Boston, MA)

William C. Wood, M.D.
Clinical Assistant Professor of Psychiatry, Weill Cornell Medicine (New York City)

Frank Yeomans, M.D., Ph.D.
Clinical Associate Professor of Psychiatry, Weill Cornell Medicine (New York City)

Kimberly A. Yonkers, M.D.
Professor and Katz Family Chair in Psychiatry, T.H. Chan School of Medicine, University of Massachusetts (Worcester, MA)

Stuart C. Yudofsky, M.D.
Distinguished Professor Emeritus, Menninger Department of Psychiatry & Behavioral Sciences, Baylor College of Medicine (Houston, TX)

Disclosure of Interests

The following contributors to this book have indicated a financial interest in or other affiliation with a commercial supporter, a manufacturer of a commercial product, a provider of a commercial service, a nongovernmental organization, and/or a government agency, as listed below:

George S. Alexopoulos, M.D.—*Advisory board:* Eisai and Janssen. *Speakers' bureau:* Otsuka.

Robert L. Findling, M.D., M.B.A.— *Research support, consulting, and/or honoraria:* Acadia, Adamas, Aevi, Afecta, Akili, Alkermes, Allergan, American Academy of Child & Adolescent Psychiatry, American Psychiatric Association Publishing, Arbor, Axsome, Daiichi-Sankyo, Emelex, Gedeon Richter, Genentech, Idorsia, Intra-Cellular Therapies, Kempharm, Luminopia, Lundbeck, Med-Avante-ProPhase, Merck, MJH Life Sciences, NIH, Neurim, Otsuka, PaxMedica, PCORI, Pfizer, Physicians Postgraduate Press, Q BioMed, Receptor Life Sciences, Roche, Sage, Signant Health, Sunovion, Supernus Pharmaceuticals, Syneos, Syneurx, Takeda, Teva, Tris, and Validus.

Joseph F. Goldberg, M.D.—*Speakers' bureau:* Abbvie, Alkermes, Axsome, Intracellular Therapies, and Sunovion. *Consultant:* BioXcel, Jazz Pharmaceuticals,

Lundbeck, Otsuka, Sunovion, and Supemus. *Royalties:* American Psychiatric Association Publishing and Cambridge University Press.

David Mataix-Cols, Ph.D.—*Royalties:* Wolters Kluwer Health (UpToDate®).

Christopher McDougle, M.D.—*Consulting:* Acadia Pharmaceuticals, Precidiag, Receptor Life Sciences, and Sage Therapeutics. *Royalties:* Oxford University Press and Springer Publishing.

Katharine A. Phillips, M.D.—*Royalties:* American Psychiatric Association Publishing (author), Guilford Publications (author), International Creative Management, Inc. (author), Oxford University Press (author), and Wolters Kluwer (UpToDate®). *Honoraria:* Informa Exhibitions (speaker at Miami Cosmetic Surgery and Aesthetic Dermatology Conference), L'Oreal (presentation for Medscape), Merck Manual (author), OCD scales (developer), other academic institutions and professional societies (speaker), and Simple and Practical Medical Education (author).

Peter V. Rabins, M.D., M.P.H.—*Royalties:* The Johns Hopkins University Press (books).

Anthony J. Rothschild, M.D.—*Grant/ research support:* Allergan, Eli Lilly (medications for a National Institutes of Health (NIH)–funded clinical trial), Janssen, National Institute of Mental Health, Otsuka, Pfizer (medications for a NIH–funded clinical trial), Praxis, and the Irving S. and Betty Brudnick Endowed Chair in Psychiatry (University of Massachusetts Medical School). *Consulting:* Janssen, Praxis, Sage Therapeutics, Xenon Pharmaceuticals, and several generic medication companies. *Royalties:* American Psychiatric Association Publishing (books), Lippincott Williams &

Wilkins (Editor-in-Chief of *Journal of Clinical Psychopharmacology*), University of Massachusetts Medical School (Rothschild Scale for Antidepressant Tachyphylaxis [RSAT®]), and Wolters Kluwer Health (UpToDate®).

Collin Shumate, M.D.—*Travel support:* APA/APAF Public Psychiatry Fellowship (funding to attend APA conferences).

Trisha Suppes, M.D., Ph.D.—*Research funding/medications for clinical grants:* Compass Pathways, Merck, National Institute on Drug Abuse, National Institutes of Health, VA Cooperative Studies Program, VA OR&D PRIME Care. *Consulting agreements/advisory boards/speaking engagements:* Merck Research Laboratories, Sunovion Pharmaceuticals. *Continuing medical education honoraria:* Clinical Education Alliance, Integrity Continuing Education, Medscape (WebMD). *Royalties:* American Psychiatric Association Publishing, Hogrefe Publishing, Jones & Bartlett, Wolters Kluwer Health (UpToDate). *Financial interests/stock ownership:* PsiloTec Health Solutions.

Holly A. Swartz, M.D.—*Royalties:* American Psychiatric Association Publishing and Wolters Kluwer (UpToDate®). *Consulting:* Clinical Education Alliance, Intracellular Therapeutics, Mediflix, Medscape/WebMD, and Physicians Postgraduate Press. *Editorial stipend:* American Psychiatric Association Publishing.

Robyn Thom, M.D.—*Research support:* Precidiag. *Royalties:* Oxford University Press.

Jennifer J. Thomas, Ph.D.—*Royalties:* Cambridge University Press and Oxford University Press.

Roger D. Weiss, M.D.—*Consulting:* Alkermes.

The following contributors indicated they have no competing financial interests or affiliations with regard to the content of this book:

Jamie Miller Abelson, M.S.W.
Stewart Adelson, M.D.
Paul S. Appelbaum, M.D.
Jonathan Avery, M.D.
Richard Balon, M.D.
John W. Barnhill, M.D.
Eugene Beresin, M.D.
Benjamin Brody, M.D.
Victoria E. Cosgrove, Ph.D.
Catherine Crone, M.D.
Anna Dickerman, M.D.
Arden D. Dingle, M.D.
Lorena Fernández de la Cruz, Ph.D.
Eve K. Freidl, M.D.
Matthew J. Friedman, M.D., Ph.D.
Richard A. Friedman, M.D.
Cynthia A. Graham, Ph.D.
Robert E. Hales, M.D., M.B.A.
Donald M. Hilty, M.D.
Thomas R. Kosten, M.D.
Peter D. Kramer, M.D.
Ryan E. Lawrence, M.D.
James L. Levenson, M.D.
Petros Levounis, M.D., M.A.

José R. Maldonado, M.D.
Katharina Meyerbröker, Ph.D.
Robert Michels, M.D.
Barbara L. Milrod, M.D.
Megan Mroczkowski, M.D.
Cheryl C. Munday, Ph.D.
Joseph F. Murray, M.D.
Maria A. Oquendo, M.D.
Brian Palen, M.D.
Julie B. Penzner, M.D.
Lauren Z. Rynar, Ph.D.
Susan Samuels, M.D.
Lorin M. Scher, M.D.
Marc A. Schuckit, M.D.
Charles L. Scott, M.D.
Charles H. Silberstein, M.D.
Daphne Simeon, M.D.
Theodore A. Stern, M.D.
William S. Stone, Ph.D.
Rosemary Tannock, Ph.D.
Ming T. Tsuang, M.D., Ph.D., D.Sc.
John T. Walkup, M.D.
Michael F. Walton, M.D.
Frank Yeomans, M.D., Ph.D.

Introduction

DSM-5-TR Clinical Cases is intended to accompany DSM-5-TR. Each of this book's 104 cases begins with a clinical vignette followed by a case discussion. The cases are organized to fit into one of the 19 core DSM-5-TR chapters. In other words, a case that features borderline personality disorder will be found in the chapter on personality disorders. In cases that feature co-occurring disorders, the case will be found in the chapter on what is considered to be the primary psychiatric disorder (although it is often true that each of the co-occurring disorders should also be the subject of clinical attention).

Each of the 133 discussants was asked to act like "an expert on the shoulder," outlining the thought process that might go into a diagnostic understanding of the patient. The limit of about 1,000 words for the combined case and discussion means that neither is exhaustive, but this same brevity allows the book to highlight the ways in which experienced clinicians efficiently convert complex clinical data into a differential diagnosis. It also allows the reader to obtain a focused learning experience in one sitting. Throughout, the reader is encouraged to actively consider the tentative diagnoses that conclude each discussion. Would you agree, disagree? Would you want more information? What sorts of co-occurring disorders might be considered? What is likely to develop in the patient during the ensuing months and years?

DSM-5-TR Clinical Cases is updated from the book of clinical cases that accompanied DSM-5. The authors, cases, and discussions are largely the same, although the book has been revised to include changes in DSM-5-TR as well as to expand its consideration of ethnicity, race, and other demographic factors.

Translated into a dozen languages, *DSM-5 Clinical Cases* was read by a variety of mental health clinicians, trainees, and students, as well as by nonprofessionals. We hope that readers will find this updated edition to be even more interesting and useful.

CHAPTER 1

Neurodevelopmental Disorders

INTRODUCTION

Robert Haskell, M.D.

In its approach to mental illness across the lifetime of a patient, DSM-5 naturally begins with the neurodevelopmental disorders. As a group, these disorders are usually first diagnosed in infancy, childhood, or adolescence. Individually, these disorders have undergone a mix of pruning, reorganization, and clarification, including one of DSM-5's most controversial changes—to the definition of and diagnostic criteria for autism.

In DSM-5-TR, autism spectrum disorder describes patients previously divided among autistic disorder, Asperger's disorder, childhood disintegrative disorder, Rett's disorder, and pervasive developmental disorder not otherwise specified. These are no longer considered to be separate clinical entities. The new criteria include 1) persistent and pervasive deficits in social communication and social interaction and 2) restricted, repetitive patterns of behavior, interests, and activities. As now defined, autism spectrum disorder (ASD) can be subcategorized by the presence or absence of intellectual impairment and/or an associated medical condition. In addition, the identification of three severity levels helps clarify the need for additional social or occupational services. For example, a patient requiring "very substantial support" might display extreme behavioral inflexibility or might possess only 20 words of intelligible speech.

Attention-deficit/hyperactivity disorder (ADHD) continues to be subdivided into two symptom dimensions (inattention and hyperactivity/impulsivity), with a core requirement being the presence of at least six symptoms from either or both of the two dimensions. For example, inattention might be noted by the presence of such behaviors as making careless mistakes, failing to follow through with homework, and losing books. Criteria for hyperactivity/impulsivity include fidgetiness, impatience, and garrulousness. The diagnosis of ADHD is generally incomplete without inclusion of dimensional specifiers (predominantly inattentive, predominantly hyperactive/impulsive, or combined). Several of these symptoms must have been present prior to age 12, a change from DSM-IV's requirement that symptoms causing impairment be present prior to age 7. Another change is a reduction in the number of symptomatic criteria for adults from six to five within a particular dimension. These latter two changes reflect evidence that "loosening" criteria allows for identification of people who have symptoms, distress, and dysfunction that are very similar to those of people already diagnosed with ADHD and who can potentially benefit from clinical attention. As is true throughout DSM-5, it is up to the clinician to diagnose only those people who meet symptomatic criteria and whose distress and dysfunction reach a relevant clinical threshold.

DSM-5 had replaced the DSM-IV term *mental retardation* with the name *intellectual disability (intellectual developmental disorder)*, and in DSM-5-TR, the order of the two names in the diagnosis has been reversed to *intellectual developmental disorder (intellectual disability)* to indicate that the first-named term is preferred. The three core criteria for this diagnosis are unchanged: deficits in intellectual function and in adaptation (in areas such as communication, work, or leisure), as well as an early age at onset. The diagnosis does not depend on formal intelligence testing; instead, DSM-5-TR invites the clinician to make an aggregate assessment of severity, from mild to profound, according to three important life domains: conceptual, social, and practical. For example, a person with severe intellectual developmental disorder might have little understanding of concepts such as time or money, might use language to communicate but not to explain, and would likely require support for all activities of daily living.

Disorders of communication first observed in childhood include language disorder (formerly divided into expressive and receptive language disorders); speech sound disorder, in which the patient displays an impaired ability to produce the phonological building blocks of words but has no congenital or acquired medical condition that explains the impairment; childhood-onset fluency disorder (stuttering); and a new diagnosis, social (pragmatic) communication disorder, in which the patient displays persistent difficulties in the social use of verbal and nonverbal communication—very likely a diagnostic home for some of the individuals who have traits of ASD but do not meet full criteria.

Specific learning disorder is a new umbrella diagnosis within DSM-5. Specifiers for reading, written expression, and mathematics are designed to help teachers and parents shine a more focused light on a child's academic needs.

The chapter on neurodevelopmental disorders culminates with the motor disorders, including developmental coordination disorder, stereotypic movement disorder, and the tic disorders. A tic is a nonrhythmic movement of short duration and sudden onset. Such movements can be divided into motor tics, such as shoulder shrugs and eyeblinks, and vocal tics, including sniffs, snorts, and the spontaneous production of a word or phrase. Tourette's disorder is the most complex of the tic disorders, describing patients who exhibit both multiple motor and at least one vocal tic for more than 1 year that cannot be explained by a medical condition or by the physiological effects of a substance such as cocaine.

Inevitably, the neurodevelopmental disorders share symptoms with a broad range of psychiatric illnesses, and clinicians must sort through the differential diagnosis with an understanding that that differential is much broader for children age 12 and under. Sometimes the neurodevelopmental disorders contribute to the emergence of other disorders; for example, a learning disorder may cause anxiety, and untreated ADHD may make a patient vulnerable to substance abuse. The cases that follow attempt to pull apart some of these diagnostic entanglements and explore the comorbidities that make the treatment of neurodevelopmental disorders among the most challenging tasks in psychiatry.

Suggested Readings

Brown TE (ed): ADHD Comorbidities. Washington, DC, American Psychiatric Publishing, 2009
Cepeda C, Gotanco L: Psychiatric Interview of Children and Adolescents. Washington, DC, American Psychiatric Association Publishing, 2019
Hansen RL, Rogers SJ (eds): Autism and Other Neurodevelopmental Disorders. Washington, DC, American Psychiatric Publishing, 2013

CASE 1.1

A Second Opinion on Autism

Catherine Lord, Ph.D.

Ashley, age 17, was referred for a diagnostic reevaluation after having carried diagnoses of autism and intellectual disability for almost all of her life. She was recently found to have Kleefstra syndrome, and the family wanted to reconfirm the earlier diagnoses and assess the genetic risk to the future children of her older sisters.

At the time of the reevaluation, Ashley was attending a special school with a focus on functional skills. She was able to dress herself, but she was not able to shower independently or be left alone in the house. She was able to decode (e.g., read words) and spell at a second-grade level but understood little of what she read. Changes to her schedule and heightened functional expectations tended to make her irritable. When upset, Ashley would often hurt herself (e.g., biting her wrist) and others (e.g., pinching and hair pulling).

In formal testing done at the time of the reevaluation, Ashley had a nonverbal IQ of 39 and a verbal IQ of 23, with a full scale IQ of 31. Her adaptive scores were somewhat higher, with an overall score of 42 (with 100 as average).

By history, Ashley first received services at age 9 months after her parents noticed significant motor delays. She walked at 20 months and was toilet trained at 5 years. She spoke her first word at age 6. She received a diagnosis of developmental delay at age 3 and of autism, obesity, and static encephalopathy at age 4. An early evaluation noted possible facial dysmorphology; genetic tests at that time were noncontributory.

Her parents indicated that Ashley knew hundreds of single words and many simple phrases. She had long been very interested in license plates and would draw them for hours. Her strongest skill was memory, and she could draw precise representations of license plates from different states. Ashley had always been very attached to her parents and sisters, and although affectionate toward babies, she showed minimal interest in other teenagers.

Ashley's family history was pertinent for a father with dyslexia, a paternal uncle with epilepsy, and a maternal male cousin with possible "Asperger's syndrome." Her siblings, both sisters, were in college and doing well.

On examination, Ashley was an overweight young woman who made inconsistent eye contact but often peered out the corner of her eye. She had a beautiful smile and would sometimes laugh to herself, but most of the time her facial expressions were subdued. She did not initiate joint attention by trying to catch another person's eyes. She frequently ignored what others would say to her. To request a preferred object (e.g., a shiny magazine), Ashley would rock from foot to foot and point. When offered an object (e.g., a small decorated box), she brought it to her nose and lips for inspection. Ashley spoke in a high-pitched voice with unusual intonation. During the interview, she used multiple words and a few short phrases that were somewhat rote but communicative, such as "I want to clean up," and "Do you have a van?"

In the months prior to the evaluation, Ashley's parents noticed that she had become increasingly apathetic. A medical evaluation concluded that urinary tract infections were the most likely cause for her symptoms, but antibiotics seemed only to make her more listless. Further medical evaluation led to more extensive genetic testing, and Ashley was diagnosed with Kleefstra syndrome, a rare genetic defect associated with multiple medical problems, including intellectual developmental disorder. The parents said they were also tested and found to "be negative."

The parents specifically wanted to know whether the genetic testing results affected Ashley's long-standing diagnoses and access to future services. Furthermore, they wanted to know whether their other two daughters should get tested for their risk of carrying genes for autism, intellectual disability, and/or Kleefstra syndrome.

Discussion

In regard to diagnosis, Ashley's cognitive testing and limited everyday adaptive skills are consistent with intellectual developmental disorder, a term in DSM-5-TR that is equivalent to "intellectual disability," which had previously been the preferred term. In addition, Ashley manifests two symptom clusters that are core to the diagnosis of autism spectrum disorder (ASD): 1) deficits in social communication and 2) restricted, repetitive patterns of behavior, interests, or activities. Ashley also fulfills the DSM-5-TR ASD requirement of having had symptoms in the early developmental period and a history of significant impairment. A fifth requirement for ASD is that the disturbances are not better explained by intellectual developmental disorder, which is a more complicated question in Ashley's case.

For many years, clinicians and researchers have debated the boundary between ASD and intellectual developmental disorders. As IQ decreases, the proportion of children and adults who meet criteria for ASD increases. Most individuals with IQs below 30 have ASD as well as intellectual developmental disorder.

For Ashley to meet DSM-5-TR criteria for both ASD and intellectual developmental disorder, the specific deficits and behaviors associated with ASD must be greater than what would ordinarily be seen in people with her overall intellectual development. In other words, if her deficits were due solely to limited intellectual abilities, she would be expected to have the social and play skills of a typical 3- to 4-year-old child. Ashley's social interaction is not at all like that of a typical preschooler, however, and never has been. She has limited facial expressions, poor eye contact, and minimal interest in peers. In comparison with her "mental age," Ashley demonstrates significant restriction in both her range of interests and her understanding of basic human emotions. Furthermore, she manifests behaviors that are not seen commonly at any age.

The heterogeneity of autism has led to significant conflict. Some argue, for example, that children with very severe intellectual developmental disorder should be excluded from the diagnosis of ASD. Others argue that more intellectually able children with ASD should be placed into their own category, Asperger syndrome. Research does not support either of these distinctions. For example, studies indicate that children with ASD symptoms and severe intellectual developmental disorder often have siblings with ASD and stronger intellectual abilities. Much remains to be known about ASD, but IQ does not appear to be the key distinguishing factor.

From a pragmatic perspective, the critical factor is whether an ASD diagnosis offers information that helps guide treatment and the availability of services. For Ashley, the ASD diagnosis encourages a focus on helping to support her in social skills and less structured environments. It calls attention to differences in her motivation and in her need for structure. The ASD diagnosis also underlines the importance of looking carefully for Ashley's cognitive strengths (e.g., rote memory and visual representation) and weaknesses (e.g., comprehension, social interaction, and an ability to adapt to change). All of these may play a large role in her efforts to live as independently as possible.

Ashley's parents are also concerned about the impact of the recent genetic testing results on Ashley's treatment and on her sisters' family planning. Hundreds of individual genes may play a role in the complex neurological issues involved in autism, but most cases of ASD lack a clear cause. Ashley's genetic condition, Kleefstra syndrome, is reliably associated with both intellectual developmental disorder and ASD symptoms. When a genetic or medical condition or environmental factor appears to be implicated, it is listed as a specifier, but the ASD diagnosis is not otherwise affected.

Knowledge of the genetic cause for Ashley's intellectual developmental disorder and ASD is important for several reasons. It reminds her physicians to look for medical comorbidities that are common in Kleefstra syndrome, such as problems with the heart and kidneys (possibly leading, for example, to her recurrent urinary tract infections). Knowledge of the genetic cause also expands informational resources by connecting Ashley's family to other families that are affected by this rare syndrome.

A particularly important aspect of this new genetic diagnosis is its effect on Ashley's sisters. In almost all reported cases, Kleefstra syndrome has occurred de novo, meaning that there is an extremely low likelihood that anyone else in her family has any abnormality in the affected gene region. On rare occasions, an unaffected parent has a chromosomal translocation or mosaicism that leads to the syndrome, but the fact that Ashley's parents were found to "be negative" implies they are not genetic carriers. Although this is not necessarily true for situations involving other autism-related genetic disorders, this particular genetic diagnosis in Ashley likely indicates that her sisters are not at greatly increased risk for having children with ASD, although they are not protected from ordinary risk. Such information can be very reassuring and useful to Ashley's sisters. The fact remains that although genetics undoubtedly plays a large role in ASD and intellectual developmental disorders, most cases cannot be reliably predicted, and diagnosis is made through ongoing, longitudinal observation during childhood.

Diagnoses

- Intellectual developmental disorder (intellectual disability), severe
- Autism spectrum disorder, with accompanying intellectual and language impairments, associated with Kleefstra syndrome

Suggested Readings

Kleefstra T, Nillesen WM, Yntema HG: Kleefstra syndrome. GeneReviews October 5, 2010

Lord C, Pickles A: Language level and nonverbal social-communicative behaviors in autistic and language-delayed children. J Am Acad Child Adolesc Psychiatry 35(11):1542–1550, 1996

Muhle RA, Reed, HE, Stratigos K, et al: The emerging clinical neuroscience of autism spectrum disorder: a review. JAMA Psychiatry 75(5):514–523, 2018

Willemsen MH, Vulto-van Silfhout AT, Nillesen WM, et al: Update on Kleefstra syndrome. Mol Syndromol 2(3–5):202–212, 2012

CASE 1.2

Temper Tantrums*

Robyn Thom, M.D.
Eugene Beresin, M.D.
Christopher McDougle, M.D.

Brandon was a 12-year-old boy brought in by his mother for psychiatric evaluation for temper tantrums that seemed to be contributing to declining school performance. The mother became emotional as she reported that things had always been difficult but had become worse after Brandon entered middle school. Shortly after starting middle school, Brandon had started complaining of stomachaches on schoolday mornings and was often reluctant to go to school.

Brandon's sixth-grade teachers reported that he was academically capable but that he had little ability to make friends. He seemed to mistrust the intentions of classmates who tried to be nice to him but attempted to befriend others who laughingly feigned interest in the toy cars and trucks that he brought to school. The teachers noted that he often cried and rarely spoke in class. In recent months, multiple teachers had heard him screaming at other boys, generally in the hallway but sometimes in the middle of class. The teachers had not identified a cause but generally had not disciplined Brandon because they assumed he was responding to provocation. He was embarrassed about these outbursts and did not want to go to swim practice because he did not want his swim friends to ask why he'd had an outburst at school.

When interviewed alone, Brandon responded with nonspontaneous mumbles when asked questions about school, classmates, and his family. When the examiner asked if he was interested in toy cars, however, Brandon lit up. He pulled several cars, trucks, and airplanes from his backpack and, while not making good eye contact, did talk at length about vehicles, using their apparently accurate names (e.g., front-end loader, B-52, Jaguar). When asked again about school, Brandon pulled out his cell phone and showed a string of text messages: "dumbo!!!!" "mr stutter"; "LoSeR"; "freak!"; "EVERYBODY HATES YOU." While the examiner read the long string of texts that Brandon had saved but apparently not previously revealed, Brandon added that other boys would whisper "bad words" to him in class and then scream in his

*The authors would like to thank Arshya Vahabzadeh, M.D., for his contributions to an earlier edition of this case.

ears in the hall. "And I hate loud noises." He also told the examiner that he sometimes wished that he had never been born.

Developmentally, Brandon spoke his first word at age 11 months and began to use short sentences by age 3. He had always been very focused on trucks, cars, and trains. According to his mother, he had always been "very shy" and had never had a best friend. As he has gotten older, it has become more apparent that he struggles with jokes and typical young adolescent banter because "he takes things so literally." Brandon's mother had long seen this behavior as "a little odd" but added that it was not much different from that of Brandon's father, a successful attorney, who had similarly focused interests. Both of them were "sticklers for routine" who "lacked a sense of humor." Brandon's mother noted that he made efforts to conceal his interest in trucks, cars, and trains outside of the home but would eagerly speak about them when encouraged. Brandon has shared with his mother that he tries to appear "normal" when interacting with peers at school, which is exhausting. He often feels nervous around peers and generally tries to avoid socializing.

On examination, Brandon was shy and generally nonspontaneous. He made below-average eye contact. His speech was coherent and goal directed. At times, Brandon stumbled over his words, paused excessively, and sometimes rapidly repeated words or parts of words. Brandon said he felt okay but added that he was scared of school, particularly when around other children. He appeared sad, brightening only when discussing his toy cars. He denied current suicidal thoughts or plans as well as homicidality. He denied psychotic symptoms. He was cognitively intact.

Discussion

Brandon presents with symptoms consistent with autism spectrum disorder (ASD). DSM-5 ASD incorporates several previously separate disorders, namely DSM-IV autistic disorder (autism), Asperger's disorder, and pervasive developmental disorder not otherwise specified. ASD is characterized by two main symptom domains: social communication deficits and a fixated set of interests and repetitive behaviors.

It is evident that Brandon has considerable difficulty in his peer social interactions. He is unable to form friendships, does not engage in interactive play, and struggles with reading social cues. People with ASD typically find it challenging to correctly interpret the relevance of facial expressions, body language, and other nonverbal behaviors. He is humorless and "takes things so literally." These symptoms meet the ASD criteria for social communication deficits.

In regard to the second ASD symptom domain, Brandon has fixated interests and repetitive behaviors that cause significant distress. He seems interested in cars and trains, has little interest in anything else, and has limited insight that other children might not share his enthusiasms. He requires "sameness," with distress arising if his routine is altered. Brandon meets both of the primary symptomatic criteria, therefore, for DSM-5 ASD.

Brandon also stumbles over words, pauses excessively, and repeats words or parts of words. These symptoms are consistent with stuttering, which is classified as one of the DSM-5 communication disorders, namely childhood-onset fluency disorder. Typically persistent and characterized by frequent repetitions or prolongations of sounds, broken words, pauses in speech, and circumlocutions, childhood-onset fluency disorder may result in significant social, academic, and occupational dysfunction.

Other DSM-5 communication disorders include difficulties in speech production (speech sound disorder), difficulty in use of spoken and written language (language disorder), and difficulty in the social uses of verbal and nonverbal communication (social [pragmatic] communication disorder). Although these difficulties are not noted in the case report, Brandon should be evaluated for each of these, because language impairments are so commonly part of ASD that they are listed as specifiers of ASD rather than as separate, comorbid diagnoses.

Many individuals with ASD have comorbid anxiety symptoms. The most common anxiety disorders in ASD are specific phobia, social anxiety disorder, and agoraphobia. In Brandon's case, signs that suggest he should be further evaluated for an anxiety disorder include his stomachaches, avoidance of social activities, and frequent feelings of embarrassment in social situations. The 25-item Parent-Rated Anxiety Scale for ASD (PRAS-ASD) is a reliable and valid scale for measuring anxiety in youth with ASD.

Prior to DSM-5, Brandon would have met criteria for Asperger's disorder, which identified a cluster of individuals with core autism features (social deficits and fixated interests) and normal intelligence. Perhaps because he shared autism spectrum symptoms with his own father, however, Brandon was viewed as "a little odd" but without problems that merited specific clinical attention. The lack of a diagnosis contributed to Brandon's having become the defenseless target of malicious bullying, a not uncommon finding in people with ASD.

Brandon has experienced passive suicidal thoughts. Individuals with ASD are at elevated risk for suicidal thoughts and completed suicide, and it will be important for Brandon to periodically receive careful safety assessments in the future. Without appropriate interventions for both his core ASD symptoms and his stuttering, Brandon is at serious risk for ongoing psychological trauma and academic derailment.

Brandon's ongoing passion for a single subject (in his case, trucks, cars, and trains) is typical for children with ASD. Brandon is sensitive to the fact that his peers no longer share his passion (if they ever did), so he hides his interest. Similarly, he wants to skip swim practice because of his earlier outburst at school. In both cases, his embarrassment is painful, but there are positives as well: Brandon is aware that his behaviors are unusual, and he wants to have friends; his insight and desire to socialize are positive prognostic factors and suggest that appropriate treatment interventions may be beneficial.

Diagnosis

- Autism spectrum disorder requiring support for deficits in social communication and for restricted, repetitive behaviors without accompanying intellectual impairment, with accompanying language impairment—childhood-onset fluency disorder (stuttering)

Suggested Readings

Matthias C, LaVelle JM, Johnson DR, et al: Exploring predictors of bullying and victimization of students with autism spectrum disorder (ASD): findings from NLTS 2012. J Autism Dev Disord 51(12):4632–4643, 2021

Scahill L, Lecavalier L, Schultz RT, et al: Development of the parent-rated anxiety scale for youth with autism spectrum disorder. J Am Acad Child Adolesc Psychiatry 58(9):887–896, 2019

Thom RP, Friedman NDB, Nasir R, Politte LC, Nowinski LA, McDougle CJ: Neurodevelopmental Disorders: Autism Spectrum Disorder, in Tasman's Psychiatry, 5th Edition. Edited
by Tasman A, Riba MB, Alarcon RD, et al. Berlin, Springer Nature, in press
Toth K, King BH: Asperger's syndrome: diagnosis and treatment. Am J Psychiatry 165(8):958–
963, 2008

CASE 1.3

Academic Difficulties

Stewart Adelson, M.D.
Rosemary Tannock, Ph.D.

Carlos was a 19-year-old Hispanic college student in his freshman year at a public
university in a large city. He was referred by his guidance counselor to the hospital's
outpatient psychiatric clinic for help with academic difficulties. Since starting college
6 months earlier, he had done poorly on tests and been unable to manage his study
schedule. His worries that he was going to flunk out of college were leading to anxiety, insomnia, poor concentration, and a general sense of hopelessness. After a particularly tough week, he told his family that he thought he should quit. His mother accompanied him to the clinic that had previously helped both Carlos and his younger
brother. The mother specifically wondered whether Carlos's "ADHD" might be causing his problems, or whether he had outgrown it.

Carlos had been seen at the same clinic when he was age 9, at which time he had
been diagnosed with attention-deficit/hyperactivity disorder (ADHD), predominantly combined type. Notes from that clinical evaluation indicated that Carlos had
been in trouble at school for not following instructions, not completing homework,
getting out of his seat, losing things, not waiting his turn, and not listening. He had
trouble concentrating except in regard to video games, which he "could play for
hours." Carlos had apparently been slow to talk, but his birth and developmental histories were otherwise normal. He repeated first grade because of behavioral immaturity and difficulty learning to read. The ease with which Carlos learned English, his
second language, was not noted. His family had emigrated to the United States from
the Dominican Republic when he was 5 years old. The family was Catholic and attended church every Sunday. Both of his parents worked in maintenance and house-
keeping at a local municipal hospital.

During the evaluation when Carlos was age 9, a psychoeducational assessment by a clinical psychologist confirmed reading problems (particularly problems in reading fluency and comprehension). Carlos did not, however, meet the school board criteria for a learning disability, which required evidence of a 20-point discrepancy between IQ and achievement scores. Thus, he was not eligible for special education services. The evaluator had noted Carlos to be eager to do well and anxious about underperforming. His anxiety was thought to be a reaction to his school difficulties and his challenges in meeting the academic expectations of his family. Carlos's pediatrician had recommended pharmacotherapy, but his parents did not want to pursue medication. They cited negative experiences with local youth who used diverted controlled substances and hung out "on the street." Instead, his mother reported taking on an extra job to pay for tutors to help her son "with concentration and reading." The eldest of four siblings, Carlos had done well with this intervention and was now the first member of his family to attend college.

The psychiatry trainee carefully reviewed Carlos's academic history; his symptoms, including the course and severity of sadness, anxiety, insomnia, and hopelessness; and his social and developmental history. She obtained collateral history from his family and school records. She used the revised DSM-5-TR Core Cultural Formulation Interview for assistance in obtaining a better understanding of Carlos's acculturation experiences, the family's past feelings about the clinic's recommendations, and what treatment interventions would be relevant and acceptable to Carlos and his family.

The psychiatry trainee learned that Carlos had a childhood history of "nervousness" identified by a neighborhood *curandera* (traditional healer) as *ataque de nervios*. The family had addressed this problem with supportive prayer and a traditional herbal tea. They had apparently not revealed this to the psychiatrist at the time, thinking he would find it irrelevant and not wishing to seem disrespectful of his authority. During these unrevealed episodes of acute anxiety, Carlos would experience trembling and agitation, palpitations, shortness of breath, dread of harm, and fear of separation from caregivers. Workup by the pediatrician had revealed no physiological cause.

Since starting college, Carlos reported that he had frequently been unable to remain focused while reading and listening to lectures. He was easily sidetracked and therefore had difficulty handing in his written assignments on time. He complained of feeling restless, agitated, and worried. He described difficulty falling asleep, poor energy, and an inability to "have fun" like his peers. He reported that the depressive symptoms went "up and down" over the course of the week and possibly influenced his problems with concentration; it was hard for him to be certain. He denied substance use.

Carlos said that he'd had some great teachers in high school who had understood him, helped him get the meaning of what he read, and allowed him to audiotape lectures and use other formats (e.g., videos, wikis, visual presentations) for final assignments. Without this support at college, he said he felt "lonely, stupid, a failure—unable to cope."

Although advised by his high school teacher to do so, Carlos had not registered with the university's student disability services office. He preferred not to be seen as different from his peers and thought he should be able to get through college by himself.

Carlos's family history was positive for ADHD in a younger brother. A cousin was reported to have had "dyslexia" and had dropped out of a local community college after one semester. His social and developmental history revealed that he had been well liked by his cluster of friends throughout school. His group consisted of boys and girls and tended to consist of kids more interested in school than in sports. Carlos denied ever having dated or been sexually active, and he also denied having any significant interest in pursuing either of these activities.

On examination, Carlos was well-groomed, polite, and soft-spoken. He wore clean jeans, a T-shirt, and a hoodie that he kept pulling down over his face. He sat quietly and hunched over. He sighed a lot and rarely made eye contact with the clinician. He often tapped his fingers and shuffled in his seat but responded appropriately to questions. His command of English appeared strong, but he spoke with a slight Spanish accent. He often mumbled and mispronounced some multisyllabic words (e.g., he said "literalchure" instead of "literature" and "intimate" when he clearly meant "intimidate"). He denied any suicidal thoughts. He appeared motivated to do better. On a follow-up interview with the psychiatry trainee, Carlos asked whether the conversations were confidential. When informed that they were, he hesitantly admitted that he felt overwhelmed by new relationships with college peers. He indicated that "in my neighborhood growing up, everybody was Dominican, but in college, I'm the only Dominican." He also quietly said that he thought he might "like guys rather than girls." He revealed two recent episodes of panic "like when I was a kid" that had occurred during social situations. He declined to go into further detail.

After these two initial sessions, the psychiatrist suggested extending the evaluation so that they could optimize a treatment strategy. She told Carlos that she wanted to better understand his mood and anxiety symptoms, as well as how he felt about being the first in his family to go to college (i.e., role transitions), and to talk a little more about his concerns about his sexual orientation. She also referred Carlos for updated psychoeducational testing. This psychoeducational reassessment confirmed that Carlos's reading and writing abilities were substantially and quantifiably below those expected for his age. That report also concluded that these learning difficulties were not attributable to intellectual developmental disorder, uncorrected visual or auditory acuity, psychosocial adversity, or lack of proficiency in the language of academic instruction. The report concluded that Carlos had specific difficulties with reading fluency and comprehension as well as spelling and written expression.

Discussion

Carlos presents with a history of ADHD that was diagnosed in childhood. He also appears to have anxiety and panic attacks that recurred in college. His earlier anxiety/panic had not been previously identified by his pediatrician (although it had been diagnosed as *ataque de nervios* and treated by a traditional healer in their community). He also appears to have a new-onset major depressive episode, mild severity, in the context of stressors surrounding acculturation, transition to college, and uncertainty about his sexual orientation.

When Carlos was first evaluated at age 9, DSM-IV criteria for ADHD required six of the nine symptoms listed in either of the two categories: inattention or hyperactivity-impulsivity (as well as an onset before age 12). He had been diagnosed as having the combined type of ADHD, indicating the specialty clinic had found at least six symptoms in each of these spheres.

Carlos now presents at age 19, and the case report indicates that he may have five different inattentive symptoms and two symptoms related to hyperactivity-impulsivity. This seems to indicate a symptomatic improvement. Partial remission of ADHD is common with age, especially in regard to hyperactivity symptoms. Under DSM-IV, Carlos's ADHD would be said to have remitted. DSM-5 has a lower threshold of five symptoms in either category, rather than six, so Carlos would continue to meet the symptomatic criteria for ADHD.

Carlos's anxiety and depression might actually be causing his inattention, however, and ADHD should not be diagnosed if an alternative explanation is more likely. Carlos does appear to have had ADHD as a child, but that earlier evaluation did not uncover the symptoms that were identified by a traditional healer as *ataque de nervios*.

In addition to trying to clarify the cause of his inattention (and whether he actually has ADHD), the ongoing assessment might also explore Carlos's perspective on being the first in his family to attend college and on his identity as "the only Dominican on campus." It would also be useful to tactfully explore issues related to sexual orientation. This might include his sexual feelings and fantasies, the triggers for his recent panic attacks, and his (and his family's) views on homosexual behavior. The case report mentions that members of Carlos's family are observant Catholics and that they sought out a traditional healer for Carlos's *ataque de nervios*. It would be useful to better understand how Carlos and his family merge aspects of their Catholicism and traditional Afro-Caribbean religions; such an understanding might inform Carlos's perspective on all of his concerns, including the anxiety, depression, and his "liking guys."

Carlos may well have mood and anxiety disorders in addition to ADHD. Academic problems are common in ADHD even in the absence of a specific learning disorder (SLD), although SLDs are also commonly comorbid with ADHD. Even before his repeat psychological testing, Carlos appeared to have multiple historical issues that increase the likelihood of an SLD. His speech was delayed in his first language, Spanish; his reading was slow in both Spanish and English; and he received (and thrived with) educational accommodations in high school. All of these suggest an SLD, as does his positive family history for learning disability.

Carlos's previous psychoeducational assessment failed to confirm a learning disorder because he did not meet the required discrepancy between IQ and achievement for diagnosis with an SLD. Based on an additional decade of evidence, DSM-5 eliminated this discrepancy criterion for SLD. This change has made it reasonable to refer older adolescent patients for reevaluation.

The repeat psychological testing indicates a moderately severe SLD. Because Carlos's learning difficulties began when he was school age and continue to cause academic impairment, he meets the DSM-5 diagnostic criteria for SLD. Documentation of both ADHD and SLD will enable Carlos to access academic accommodations that should allow him to more robustly pursue his college studies.

Diagnoses

- Major depressive disorder, mild, single episode
- History of panic disorder; rule out current

- History of attention-deficit/hyperactivity disorder, with predominantly inattentive presentation, of mild to moderate severity; rule out current
- Specific learning disorder affecting the domains of reading (both fluency and comprehension) and written expression (spelling and organization of written expression), all currently of moderate severity

Suggested Readings

Adelson SL, American Academy of Child and Adolescent Psychiatry (AACAP) Committee on Quality Issues (CQI): Practice parameter on gay, lesbian, or bisexual sexual orientation, gender nonconformity, and gender discordance in children and adolescents. J Am Acad Child Adolesc Psychiatry 51(9):957–974, 2012

Aggarwal NK, Lewis-Fernández R: An introduction to the Cultural Formulation Interview. Focus 18(1):77–82, 2020

Morgan PL, Staff J, Hillemeier MM, et al: Racial and ethnic disparities in ADHD diagnosis from kindergarten to eighth grade. Pediatrics 132(1):85–93, 2013

Pham AV, Riviere A: Specific learning disorders and ADHD: current issues in diagnosis across clinical and educational settings. Curr Psychiatry Rep 17(6):38, 2015

CASE 1.4

School Problems

Arden D. Dingle, M.D.

Daphne, a 13-year-old in the ninth grade, was brought for a psychiatric evaluation because of academic and behavioral struggles. She had particular difficulty starting and completing schoolwork and following instructions, and she had received failing grades in math. When prompted to complete tasks, Daphne became argumentative and irritable. She had become increasingly resistant to attending school, asking to stay home with her mother. These difficulties had been evident since early childhood but had worsened significantly this year. Because Daphne had become increasingly distressed, her parents have been less insistent on making her do any activity that upsets her.

Psychological testing indicated that Daphne had above-average intelligence, age-appropriate achievement in all subjects except math, and some difficulties in visuospatial skills. The test results were shared with the school, which offered additional tutoring. Daphne attended only a few sessions, stating that they were not helpful. Her parents talked to the school counselors and Daphne's teachers, asking for more services. They were told repeatedly that Daphne needed to be more assertive and ask for help. Several teachers commented that Daphne should be more motivated and try harder. Several years earlier, her pediatrician had diagnosed ADHD and prescribed a stimulant. She took the medication for a week, but her parents stopped giving it to her because she seemed agitated.

At home, Daphne's parents' close supervision of her homework often led to arguments with crying and screaming. Her behavior and attitude were noticeably better when she was out of school. She had two long-standing friends but had made no new close friends for several years. In groups with other children, she preferred to play with those younger than she. When her friends chose the activity or did not follow her rules, she tended to withdraw. She was generally quiet in groups and in school but more interactive with family members and individuals she knew well.

Since early childhood, Daphne has had difficulty falling asleep, requiring a nightlight and parental reassurance. Recognizing that Daphne was easily upset by change, her parents rarely forced her into new activities. She did well during the summer, which she spent with her grandparents. Her parents reported no particular traumas, stressors, or developmental or medical problems. Daphne had started her menses about 2 months prior to the evaluation. Her family history was pertinent for multiple first- and second-degree relatives with mood, anxiety, or learning disorders.

At first meeting, Daphne was shy and tense. Her eye contact was poor, and she had difficulty talking about anything other than her plastic horse collection. Within 15 minutes, she became more comfortable, revealing that she disliked school because the work was too hard. She thought that other children did not seem to like her because she was stupid and was not into clothes and dating. Sometimes they made fun of her and would start laughing whenever the teacher called on her. There were several peers who had similar interests in animals and seemed okay. She has been eating lunch with them but found it hard to relax and to believe that they really wanted to be friends. Daphne was always afraid of making mistakes, getting bad grades, and disappointing everyone. Often, she was so preoccupied with what to say or do next that she did not pay attention to her peers or teachers. She frequently was unable to make a decision for fear of not being right. Daphne was unable to identify any personal strengths or any aspect of her life that was going well. She wished she had more friends and that she was smarter. As long as she could remember, she had always felt this way. These difficulties made her sad, but she denied persistent depressive feelings or suicidal thoughts. She appeared anxious but brightened when discussing her horse figurine collection, her longtime friends, and her family.

Discussion

Daphne has symptoms of inattention, anxiety, academic difficulties, limited peer relationships, and poor self-esteem that are causing distress and impaired functioning. Biologically, Daphne is experiencing the hormonal changes of puberty against the backdrop of a family history of mood, anxiety, and learning disorders. Psychologically, Daphne is living with the belief that she is inadequate, probably connected with her ongoing academic and social difficulties. Developmentally, Daphne's emotional and social functioning appears to be somewhat delayed, with younger-than-expected interests and coping strategies. Socially, Daphne has a supportive family environment that has emphasized protecting her, possibly interfering with the acquisition of skills related to independence and autonomy. Meanwhile, the educational system has not provided the necessary support for Daphne to succeed.

Daphne's academic problems can be explained in part by a specific learning disorder in mathematics. She has persistent difficulties with math, supported by testing that showed her performance to be below her intellectual level and chronological age. Her achievement in other academic subjects and her level of adaptive functioning generally appear to be age appropriate, indicating that her global intelligence and adaptive functioning are normal and that she does not have an intellectual developmental disorder.

It can be difficult to distinguish between anxiety and mood disorders in children Daphne's age. In this case, an anxiety disorder is more likely because Daphne's symptoms have been chronic and persistent rather than episodic, which depressive symptoms often are. Daphne's sadness is related to her sense of failure and worry about her competence. With the exception of a sleep disturbance, she does not have neurovegetative symptoms. Her difficulty with falling asleep appears anxiety based, as do her social ineptitude, reluctance to comply with school demands, and overreaction when faced with unwelcome tasks. In addition to her anxiety about her capabilities, Daphne appears to have concerns about security, which may explain her tense appearance. Daphne manages her anxieties by avoiding or controlling activities. Although some of her concerns are consistent with other anxiety disorders, such as social anxiety disorder or separation anxiety disorder, Daphne's worries extend beyond those domains. Given the pervasiveness of her anxiety, the most appropriate diagnosis is generalized anxiety disorder (GAD).

GAD is characterized by persistent, excessive anxiety and worry. Symptom criteria include restlessness, poor concentration, irritability, muscle tension, sleep disturbance, and being easily fatigued. Although three of six criteria are required for adults, a GAD diagnosis can be made in children with only one symptom in addition to the excessive anxiety and worry.

Social difficulties are common among children and adolescents, particularly those with psychiatric disorders. Daphne's issues are related to her anxiety about being competent and likable. Her academic struggles and anxiety have impeded her development, making her emotionally and socially immature.

Her immaturity might suggest an autism spectrum disorder. She does have difficulty initiating social interactions and engaging in reciprocity with peers (with poor eye contact notable on examination), but Daphne does not have the communication difficulties, rigidity, or stereotyped behaviors associated with autism. Her behavior improves with familiarity, and she expresses interest in her peers.

Daphne's language, speech, and communication skills seem developmentally appropriate, making disorders in these areas unlikely.

Oppositional defiant disorder might also be considered because Daphne is resistant and uncooperative in school and at home when it comes to her academic work. However, this attitude and behavior do not carry over to other situations, and her behaviors do not meet oppositional defiant disorder's requirements for symptom level and frequency. They are better conceptualized as a manifestation of anxiety and an attempt at its management.

Inattention is a symptom that occurs in a variety of diagnoses. Individuals with ADHD have problems with attention, impulsivity, and/or hyperactivity that occur in multiple settings prior to age 12 and cause significant impairment. Although Daphne has several symptoms consistent with inattention, these seem confined to school settings. She also does not appear to have significant problems with behaviors related to impulsivity or activity regulation. ADHD should remain a diagnostic possibility, but other diagnoses better account for Daphne's difficulties.

The environmental contributions to Daphne's problems should not be minimized. Her central psychiatric diagnoses—a specific learning disorder in mathematics and GAD—do not appear to have been adequately addressed either at home or at school. With more adequate services, Daphne would likely feel less anxiety and emotional distress and be far more likely to succeed in her course work and to stay on track developmentally.

Although the case report indicates that Daphne's diagnosis and treatment were delayed, we do not know much about her demographic background. In general, we know that learning disorders in children often go unidentified, especially for children whose families are poor, members of historically marginalized groups, immigrants, or living in adverse circumstances. Daphne's parents tried to advocate for a more thorough diagnosis (and treatment), with little apparent success. Their efforts to shield Daphne from stress were well meaning but might have prevented her from gaining successful experiences and contributed to her sense of incompetence.

It would be useful to better understand Daphne's perspective on her anxiety, her academic performance, and anything else that she finds interesting or problematic. She has experienced negative, critical comments that might have escalated to bullying and harassment. An evaluation that looks specifically for these common experiences is likely not only to find additional problems but also to be felt as empathic by patients who might otherwise quietly hold on to private shames.

Diagnoses

- Specific learning disorder (mathematics)
- Generalized anxiety disorder

Suggested Readings

Burenkova OV, Naumova OY, Grigorenko EL: Stress in the onset and aggravation of learning disabilities. Dev Rev 61:100968, 2021

Creswell C, Waite P, Hudson J: Practitioner review: anxiety disorders in children and young people—assessment and treatment. J Child Psychol Psychiatry 61(6):628–643, 2020

Fletcher JM, Grigorenko EL: Neuropsychology of learning disabilities: the past and the future. J Int Neuropsychol Soc 23(9–10):930–940, 2017

Grigorenko EL, Compton DL, Fuchs LS, et al: Understanding, educating, and supporting children with specific learning disabilities: 50 years of science and practice. Am Psychol 75(1):37, 2020

Strawn JR, Lu L, Peris TS, et al: Research review: pediatric anxiety disorders—what have we learnt in the last 10 years? J Child Psychol Psychiatry 62(2):114–139, 2021

CASE 1.5

Fidgety and Distracted

Robert Haskell, M.D.
John T. Walkup, M.D.

Ethan, a 9-year-old boy, was referred to a psychiatric clinic by his teacher, who noticed that his attention was flagging. At that time, Ethan was a fourth grader at a private regular-education school for boys. The teacher told Ethan's parents that although Ethan had been among the best students in his class in the fall, his grades had slipped during the spring semester. He tended to get fidgety and distracted when the academic work became more challenging, and the teacher suggested the parents seek neuropsychiatric testing for him.

At home, Ethan's mother explained, he seemed more emotional of late: "He just looks weepy sometimes, which is unusual for him." She denied any difficulties at home, and she described her husband, son, 8-year-old daughter, and herself as a "happy family." She had noticed, however, that Ethan seemed uneasy about being left alone. He had become "clingy," often following his parents around the house, and he hated being in any room by himself. Ethan had also started climbing into bed with his parents in the middle of the night, something he had never done in the past. Although Ethan had a few good friends in the neighborhood and at school and was glad to have other kids come to his house, he refused to go on sleepovers.

Ethan's mother agreed that he appeared more fidgety. She had noticed that he often seemed to be shrugging his shoulders, grimacing, and blinking, which she took to be a sign of anxiety. These movements worsened when he was tired or frustrated, and they diminished in frequency during calm, focused activities such as clarinet practice or homework, especially when she was helping him.

His mother also mentioned that Ethan had suddenly become "superstitious." Whenever he stepped through a doorway, he would go back and forth until he touched both doorjambs with his hands simultaneously, twice in rapid succession. She hoped that Ethan's more conspicuous habits would subside by summer, when the family took its annual vacation. She felt that it was the right year for Disneyland, but Ethan's father had suggested taking him on a fishing trip ("just the boys") while mother and daughter visited relatives in New York City.

Ethan's mother recalled her son as an "easy child, but sensitive." He was the product of a planned, uncomplicated pregnancy and met all his developmental milestones on time. He had no history of medical problems or recent infections, but his mother mentioned that he had begun to make frequent visits to the school nurse's office complaining of stomachaches.

On examination, Ethan was a slightly built boy with fair, freckly skin and blond hair. He was somewhat fidgety, tugging at his pants and shifting in his seat. Hearing his mother talk about his new movements seemed to provoke them, and the examiner noted that Ethan also occasionally blinked tightly, rolled his eyes, and made throat-clearing noises. Ethan said that he sometimes worried about "bad things" happening to his parents. His concerns were vague, however, and he seemed to fear only that burglars might break into their house.

Discussion

Ethan presents with declining school performance, which his family seems to attribute to a cluster of anxiety symptoms that are of relatively recent onset. He is uneasy with solitude and reluctant to attend sleepovers, has fears that bad things will happen to his parents, and makes frequent trips to the school nurse. He appears to meet criteria for DSM-5 separation anxiety disorder, the symptoms of which need only persist for 1 month in children and adolescents.

Ethan's mother also points out that he has become more fidgety. She links his shoulder shrugging, grimacing, and blinking to this recent onset of separation anxiety. Neither the parents nor the teacher appears to recognize these movements as tics, which are nonrhythmic movements of short duration and sudden onset. Ethan appears to have a variety of tics, including those observed by the interviewer: some motor (blinks, shoulder rolls) and some vocal (chirps, grunts, throat clearing, sniffs, clicks). Tics can be simple, meaning that they last only milliseconds, or complex, which are of longer duration or consist of a chain or sequence of movements. Although tics may vary broadly throughout the course of a tic disorder, they tend to recur in a specific repertoire during any given period of the illness.

The specific tic disorder (if any) is determined by the type and duration of movements. In Tourette's disorder, both motor and vocal tics must be present, whereas in persistent (chronic) motor or vocal tic disorder, only motor or vocal tics are present. Ethan has a mixture of tics, but at this point they have been present for only about 6 months—not the minimum of 1 year required for either Tourette's disorder or persistent tic disorder. Therefore, Ethan is diagnosed with provisional tic disorder.

Tics occur in 15%–20% of children, and it appears that 0.6%–1.0% develop Tourette's disorder. On average, tics emerge between ages 4 and 6, reach peak severity by age 10–12, and generally decline in severity during adolescence. Tics first observed in adulthood were very likely present but unnoticed in childhood. Tics are typically worsened by anxiety, excitement, and exhaustion and abate during calm, focused activity—which is why that fishing trip with dad may be Ethan's best bet for a summer vacation.

Anxiety likely explains Ethan's inattention in the classroom. Although attention-deficit/hyperactivity disorder, inattentive subtype, cannot be ruled out, it seems more probable that tics and anxiety have taken Ethan off task, as he has no early history of inattention or hyperactivity. His success in the fall semester all but rules out a learning disorder, so no testing is indicated. (As a rule, testing should always follow the treatment of a confounding problem such as anxiety.)

Ethan does manifest rituals in the doorway, which suggests OCD, which is an illness that often co-occurs with both anxiety and tic disorders. Although that possibility might be further explored, a diagnosis of OCD—like that of other psychiatric disorders—requires not only symptoms but also a clinical evaluation that finds the symptoms are distressing or impairing. Without additional information as to whether the rituals have an impact on him, Ethan would not meet criteria for OCD.

Diagnoses

- Provisional tic disorder
- Separation anxiety disorder

Suggested Readings

Martino D, Ganos C, Pringsheim TM: Tourette syndrome and chronic tic disorders: the clinical spectrum beyond tics. Int Rev Neurobiol 134:1461–1490, 2017

Olfson M, Crystal S, Gerhard T, et al: Patterns and correlates of tic disorder diagnoses in privately and publicly insured youth. J Am Acad Child Adolesc Psychiatry 50(2):119–131, 2011

Plessen KJ: Tic disorders and Tourette's syndrome. Eur Child Adolesc Psychiatry 22 (suppl 1):S55–S60, 2013

Walkup JT, Ferrão Y, Leckman JF, et al: Tic disorders: some key issues for DSM-V. Depress Anxiety 27:600–610, 2010

CHAPTER 2

Schizophrenia Spectrum and Other Psychotic Disorders

INTRODUCTION

John W. Barnhill, M.D.

Schizophrenia is the prototypical psychotic disorder. Not only is it the most common psychosis, but schizophrenia tends to involve abnormalities in all five of the emphasized symptom domains: hallucinations, delusions, disorganized thinking (speech), grossly disorganized or abnormal motor behavior (including catatonia), and negative symptoms. Like the DSM-5 neurodevelopmental disorders, schizophrenia is viewed as a neuropsychiatric disorder with complex genetics and a clinical course that tends to begin during a predictable stage of development. Whereas the neurodevelopmental disorders tend to begin during childhood, symptoms of schizophrenia tend to develop during late adolescence and early adulthood.

The schizophrenia diagnosis underwent some minor revisions in DSM-5. For example, because of their limited diagnostic stability, low reliability, and poor validity, schizophrenia subtypes were eliminated. These subtypes had included such categories as disorganized, paranoid, and residual types of schizophrenia.

Long associated with schizophrenia, catatonia remains one of the potential diagnostic criteria for most of the psychotic diagnoses, including schizophrenia, but it can also be designated as a specifier for other psychiatric and nonpsychiatric medical conditions, including depressive and bipolar disorders. "Other specified catatonia" can

21

also be diagnosed when criteria are either uncertain or incomplete for either the catatonia or the comorbid psychiatric or nonpsychiatric medical condition.

The DSM-5 schizophrenia diagnosis continues to require persistence of two of five symptomatic criteria (delusions, hallucinations, disorganized speech, disorganized behavior or catatonia, and negative symptoms). One pertinent change in DSM-5 was the elimination of a special status for particular types of delusions and hallucinations, any one of which would previously have been adequate to fulfill symptomatic criteria for schizophrenia. A second change was the requirement for one of the two symptomatic criteria to be a positive symptom, such as delusions, hallucinations, or disorganized thinking.

On the basis of recent research, DSM-5-TR has expanded its discussion of the impacts of stress and early life experience on the development of schizophrenia. For example, early trauma and neglect appear to be associated with both increased rates and increased severity of schizophrenia. Similarly, asylum seekers may have higher rates, as might members of ethnic minority groups when they live in areas with lower proportions of ethnic groups. Most often implicated in these rates of schizophrenia are various sorts of trauma, including discrimination, stigmatization, and reduced levels of social support.

Criteria for schizoaffective disorder were tightened in DSM-5. As was the case in DSM-IV, a diagnosis of schizoaffective disorder requires that the patient meet criteria for schizophrenia and have symptoms of either major depressive or bipolar disorder concurrent with having active symptoms of schizophrenia. Also, as was the case previously, there must have been a 2-week period of delusions or hallucinations without prominent mood symptoms. The significant change in DSM-5 was that criteria for a major mood disorder must have been met for the majority of the total duration of the active and residual phases of the overall illness. Therefore, the schizoaffective diagnosis requires more attention to the longitudinal course than was previously the case. Furthermore, the diagnostic requirement that major mood symptoms be present during most of the course of the psychotic disorder (including both the active and the residual phases) is expected to lead to a significant reduction in the number of people who meet criteria for schizoaffective disorder.

Delusional disorder remains focused on the presence of delusions in the absence of other active symptoms of schizophrenia, depressive or bipolar disorders, and pertinent substance use. Bizarre delusions are now included as symptomatic criteria for delusional disorder, whereas delusions that are considered to be part of body dysmorphic disorder (BDD) and obsessive-compulsive disorder (OCD) should not lead to a delusional disorder diagnosis but rather to a primary diagnosis of either BDD or OCD, along with the "absent insight/delusional beliefs" specifier.

Brief psychotic disorder and schizophreniform disorder remained essentially unchanged in DSM-5. They are distinguished from schizophrenia primarily on the basis of the duration of symptoms, with brief psychotic episode referring to people who have symptoms for less than 1 month, and schizophreniform referring to people who have symptoms lasting 1–6 months. DSM-5-TR does discuss evidence indicating that brief psychotic episode often has a favorable prognosis, despite relapse rates that may be higher than 50%. Similarly, although most people with a provisional schizophreniform diagnosis go on to receive a schizophrenia or schizoaffective disorder diagnosis, one-third appear to recover within that 6-month window.

Not specifically discussed in this text are cases that involve atypical or incomplete presentations or situations such as the emergency room setting, where information is often incomplete. Within DSM-5, these diagnostic categories are referred to as "other specified schizophrenia spectrum and other psychotic disorder," "unspecified catatonia," and "unspecified schizophrenia spectrum and other psychotic disorder."

The "other specified" and "unspecified" categories reflect the reality that humans' thoughts, feelings, and behaviors lie on a continuum, as do their disorders, and are provided as diagnostic options throughout much of DSM-5. These diagnostic gray zones are especially pertinent in regard to schizophrenia spectrum illness. For many people who end up with a chronic illness such as schizophrenia or schizoaffective disorder, there exists a period of time in which they begin to show symptoms but are not yet diagnosed. It had been proposed that this issue be addressed in DSM-5 by creating a new diagnosis, *attenuated psychosis syndrome*. Psychiatrists are not yet able to robustly predict which patients are most likely to go on to develop full-blown psychotic symptoms, but accurate prediction is important enough that the syndrome is mentioned in two places. First, attenuated psychosis syndrome can be used as a specifier within this chapter of DSM-5, where it would be listed as "other specified schizophrenia spectrum and other psychotic disorder (attenuated psychosis syndrome)." The condition is also discussed in more detail in the "Conditions for Further Study" chapter in DSM-5 Section III.

Suggested Readings

Bailey T, Alvarez-Jimenez M, Garcia-Sanchez AM, et al: Childhood trauma is associated with severity of hallucinations and delusions in psychotic disorders: a systematic review and meta-analysis. Schizophr Bull 44:1111–1122, 2018

Bromet EJ, Kotov R, Fochtmann LJ, et al: Diagnostic shifts during the decade following first admission for psychosis. Am J Psychiatry 168(11):1186–1194, 2011

Fusar-Poli P, Cappucciati M, Bonoldi I, et al: Prognosis of brief psychotic episodes: a meta-analysis. JAMA Psychiatry 73(3):211–220, 2016

Lieberman JA, Stroup TS, Perkins DO, Dixon LB (eds): American Psychiatric Association Publishing Textbook of Schizophrenia. Washington, DC, American Psychiatric Association Publishing, 2020

CASE 2.1

Emotionally Disturbed

Carol A. Tamminga, M.D.

Felicia Allen was a 32-year-old single woman brought to the emergency room (ER) by police after she apparently tried to steal a city bus in Chicago. Because she appeared to be an "emotionally disturbed person," a psychiatry consultation was requested.

According to the police report, Ms. Allen threatened the driver with a knife, took control of the almost empty city bus, and crashed it. A more complete story was elicited from a friend of Ms. Allen's who had been on the bus but who had not been arrested. According to her, they had boarded the bus on their way to a nearby shopping mall. Ms. Allen became frustrated when the driver refused her dollar bills, instead demanding exact change. She looked in her purse, but instead of finding exact change, she pulled out a kitchen knife that she carried for protection. The driver fled, so she got into the empty seat and drove the bus across the street into a nearby parked car.

On examination, Ms. Allen was a handcuffed, heavyset young woman with a bandage on her forehead. She fidgeted and rocked back and forth in her chair. She appeared to be mumbling to herself. When asked what she was saying, the patient made momentary eye contact and just repeated, "Sorry, sorry." She did not respond to other questions.

More information was elicited from a psychiatrist who had come to the ER soon after the accident. He said that Ms. Allen and her friend were longtime residents at the state psychiatric hospital where he worked. They had just begun to take passes every week as part of an effort toward social remediation; it had been Ms. Allen's first bus ride without a staff member.

According to the psychiatrist, Ms. Allen had received a diagnosis of "childhood-onset, treatment-resistant paranoid schizophrenia." She had started hearing voices by age 5 years. Big, strong, intrusive, and psychotic, she had been hospitalized almost constantly since age 11. Her auditory hallucinations generally consisted of a critical voice commenting on her behavior. Her thinking was concrete, but when relaxed she could be self-reflective. She was motivated to please and recurrently said her biggest goal was to "have my own room in my own house with my own friends." The psychiatrist said that he was not sure what had caused her to pull out the knife. She had not been hallucinating lately and had been feeling less paranoid, but he wondered if she had been more psychotic than she had let on. It was possible that she was just impatient and irritated. The psychiatrist also believed that she had spent almost no period of life developing normally and so had very little experience with the real world.

Ms. Allen had been taking clozapine for 1 year, with good resolution of her auditory hallucinations. She had gained 35 pounds on the clozapine, but she had less trouble getting out of bed in the morning and was functioning at a higher level. She was hoping to get a job and live more independently, and the bus trip had been intended as a step in that direction. Because of these improvements and goals, she had insisted on continuing to take the clozapine despite the weight gain.

Discussion

Stealing a city bus is not reasonable, and it reflects Ms. Allen's concrete characteristic of thought and her inability to deal effectively with the world. Her cognitive dysfunction causes her to behave bizarrely. She mumbles and talks to herself, suggesting auditory hallucinations. She lives in a state mental hospital, suggesting severe, persistent mental illness.

DSM-5 schizophrenia requires at least two of five symptoms: delusions, hallucinations, disorganized speech, disorganized or abnormal behavior, and negative symptoms. Functioning must be impaired, and continuous signs of the illness must persist for at least 6 months. Even without any more information about Ms. Allen's history, the diagnosis of schizophrenia is clear.

Ms. Allen's psychosis began when she was a child. Early-onset symptoms are often unrecognized because children tend to view their psychotic experience as "normal." Identifying the symptom (e.g., hearing voices that are not there) and associating this with a milestone (e.g., going to a certain grade or school) can help the adult patient retrospectively identify symptom onset. Although the symptoms and treatments are similar for both, childhood-onset schizophrenia is often more severe than adult-onset schizophrenia. Early psychotic symptoms are impairing in and of themselves, but they also deprive the young person of the social learning and cognitive development that take place during critical childhood years.

Ms. Allen's behavior on the bus likely reflects not only the psychosis and cognitive dysfunction that are part of schizophrenia but also her diminished experience in real-life social settings. In addition to treating her psychotic symptoms with clozapine, her psychiatric team appears to be trying to remediate her losses by connecting her to a "friend" and organizing the shopping trip. The treatment team is also quite active and involved, as reflected by the psychiatrist's almost immediate presence in the ER after the bus incident.

Schizophrenia is a heterogeneous disorder, affecting multiple domains. It is likely that there are multiple schizophrenias, differentiated by as-yet unknown markers. Because of insufficient evidence about validity, DSM-5 did away with categories such as schizophrenia, paranoid type. Instead, DSM-5 outlines several ways in which the diagnosis can be subtyped. One way is by overall activity and chronicity of symptoms (e.g., single vs. multiple episodes; in acute episode, in partial remission, in full remission). Another way to categorize is by assessing the severity of each of the five core schizophrenia symptoms, using a 0–4 scale.

For example, Ms. Allen was able to try to travel with a "friend," and her hospital-based psychiatrist did arrive in the ER very quickly. These might reflect an engaged, active treatment program, but when combined with her apologetic attitude and her stated efforts toward independence, they likely indicate a relative lack of negative symptoms such as anhedonia, reduced social networks, and alogia. Such activity-driven behavior is unusual in patients with schizophrenia and suggests that she is not depressed. It is hard to judge Ms. Allen's cognitive capacity without testing. Her obvious concrete thinking is represented by a failure to understand the process of paying for her bus ride or abstracting behavioral clues. Whether she has the additional characteristics of a schizophrenia-like working memory disorder or attentional dysfunction is hard to tell from this vignette, but she should be tested. Cognitive training and remediation may be specifically helpful, and cognition may be tested repeatedly using a scale such as the Brief Assessment of Cognition in Schizophrenia.

In addition to assessing the extent of positive symptoms, it is crucial for the field of psychiatry to better understand, categorize, and follow the negative symptoms and cognitive dysfunctions of schizophrenia. Whereas the most effective interventions for schizophrenia have long revolved around the antipsychotic medications that ameliorate positive symptoms, future treatments will likely focus increasingly on the specific behavioral, cognitive, and emotional disturbances that are also an integral part of schizophrenia.

Diagnosis

- Schizophrenia, multiple episodes, currently in acute episode

Suggested Readings

Heckers S, Barch DM, Bustillo J, et al: Structure of the psychotic disorders classification in DSM 5. Schizophr Res 150(1):11–14, 2013

Lieberman JA, Stroup TS, Perkins DO, Dixon LB (eds): American Psychiatric Association Publishing Textbook of Schizophrenia. Washington, DC, American Psychiatric Association Publishing, 2020

Tandon R, Gaebel W, Barch DM, et al: Definition and description of schizophrenia in the DSM-5. Schizophr Res 150(1):3–10, 2013

CASE 2.2

Increasingly Odd

William S. Stone, Ph.D.
Ming T. Tsuang, M.D., Ph.D., D.Sc.

Gregory Baker was a 20-year-old African American man who was brought to the emergency room (ER) by the campus police of the university from which he had been suspended several months earlier. The police had been called by a professor who reported that Mr. Baker had walked into his classroom shouting, "I am the Joker, and I am looking for Batman." When Mr. Baker refused to leave the class, the professor contacted security.

Although Mr. Baker had much academic success as a teenager, his behavior had become increasingly odd during the past year. He quit seeing his friends and spent most of his time lying in bed staring at the ceiling. He lived with several family members but rarely spoke to any of them. He had been suspended from college because of lack of attendance. His sister said that she had recurrently seen him mumbling quietly to himself and noted that he would sometimes, at night, stand on the roof of their home and wave his arms as if he were "conducting a symphony." He denied having any intention of jumping from the roof or having any thoughts of self-harm, but claimed that he felt liberated and in tune with the music when he was on the roof. Although his father and sister had tried to encourage him to see someone at the university's student health clinic, Mr. Baker had never seen a psychiatrist and had no prior hospitalizations.

During the prior several months, Mr. Baker had become increasingly preoccupied with a female friend, Anne, who lived down the street. While he insisted to his family that they were engaged, Anne told Mr. Baker's sister that they had hardly ever spoken and certainly were not dating. Mr. Baker's sister also reported that he had written many letters to Anne but never mailed them; instead, they just accumulated on his desk.

His family said that they had never known him to use illicit substances or alcohol, and his toxicology screen was negative. When asked about drug use, Mr. Baker appeared angry and did not answer.

On examination in the ER, Mr. Baker was a well-groomed young man who was generally uncooperative. He appeared constricted, guarded, inattentive, and preoccupied. He became enraged when the ER staff brought him dinner. He loudly insisted that all of the hospital's food was poisoned and that he would only drink a specific type of bottled water. He was noted to have paranoid, grandiose, and romantic delusions. He appeared to be internally preoccupied, although he denied hallucinations. Mr. Baker reported feeling "bad" but denied depression and did not show disturbances in his sleep or appetite. He was adequately oriented to person and place but less so to time. He spoke articulately but refused formal cognitive testing. His insight and judgment were deemed to be poor.

Mr. Baker's grandmother had died in a state psychiatric hospital, where she had lived for 30 years. Her diagnosis was unknown. Mr. Baker's mother was reportedly "crazy." She had abandoned the family when Mr. Baker was young, and he was raised by his father and paternal grandmother.

Ultimately, Mr. Baker agreed to sign himself into the psychiatric unit, stating, "I don't mind staying here. Anne will probably be there, so I can spend my time with her."

Discussion

Mr. Baker's case involves an all-too-familiar scenario in which a high-functioning young man undergoes a significant decline. In addition to having paranoid, grandiose, and romantic delusions, Mr. Baker appears to be responding to internal stimuli (i.e., auditory hallucinations) and demonstrating negative symptoms (lying in bed all day). These symptoms have persisted and intensified over the past year. The history does not indicate medications, substances of abuse, or other medical or psychiatric disorders that could cause these symptoms. Therefore, he meets DSM-5 criteria for schizophrenia. Although a family history of psychiatric illness is not a requisite for the diagnosis, Mr. Baker's mother and grandmother appear to have also experienced major mental disorders.

Schizophrenia is, however, a heterogeneous disorder. For example, Mr. Baker's most prominent psychotic symptoms are delusions. Another person with schizophrenia might present most prominently with disorganization of speech and behavior and without any delusions. DSM-5 tries to address this heterogeneity by encouraging a dimensional viewpoint rather than a categorical one. In other words, instead of clarifying whether a patient has "paranoid" or "disorganized" schizophrenia, DSM-5 encourages assessment of a variety of specifiers. One important specifier, the course specifier, requires a longitudinal assessment to determine whether this is a first episode or one of multiple episodes, and whether it is an acute episode, in partial remission, or in full remission.

DSM-5 encourages specific ratings of symptoms. For example, is the current episode accompanied by catatonia? On a 5-point scale (from 0 to 4), how severe is each of the five cardinal schizophrenia symptoms? DSM-5 also encourages an assessment of cognition, mania, and depression domains. For example, some of Mr. Baker's behaviors (e.g., interrupting a class to proclaim his identity as the Joker) may seem to be symptomatic of mania, but they are unaccompanied by disturbances in sleep, mood, or level of activity. Similarly, Mr. Baker said he felt "bad" but not depressed. These clinical observations likely distinguish Mr. Baker from other subcategories of people with schizophrenia. As noted, Mr. Baker refused cognitive assessment. Although it would not have contributed to the formal diagnosis, cognitive deficits, like negative symptoms, contribute strongly to individual differences in schizophrenia and to differences in clinical outcomes and functional capacities.

The schizophrenia diagnosis can be made without assessing these severity specifiers. Nevertheless, the use of dimensional ratings improves the ability to assess Mr. Baker for the presence of core symptoms of schizophrenia in a more individualized manner. The inclusion of dimensions that cut across diagnostic categories will facilitate the development of a differential diagnosis that includes bipolar disorder and schizoaffective disorder. These assessments may clarify Mr. Baker's functional prognosis in major life roles (e.g., living arrangement or occupational status). Finally, repeated dimensional assessments may facilitate a longitudinal understanding of Mr. Baker's symptomatology, development, and likely responses to treatment.

Diagnosis

- Schizophrenia, first episode, currently in acute episode

Suggested Readings

Andreasen NC: The core dimensions of schizophrenia, in New Oxford Textbook of Psychiatry, 3rd Edition. Edited by Geddes JR, Andreasen NC, Goodwin GM. New York, Oxford University Press, 2020, pp 565–573

Green MF, Horan WP, Lee J: Nonsocial and social cognition in schizophrenia: current evidence and future directions. World Psychiatry 18(2):146–161, 2019

Stone WS, Faraone SV, Tsuang MT: Schizoaffective and schizotypal disorders/acute and transient psychotic disorders, in New Oxford Textbook of Psychiatry, 3rd Edition. Edited by Geddes JR, Andreasen NC, Goodwin GM. New York, Oxford University Press, 2020, pp 609–618

CASE 2.3

Hallucinations of a Spiritual Nature

Lianne K. Morris Smith, M.D.

Dolores Malaspina, M.D., M.P.H.

Hakim Coleman was a 25-year-old U.S. Army veteran turned community college student who presented to the emergency room (ER) with his girlfriend and sister. On examination, he was a tall, slim, and well-groomed young man with glasses. He spoke softly, with an increased latency of speech. His affect was blunted except when he became anxious while discussing his symptoms.

Mr. Coleman stated that he had come to the ER at his sister's suggestion. He said he could use a "general checkup" because of several days of "migraines" and "hallucinations of a spiritual nature" that had persisted for 3 months. His headache involved "sharp, shooting" sensations in various bilateral locations in his head and a "ringing" sensation along the midline of his brain that seemed to worsen when he thought about his vices.

Mr. Coleman described his vices as being "alcohol, cigarettes, disrespecting my parents, girls." He denied guilt, anxiety, or preoccupation with any of his military duties during his tour in Iraq, although his sister shared that Hakim's military responsibilities were of a confidential nature. He had joined an evangelical church 4 months earlier in the context of being "riddled with guilt" about "all the things I've done." Three months earlier, he began "hearing voices trying to make me feel guilty" most days. The last auditory hallucination had been the day before. During these past few months, he became withdrawn and noticed that strangers were commenting on his past sins.

Mr. Coleman believed that his migraines and guilt might be due to alcohol withdrawal. He had been drinking three or four cans of beer most days of the week for several years until he "quit" 4 months earlier after joining the church. He still drank "a beer or two" every other week but felt guilty afterward. He denied alcohol withdrawal symptoms such as tremor and sweats. He had smoked cannabis up to twice monthly for years but completely quit when he joined the church. He denied using other illicit drugs except for one uneventful use of cocaine 3 years earlier. He sometimes would sleep only a few hours and did report some nightmares. Otherwise, Mr. Coleman denied depressive, manic, or psychotic symptoms and violent ideation.

Regarding PTSD, Mr. Coleman's score on the 20-item self-administered PTSD Checklist for DSM-5 was below the cutoff score (between 31 and 33 out of 80) that would indicate probable PTSD in veterans. He denied that his military experience was unusually or especially frightening, horrible, or traumatic. Regarding other stressors, he felt overwhelmed by his current responsibilities, which included attending school and near-daily church activities. He had been a straight-A student at the start of the school year but was now receiving Bs and Cs.

The patient's girlfriend and sister were interviewed separately. They agreed that Mr. Coleman had become socially isolative and quiet, after having previously been fun and outgoing. He had also never been especially religious prior to this episode. His sister believed that Mr. Coleman had been "brainwashed" by the church. His girlfriend, however, had attended services with Mr. Coleman. She reported that several members of the congregation had told her they had occasionally talked to new members who felt guilt over their prior behaviors, but none who had ever hallucinated, and they were worried about him.

A physical examination of the patient, including a neurological screen, was unremarkable, as were routine laboratory testing, a blood alcohol level, and urine toxicology. A noncontrast head computed tomography (CT) scan was normal.

Discussion

The differential diagnosis for a young military veteran with new-onset psychosis and a history of substance use disorder is broad. The primary possibilities include an independent psychotic disorder, PTSD, a mood disorder with psychotic features, a substance-induced psychotic disorder, a psychotic disorder due to another medical condition, and a cultural syndrome.

Although his veteran status and some symptoms suggest PTSD, it is important to recognize that schizophrenia and PTSD are highly comorbid, with a number of symptoms occurring in both diagnoses. There can be substantial confusion between independent psychotic disorders and PTSD, with underidentification of psychotic disorders, which can also be precipitated by trauma. PTSD may include flashbacks that have a hallucinatory quality, and hypervigilance may reach paranoid proportions. At the same time, a diagnosis of PTSD requires a traumatic event and a cluster of characteristic symptoms. For Mr. Coleman, however, psychotic symptoms are predominant, and—despite his serving in a military zone—he denies significant traumatic experiences.

Mr. Coleman appears to warrant a diagnosis of schizophreniform disorder, a diagnosis that differs from schizophrenia in two substantive ways: the total duration of schizophreniform illness—including prodrome, active, and residual phases—is greater than 1 month but less than 6 months. Unlike schizophrenia, there is no criterion that mandates social or occupational impairment. For both schizophreniform disorder and schizophrenia, the patient must meet at least two of five symptomatic criteria. Mr. Coleman describes hallucinations ("hearing voices trying to make me feel guilty") and negative symptoms (blunted affect, avolition, social isolation). The case report does not mention delusions or disorganization of either speech or behavior.

Not relevant to DSM-5 criteria, but of interest, is that Mr. Coleman reports two Schneiderian symptoms besides auditory hallucinations: ideas of reference and possible cenesthetic hallucinations based on his description of his atypical headaches ("ringing" in his brain).

Multiple other disorders should be considered before concluding with a schizophrenia spectrum disorder. For example, Mr. Coleman specifically denies prominent depression and mania, both of which can cause psychotic symptoms. A variety of medical conditions can also cause psychosis, but these also seem to not pertain to Mr. Coleman's situation.

The patient himself is convinced that his symptoms are due to alcohol. Alcohol can indeed cause psychotic symptoms, whether during acute intoxication, after heavy prolonged use, or during acute withdrawal, but Mr. Coleman's recent drinking appears to have been modest, perhaps "a beer or two" every other week. He denies ever having had symptoms of withdrawal or other complications. His hallucinations began months after he cut back on his alcohol use, and the psychotic symptoms persisted for months. Additionally, his laboratory tests, including a hepatic panel and complete blood count, were normal, which would be unusual in patients with the sort of chronic alcohol use that usually accompanies alcohol-induced psychosis or significant withdrawal.

Mr. Coleman's chronic cannabis use could potentially be implicated in the development of psychosis, but his cannabis use has been only sporadic, and he apparently had not used cannabis for several months prior to the onset of hallucinations. His history is confirmed by a negative toxicology screen, which, in a moderate to heavy user, would likely be positive for 1–4 weeks after cessation.

It would appear that Mr. Coleman's concerns about alcohol and cannabis are linked to hyper-religious guilt rather than an actual substance use disorder. The possibility of another medical condition was considered, but his normal laboratory testing and physical examination results provided no such evidence.

Schizophreniform disorders last at least 1 month but less than 6 months. In regard to Mr. Coleman, his initial 1–2 months of religious preoccupation and guilty ruminations would be considered a prodromal phase. The 3 months preceding presentation to the ER would represent the active phase of psychosis. Because Mr. Coleman's psychotic symptoms have lasted 4–5 months but are ongoing, he would be said to have provisional schizophreniform disorder. Obviously, everyone who goes on to develop schizophrenia has a 6-month period in which they could be said to have schizophreniform disorder, but about one-third of people with schizophreniform disorder do not go on to develop schizophrenia or schizoaffective disorder.

Three other diagnostic possibilities that deserve mention are PTSD, a dissociative disorder, and a shared cultural syndrome. The case does not go into depth about Mr. Coleman's military experience, but even if he denies experiencing trauma, the experience of being in an active war zone can be a traumatic exposure in itself. He did not report symptomatic features of PTSD, but it is not clear whether the evaluation systematically searched for such symptoms. Given that avoidance is a cardinal feature of PTSD—making it less likely that he would spontaneously report the symptoms without being prompted—it would be useful to tactfully explore the possibility of PTSD in all people at elevated risk.

Mr. Coleman's family members indicate that his symptoms began around the time of his initiation into an evangelical church and worry that he has been "brainwashed." DSM-5 includes a possibly pertinent category, listed under "other specified dissociative disorders," within the chapter on dissociative disorders. This disorder is reserved for individuals who experience an identity disturbance due to prolonged and coercive persuasion in the context of such experiences as long-term political imprisonment or recruitment by cults.

It is also possible that Mr. Coleman's unusual beliefs are a nonpathological manifestation of religious beliefs that he shares with other members of his church.

It appears that his psychotic symptoms began prior to his entry into the church and may have motivated him to join a church that had previously not been of interest to him. In addition, although he attended church frequently, there is no evidence that he joined a cult or particularly manipulative religious sect. Furthermore, other congregants viewed his hallucinations as aberrant, implying that his views are not part of a shared cultural or religious mindset.

The initial diagnosis of provisional schizophreniform disorder is temporary. Longitudinal follow-up will clarify whether Mr. Coleman's symptoms attenuate or progress to a chronic psychotic illness.

Diagnosis

- Schizophreniform disorder (provisional)

Suggested Readings

Bromet EJ, Kotov R, Fochtmann LJ, et al: Diagnostic shifts during the decade following first admission for psychosis. Am J Psychiatry 168(11):1186–1194, 2011

Heckers S, Barch DM, Bustillo J, et al: Structure of the psychotic disorders classification in DSM 5. Schizophr Res 150(1):11–14, 2013

O'Conghaile A, DeLisi LE: Distinguishing schizophrenia from posttraumatic stress disorder with psychosis. Curr Opin Psychiatry 28(3):249–255, 2015

Prins A, Bovin MJ, Smolenski DJ, et al: The Primary Care PTSD Screen for DSM-5 (PC-PTSD-5): development and evaluation within a veteran primary care sample. J Gen Intern Med 31(10):1206–1211, 2016

Wortmann JH, Jordan AH, Weathers FW, et al: Psychometric analysis of the PTSD Checklist-5 (PCL-5) among treatment-seeking military service members. Psychol Assess 28(11):1392–1403, 2016

CASE 2.4

Mind Control

Rajiv Tandon, M.D.

Itsuki Daishi was a 23-year-old engineering student from Japan who was referred to his university student mental health clinic by a professor who had become concerned about his irregular class attendance. When they had met to discuss his declining performance, Mr. Daishi had volunteered to the professor that he was distracted by the "listening devices" and "thought control machines" that had been placed in his apartment.

While initially wary of talking to the psychiatrist, Mr. Daishi indicated that he was relieved to finally get a chance to talk in a room that had not yet been bugged. He said that his problems began 3 months earlier, after he returned from a visit to Japan. He said his first indication of trouble was when a classmate sneezed and grinned at him in an odd way. Later that same week, he noticed two strangers lurking suspiciously outside his apartment.

Mr. Daishi decided that those lurking strangers had installed tiny mind-control devices throughout his apartment, devices that were intended to weaken his resolve and prepare him for an onslaught of misinformation from Fox News reporters who intended to convert him into being a follower of Donald Trump. After weakening his resolve, Mr. Daishi found himself only able to watch Fox News, and he then found that those television reporters began to relentlessly comment indirectly and critically about him. He soon came to the conclusion that they had targeted him because of his "superior intelligence" and because he would soon become the prime minister of Japan. He concluded that the Trump Republicans wanted an ally in Tokyo. Mr. Daishi indicated that he was trying to stay strong, but it was difficult to keep the reporters from putting ideas into his head.

Mr. Daishi reported that he became increasingly vigilant, fearing that everyone at school and in his apartment complex was "in on the plot." He slept little, became withdrawn, and stopped attending classes, but he did continue to eat and maintain his personal hygiene.

He denied feeling elated or euphoric. He described his level of energy as "okay" and his thinking as clear "except when they try to put ideas into my head." He admitted to feeling extremely fearful for several hours on one occasion during his recent trip to Japan. At that time, he had smoked "a lot of pot" and began hearing strange sounds and believing that his friends were laughing at him. He denied any cannabis consumption since his return to the United States and denied ever having experimented with any other substances, saying that he generally would not even drink alcohol. He denied all other history of auditory or visual hallucinations.

When Mr. Daishi's uncle, listed as his local guardian, was contacted, he described his nephew as a healthy, intelligent, and somewhat shy boy without any prior history of any major psychiatric illness. He described Mr. Daishi's parents as very loving and supportive, although his father "might be a little stern." There was no family history of any major mental illness.

On examination, Mr. Daishi was well groomed and cooperative, with normal psychomotor activity. His speech was coherent and goal directed. He described his mood as "afraid." The range and mobility of his affective expression were normal. He denied any ideas of guilt, suicide, or worthlessness. He was convinced that he was being continuously monitored and that there were "mind control" devices in his apartment. He denied hallucinations. His cognitive functions were generally within normal limits. He appeared to have no insight into his beliefs.

On investigation, Mr. Daishi's laboratory test results were normal, his head computed tomography scan was unremarkable, and his urine drug screen was negative for any substances of abuse.

Discussion

Mr. Daishi meets criteria for delusional disorder, which requires one or more delusions that persist for longer than 1 month but no other psychotic symptoms. Most of Mr. Daishi's delusions are persecutory and related to monitoring devices. He has delusions of reference (a classmate sneezing and grinning at him), persecution (television reporters, mind-control devices), and thought insertion (reporters putting ideas into his head). He warrants the "mixed type" specifier because of his grandiosity (his "superior intelligence" and plan to become prime minister of Japan) and reduced sleep, but he has no other symptoms of mania.

Other psychotic disorders should also be considered. The 3-month duration of symptoms is too long for brief psychotic disorder (no longer than 1 month) and too brief for schizophrenia (no briefer than 6 months) but is an appropriate duration for schizophreniform disorder (between 1 and 6 months' duration). Mr. Daishi does not appear, however, to have a second symptom (e.g., hallucinations, negative symptoms, or disorganization) as required for a schizophreniform diagnosis. In DSM-IV, a single bizarre delusion—the delusion of thought insertion—would have been adequate to meet symptomatic criteria for schizophreniform disorder (or schizophrenia), but bizarre delusions no longer receive special treatment among the DSM-5 schizophrenia spectrum disorders.

The absence of manic or major depressive mood symptoms excludes a diagnosis of bipolar disorder (with psychotic features), major depressive disorder (with psychotic features), or schizoaffective disorder.

Two environmental factors may also be pertinent to Mr. Daishi's delusions. For one, his long flight from Japan, with associated jet lag and sleep deprivation, may have triggered mania and psychosis. Second, the psychosis appears to have developed around the time that he used cannabis, a drug that can trigger psychotic symptoms when used alone and when adulterated with another substance such as phencyclidine. If evaluated for psychosis immediately after the flight or his use of cannabis, either (or both) might be considered in the diagnosis. Mr. Daishi's symptoms have persisted, however, for more than a month after either of those putative triggers. Jet lag was specifically removed from DSM-5 as a subtype of circadian rhythm sleep-wake disorders because its effects tend to be mild and short-lived. In addition, DSM-5 and DSM-5-TR specifically exclude the diagnosis of substance-induced psychotic disorder when symptoms persist for a substantial period of time (e.g., 1 month) following discontinuation of the substance.

Diagnosis

• Delusional disorder, mixed type

Suggested Readings

Muñoz-Negro JE, Ibanez-Casas I, de Portugal E, et al: A dimensional comparison between delusional disorder, schizophrenia and schizoaffective disorder. Schizophr Res 169(1–3):248–254, 2015

Nisbett RE: The Geography of Thought: How Asians and Westerners Think Differently—and Why. New York, Free Press, 2003

Peralta V, Cuesta MJ: Characteristics and clinical correlates of dimensions of delusional experience in schizophrenia and delusional disorder. Schizophr Res 176(2–3):404–410, 2016

Tandon R, Carpenter WT: DSM-5 status of psychotic disorders: 1 year prepublication. Schizophr Bull 38(3):369–370, 2012

CASE 2.5

Sad and Psychotic

Anthony O. Ahmed, Ph.D.

John Evans was a 25-year-old single, unemployed white man who had been seeing a psychiatrist for several years for management of psychosis, depression, anxiety, and abuse of marijuana and alcohol.

After an apparently normal childhood, Mr. Evans began to show dysphoric mood, anhedonia, low energy, and social isolation by age 15 years. At about the same time, Mr. Evans began to drink alcohol and smoke marijuana every day. In addition, he developed recurrent panic attacks, marked by a sudden onset of palpitations, diaphoresis, and thoughts that he was going to die. When he was at his most depressed and panicky, he twice received a combination of sertraline 100 mg/day and psychotherapy. In both cases, his most intense depressive symptoms lifted within a few weeks, and he discontinued the sertraline after a few months. Between episodes of severe depression, he was generally seen as sad, irritable, and amotivated. His school performance declined around tenth grade and remained marginal throughout the rest of high school. He did not attend college as his parents had expected him to, but instead lived at home and did odd jobs in the neighborhood.

Around age 20, Mr. Evans developed a psychotic episode in which he had the conviction that he had murdered people when he was 6 years old. Although he could not remember who these people were or the circumstances, he was absolutely convinced that this had happened, something that was confirmed by continuous voices accusing him of being a murderer. He also became convinced that other people would punish him for what had happened, and thus he feared for his life. Over the ensuing few weeks, he became guilt-ridden and preoccupied with the idea that he should kill himself by slashing his wrists, which culminated in his being psychiatrically hospitalized.

Although he was predominantly anxious on admission, Mr. Evans soon became very depressed, with prominent anhedonia, poor sleep, and decreased appetite and concentration. With the combined use of antipsychotic and antidepressant medications, both the depression and the psychotic symptoms remitted after 4 weeks. Therefore, the total duration of the psychotic episode was approximately 7 weeks, 4 of which were also characterized by major depressive disorder. Mr. Evans had been hospitalized with the same pattern of symptoms two additional times before age 22, and each of these episodes started with several weeks of delusions and hallucinations related to his conviction that he had murdered someone when he was a child, followed by severe depression lasting an additional month. Both relapses occurred while he was apparently adherent to reasonable dosages of antipsychotic and antidepressant medications. During the 3 years prior to this evaluation, Mr. Evans had been adherent to clozapine and had been without hallucinations and delusions. He had also been adherent to his antidepressant medication and supportive psychotherapy, although his dysphoria, irritability, and amotivation never completely resolved.

Mr. Evans's history was significant for marijuana and alcohol misuse that began at age 15. Before the onset of psychosis at age 20, he smoked several joints of marijuana almost daily and binge-drank on weekends, with occasional blackouts. After the onset of the psychosis, he decreased his marijuana and alcohol use significantly, with two several-month-long periods of abstinence, yet he continued to have psychotic episodes up through age 22. He started attending Alcoholics Anonymous and Narcotics Anonymous groups, achieved sobriety from marijuana and alcohol at age 23, and had remained sober for the 2 years prior to this evaluation.

Discussion

Mr. Evans has struggled with depression and anxiety since adolescence, worsened by frequent use of marijuana and alcohol. At first, his treaters diagnosed him with depression and panic disorder and treated him accordingly. He did not enter college, as his family had expected, and he has not been employed since graduation from high school. At age 20, psychosis emerged and he required psychiatric hospitalization.

His major psychotic symptom is paranoia, with persecutory delusions and paramnesias of homicide. The delusions are worsened by auditory hallucinations, which he experiences as confirmation of his delusions. The delusions and hallucinations occurred almost daily between ages 20 and 22, until they resolved with clozapine treatment. Although he reports difficulties with memory, he has not displayed marked cognitive impairment or disorganization of thought. He is socially isolated and minimally able to interact with others. The extent, severity, and duration of his psychotic symptoms are consistent with the diagnosis of a schizophrenia spectrum disorder.

Mr. Evans's psychosis emerged after several years of depression, anxiety, and panic attacks. Since the onset of his psychotic illness, he has experienced multiple episodes of depression, which emerge after periods of delusion and hallucinations and feature overwhelming guilt, prominent anhedonia, poor sleep, and occasional bursts of irritability. He tends to become suicidal when psychosis and depression intensify.

Mr. Evans meets criteria for DSM-5 schizoaffective disorder. He has had an uninterrupted period in which his major depressive symptoms were concurrent with his schizophrenia symptoms. He has had several-week periods of hallucinations and delusions without prominent mood symptoms. Since the onset of the active and residual portions of his schizophrenia, the major depressive symptoms have been present most of the time.

Mr. Evans also used marijuana and alcohol for 8 years. Although these might have contributed to the emergence of his mood and psychotic symptoms, he continued to experience significant delusions, hallucinations, and depression between ages 20 and 22, when he stopped using marijuana and alcohol for several months. An alcohol- or marijuana-induced depressive, anxiety, or psychotic disorder might have been considered at various times in Mr. Evans's life, but the persistence of his mood and psychotic symptoms for months after the discontinuation of marijuana and alcohol indicates that he does not have a substance-induced psychiatric disorder.

His response to treatment with antipsychotic, antidepressant, and mood-stabilizing medication is typical: several unsuccessful treatments with antipsychotic drugs, the need for combined treatment during periods of exacerbations, and unsuccessful attempts to taper either the antidepressant or the antipsychotic medication.

One complicating factor in regard to diagnosing schizoaffective disorder is the reality that although DSM-5 requires that the mood disorder be present for the majority of the active and residual phases of the schizophrenia, mood and psychotic disorders tend to vary significantly in regard to treatment response and clinical course. For example, whereas depressive and bipolar disorders tend to run in cycles, schizophrenia—once it unfolds—tends to persist. Furthermore, depressive and bipolar disorders tend to be more amenable to treatment than schizophrenia, especially because the diagnostic time frame for the latter includes the residual phase of schizophrenia, which can be largely resistant to psychiatric interventions. It remains to be seen how this tightening of the criteria for schizoaffective disorder will affect the identification and treatment of this cluster of patients.

Diagnoses

- Schizoaffective disorder, depressive type
- Alcohol use disorder, in remission
- Cannabis use disorder, in remission

Suggested Reading

Heckers S: Diagnostic criteria for schizoaffective disorder. Expert Rev Neurother 12(1):1–3, 2012

Lintunen J, Taipale H, Tanskanen A, et al: Long-term real-world effectiveness of pharmacotherapies for schizoaffective disorder. Schizophr Bull 47(4):1099–1107, 2021

Livingstone K, Harper S, Gillanders D: An exploration of emotion regulation in psychosis. Clin Psychol Psychother 16(5):418–430, 2009

Veras AB, Cougo S, Merira F, et al: Schizophrenia dissection by five anxiety and depressive subtype comorbidities: clinical implications and evolutionary perspective. Psychiatry Res 257:172–178, 2017

CASE 2.6

Psychosis and Cannabis

Melissa Nau, M.D.
Heather Warm, M.D.

Kevin Foster, a 32-year-old married white man with a history of bipolar disorder, was brought to the emergency room (ER) by police after his wife called 911 to report that he was threatening to jump out of their hotel window.

At the time of the episode, Mr. Foster and his wife were on vacation, celebrating their fifth anniversary. To commemorate the event, they decided to get tattoos. Afterward, they went to a nearby park, where Mr. Foster bought and smoked a marijuana cigarette. During the ensuing hour, Mr. Foster began to believe that the symbols in his tattoo had mysterious meaning and power. He became convinced that the tattoo artist was conspiring with others against him and that his wife was cheating on him. After returning to the hotel, the patient searched his wife's phone for evidence of her infidelity and threatened to jump out the window. The patient's wife, an ER physician, successfully convinced the patient to go to sleep, thinking that the episode would resolve.

The following day, the patient remained paranoid and delusional. He again threatened to jump out the window, and indicated that he would have no choice but to kill his wife the next time she slept. She called 911, and her husband was brought to the ER of a large nearby hospital. Later that day, he was admitted to an acute inpatient psychiatric unit with a diagnosis of unspecified psychotic disorder.

Mr. Foster had smoked cannabis sporadically from age 18 but began to smoke daily 5 years prior to this admission. In the past year, his cannabis use had steadily increased; previously he had been smoking once per day, but more recently his use had increased to three times a day, beginning when he awoke. He noted that he has begun to feel "anxious" when not under the influence of cannabis and believed his thrice-daily use helped him "even out." The patient and his wife denied that he had ever used other illicit substances, and the patient indicated that he rarely drank alcohol. Until 1 year earlier, he had never seen a psychiatrist or been viewed by his friends and family as having significant psychiatric issues.

In the past year, however, Mr. Foster had been hospitalized four times for psychiatric problems. He had been hospitalized twice with classic manic symptoms and once for a suicidal depression. In addition, 7 months prior to this presentation, the patient had been hospitalized for a 6-week episode of cannabis-induced psychosis, which responded well to risperidone. At that time, his main symptom was paranoia.

Two months prior to this admission, he entered a 1-month inpatient substance abuse treatment program for cannabis use disorder. Until the weekend of this admission, he had continued to smoke marijuana but had not used alcohol or any other substances since discharge from the rehabilitation facility. He had also been functioning well while taking lithium monotherapy for 3 months.

Mr. Foster had been steadily employed as a film editor since graduating from college. His father had a bipolar disorder, and his paternal grandfather committed suicide via gunshot but with an unknown diagnosis.

On the second day of hospitalization, Mr. Foster began to realize that his wife was not cheating on him and that the symbols in his tattoo were not meaningful. By the third day, he spontaneously said the paranoia was the result of cannabis intoxication. He declined further risperidone but continued lithium monotherapy. He was discharged with an appointment to follow up with his outpatient psychiatrist.

Discussion

Soon after smoking a marijuana cigarette, Mr. Foster began to believe that the symbols of his new tattoo had mysterious meaning and power. Within hours, he became paranoid about the tattoo artist and delusionally jealous. He threatened to kill himself and his wife. He was admitted to a psychiatric unit. The psychotic symptoms cleared within a few days, and the patient regained appropriate insight. This symptom trajectory fits DSM-5 substance/medication-induced psychotic disorder, which requires delusions or hallucinations that develop during, or soon after, substance intoxication or withdrawal (or after exposure to or withdrawal from a medication).

An additional DSM-5 diagnostic criterion for cannabis-induced psychotic disorder revolves around whether Mr. Foster's delusions might not be better explained by an independent psychotic disorder such as schizophrenia or psychotic symptoms within depression or mania. His symptoms resolved within 3 days, which is typical for a cannabis-induced psychosis but not for an independent psychotic disorder. The rapid resolution of symptoms would support the likelihood that the cannabis caused his symptoms.

Mr. Foster's psychiatric history complicates the diagnosis in two different ways. First, of the four psychiatric hospitalizations Mr. Foster has had in the past year, one was for paranoid delusions in the context of cannabis use, leading to a 6-week hospitalization. The duration of the actual paranoid delusions is not entirely clear, but they appear to have lasted far longer than would be typical for a cannabis-induced psychosis. DSM-5 specifically cautions that persistence of a psychosis beyond 1 month after the exposure implies that the psychosis may be independent rather than substance induced.

Second, of Mr. Foster's three other psychiatric hospitalizations, two were for "classic" mania and one was for "suicidal depression." It is not clear whether paranoia or psychosis was part of these episodes. DSM-5 points out that a history of recurrent non-substance-related psychotic episodes would make a substance-induced psychosis less likely.

It is not clear whether these psychiatric episodes can be brought together under a single diagnostic umbrella. For example, Mr. Foster could have bipolar disorder with recurrent episodes of depression and mania. The cannabis might help him sleep—

which might reduce the mania—but could possibly trigger episodes. If manic and depressive episodes (with or without psychosis) are triggered by a substance but symptoms persist for an extended period of time, then the most accurate diagnosis would be the bipolar disorder. This would be especially true if similar symptoms develop in the absence of substance use. Mr. Foster has a family history significant for bipolar disorder, which could further support such a diagnosis. On the other hand, Mr. Foster did not endorse any mood symptoms during this most recent psychotic episode, and psychotic symptoms resolved within 2–3 days. This history would seem to indicate that although Mr. Foster has historically met criteria for bipolar disorder, it seems to be currently in remission.

Additionally, his recurrent and increasing cannabis use despite adverse consequences (e.g., psychotic episodes requiring hospitalization) suggests a diagnosis of cannabis use disorder, moderate. We can presume that during his hospitalizations he was counseled on the need to cut back his use; however, we see no evidence of this. Furthermore, his use has increased over the past year, with feelings of withdrawal when not using.

Multiple schizophrenia spectrum disorders might be considered. Given a 3-day duration of symptoms, however, most diagnoses are quickly eliminated as possibilities. In addition, Mr. Foster appears to have only one affected domain (delusions). Delusional disorder involves only delusions, but the minimum duration is 1 month. Brief psychotic disorder also requires only one of the four primary schizophrenia spectrum symptoms (such as delusions), but it does require an evaluation as to whether the precipitant might be a substance or medication.

At the moment, then, a cannabis-induced psychotic disorder appears to be the most likely diagnosis for Mr. Foster's particular episode. Clarification might be possible through more thorough investigation of prior medical records, but even more helpful will be ongoing, longitudinal follow-up.

Diagnoses

- Cannabis-induced psychotic disorder
- Bipolar I disorder, in remission
- Cannabis use disorder, moderate

Suggested Readings

Caton CL, Hasin DS, Shrout PE, et al: Stability of early-phase primary psychotic disorders with concurrent substance use and substance-induced psychosis. Br J Psychiatry 190:105–111, 2007

Ekleberry S: Treating Co-Occurring Disorders: A Handbook for Mental Health and Substance Abuse Professionals. Binghamton, NY, Haworth, 2004

Grant BF, Stinson FS, Dawson DA, et al: Prevalence and co-occurrence of substance use disorders and independent mood and anxiety disorders: results from the National Epidemiologic Survey on Alcohol and Related Conditions. Arch Gen Psychiatry 61(8):807–816, 2004

Pettinati HM, O'Brien CP, Dundon WD: Current status of co-occurring mood and substance use disorders: a new therapeutic target. Am J Psychiatry 170(1):23–30, 2013

Starzer MSK, Nordentoft M, Hjorthøj C: Rates and predictors of conversion to schizophrenia or bipolar disorder following substance-induced psychosis. Am J Psychiatry 175(4):343–350, 2018

CASE 2.7

Flea Infestation

Julie B. Penzner, M.D.

Lara Gonzalez, a 51-year-old divorced freelance journalist, brought herself to the emergency room requesting dermatological evaluation for flea infestation. When no corroborating evidence was found on skin examination and the patient insisted that she was unsafe at home, she was admitted to an inpatient psychiatric service with "unspecified psychotic disorder."

Her concerns began around 1 week prior to presentation. To contend with financial stress, she had taken in temporary renters for a spare room in her home and had begun pet sitting for some neighbors. Under these conditions, she perceived tiny insects burrowing into her skin and walls and covering her rugs and mattress. She had spent the 36 hours prior to presentation frantically cleaning her home, fearing that her tenants would not pay if they saw the fleas. She showered repeatedly, using shampoos meant to treat animal infestations, and she consulted three different exterminators, although none found evidence of fleas. She threw away a bag of clothing, believing she heard fleas "rustling and scratching inside." She bought replacement clothes that she kept in their own trash bag, thereby spending almost all of her savings, which worsened her preexisting financial strain.

Aside from her concerns about infestation, Ms. Gonzalez denied symptoms of depression, mania, and suspiciousness. She denied using any drugs or alcohol. No one in her family had a history of psychiatric illness. Ms. Gonzalez had been diagnosed with depression in college and briefly treated with an antidepressant. She had no relevant medical problems.

Her worries about infestation began in the setting of her sister's diagnosis with invasive cancer, the onset of her own menopause, financial strain that was likely forcing her to move from the United States back to Argentina (her country of origin), and a recent breakup with her boyfriend. At baseline, she described herself as an obsessive person who had always had "contamination phobias" that historically worsened during times of anxiety.

On mental status examination, Ms. Gonzalez was calm and easily engaged, with normal relatedness and eye contact. She offered up a small plastic bag containing "fleas and larvae" that she had collected in the hospital while awaiting evaluation. Inspection of the bag revealed lint and plaster. Her speech had an urgent quality to it, and she described her mood as "sad right now." She was tearful intermittently but otherwise smiling reactively. Her thoughts were overly inclusive and intensely focused on fleas. She expressed belief that each time a hair fell out of her head, it would morph into larvae. When crying, she believed an egg came out of her tear duct. She was not suicidal or homicidal. She expressed an unshakable belief that lint was larvae, and that she was infested. She denied hallucinations. Cognition was intact. Her insight was impaired, but her judgment was deemed reasonably appropriate.

Dermatological examination revealed no insects or larvae embedded in Ms. Gonzalez's skin. Results of neurological examination, head computed tomography scan, laboratory tests, and toxicology data were normal. She was discharged from the emergency room on a low-dose antipsychotic medication and seen weekly for supportive psychotherapy. Her preoccupation improved within days and resolved entirely within 2 weeks. She developed enough insight to refer to her belief that fleas were in her skin as a "crazy thought." She attributed her "break from reality" to multiple stressors, and was able to articulate that she relied on her delusion as a way to distract herself from real problems. Her family corroborated her quick return to baseline.

Discussion

Ms. Gonzalez's delusions with quick return to full premorbid functioning suggest a diagnosis of brief psychotic disorder with marked stressors. Formerly called "brief reactive psychosis," a brief psychotic disorder (with or without marked stressors) may not be diagnosed until return to baseline has occurred. The differential diagnosis of this condition is important.

At the time of presentation, the patient was diagnosed with "unspecified psychotic disorder," a term often used when psychosis is present but information is incomplete. Only after her symptoms rapidly resolved could she be diagnosed with a brief psychotic disorder. Ms. Gonzalez's insight returned quite quickly, and she was able to link her symptoms to antecedent stressors. Although treatment is likely to shorten the duration of an acute psychotic episode, DSM-5 specifically does not factor treatment into the requirement that the episode last less than 1 month.

It is worth noting that stressors can be positive (e.g., marriage, new job, new baby) or negative, as in Ms. Gonzalez's case. A favorable prognosis is often associated with a history of good premorbid functioning, significant acute stressors, and a lack of family or personal history of psychiatric illness. Stressors can also be medical; two recent case reports have described brief psychotic disorder associated with COVID-19 and related quarantine.

Ms. Gonzalez's sleeplessness, behavioral agitation, and premorbid depressive history might also suggest a bipolar episode, but there are no other symptoms to support this diagnosis. Similarly, her delusional obsession with flea infestation suggests a possible delusional disorder, but Ms. Gonzalez's symptoms resolved far too quickly for this to be likely. If her preoccupation with infestation were to persist for a month, as often happens, she would likely warrant a DSM-5 diagnosis of delusional disorder, somatic subtype; such a diagnosis might also be referred to as "delusional parasitosis."

Patients with personality disorders can have "micropsychoses," but Ms. Gonzalez does not appear to have a personality disorder or a particular personality vulnerability. Malingering and factitious disorder appear unlikely, as do delirium and other medically mediated illnesses.

Brief psychotic episodes have a low prevalence in the population, which could indicate that brief psychoses are unusual. It could also indicate that people with a very short duration of psychotic symptoms may not seek psychiatric help. The brevity and unpredictability of symptoms also makes it difficult to do research and for any particular clinician or institution to develop an expertise. Brief psychotic episodes are also noted to have a relatively low stability over time, which makes sense given that—unlike schizophrenia—brief psychotic episodes are, by definition, of short duration and cannot even be diagnosed without both remission of symptoms and careful follow-up.

Diagnosis

- Brief psychotic disorder with marked stressors

Suggested Readings

Haddad PM, Al Abdulla M, Latoo J, et al: Brief psychotic disorder associated with quarantine and mild COVID-19. BMJ Case Rep 13(12):e240088, 2020

Jørgensen P, Bennedsen B, Christensen J, Hyllested A: Acute and transient psychotic disorder: comorbidity with personality disorder. Acta Psychiatr Scand 94(6):460–464, 1996

Salvatore P, Baldessarini RJ, Tohen M, et al: McLean-Harvard International First-Episode Project: two-year stability of DSM-IV diagnoses in 500 first-episode psychotic disorder patients. J Clin Psychiatry 70(4):458–466, 2009

Smith CM, Komisar JR, Mourad A, Kincaid BR: COVID-19-associated brief psychotic disorder. BMJ Case Rep 13(8):e236940, 2020

CHAPTER 3

Bipolar and Related Disorders

INTRODUCTION

John W. Barnhill, M.D.

Bipolar disorders feature a distinct period of mania or hypomania. For example, a patient might develop a relatively acute onset of euphoria, diminished need for sleep, grandiosity, pressured speech, racing thoughts, and a variety of behavioral indiscretions. Absent complicating factors, such a patient would likely be readily identified as having a manic episode as part of bipolar I disorder.

Complicating factors abound in diagnosing bipolar and related disorders, however, which is one reason that this chapter features an abundance of cases. Most of the complications relate to symptom evaluation. DSM-5 identified seven symptoms that tend to cluster in bipolar I disorder, and the diagnosis of mania requires three of these symptoms. Each of the symptoms requires clinical judgment in regard to both duration and intensity, and certain problems, such as "distractibility" and "reduced need for sleep," are not always obvious during a clinical evaluation. A diagnosis of mania requires that symptoms from this cluster persist for most of the day, every day, for at least a week. This standard requires an accurate history, which can be difficult to obtain from any patient, but particularly from a patient who may have little insight into the presence of a psychiatric problem (as is often the case for individuals with bipolar disorder). An accurate bipolar history is even more difficult to obtain when the presenting symptom is depression, and manic symptoms might not have been present for many years. Half of patients with bipolar disorder use illicit substances, which can complicate the presentation, diagnosis, and treatment. Depression is so commonly found in bipolar disorder that the disorder was previously called "manic depression." The relationship between the two mood states is not always clear, however, which is one reason that bipolar and related disorders were shifted into a separate chapter in DSM-5. As it turns out, depression can be absent in bipolar disorder, but it can also be the dominant mood state in regard to both frequency and intensity of symptoms. Mood can oscillate between the two poles of depression and mania, or the two can coexist (e.g., a mood episode with mixed features). The relationship between the depressive and manic symptoms is made even more complicated by the reality that patients are more likely to spontaneously complain about dysphoria than about euphoria.

Finally, as is generally the case for disorders throughout DSM-5, a bipolar diagnosis requires impairment. Some of the core symptoms of mania—increased activity, euphoria, and talkativeness—can lead to *increased* effectiveness and pleasure, at least in the short term, which further complicates the assessment.

DSM-5 addressed these uncertainties by describing multiple syndromes within the bipolar spectrum. For example, diagnoses of mania and hypomania both require "three of seven listed criteria, most of the day, nearly every day." However, mania requires at least one episode lasting at least 7 days, whereas hypomania requires only a 4-day duration. Instead of requiring a marked impairment in social or occupational functioning, as specified for mania, hypomania requires an unequivocal change from baseline that is observable by others. These criteria take into consideration the reality that manic and hypomanic patients often lack insight, and the criteria emphasize that hypomania is less severe than mania. Hypomania is a key feature of DSM-5 bipolar II disorder. A second distinguishing feature of bipolar II disorder is the requirement for at least one major depressive episode at a time when hypomanic symptoms are not present. This requirement is in contrast to bipolar I disorder, which does not require the historical presence of depression.

Other patients may have classic manic or hypomanic symptoms but with an apparent physiological precipitant. For example, a patient may have developed manic symptoms immediately after receiving prednisone, a steroid, for a flare-up of systemic lupus erythematosus (lupus). In this case, the clinician might conclude that the patient has bipolar disorder, which would presumably warrant a mood-stabilizing medication. Alternatively, the patient may have had a fairly common reaction to steroids and warrant a diagnosis of medication-induced bipolar disorder (a disorder commonly and inaccurately labeled "steroid psychosis"); if so, a likely treatment would be reduction of the steroid medication. The patient's symptoms may, however, be best conceptualized as neuropsychiatric lupus, which in DSM-5 would be called bipolar disorder due to another medical condition. In that case, however, the patient might be best treated by an *increase* in steroids. One reason that the bipolar diagnosis is so hotly contested is that making the correct diagnosis is vitally important for patient care.

The bipolar spectrum also includes clusters of individuals whose mania-related symptoms are significant but who do not meet criteria for bipolar I or II disorder by virtue of the number or duration of symptoms. For example, some patients have a chronic course of alternating hypomanic and subthreshold depressive symptoms. To reach the diagnostic threshold for DSM-5 cyclothymic disorder, these symptoms need to be distressing and persistent (more days than not for at least 2 years—1 year in ado-lescents—with no more than 2 months without symptoms), and the individual should never have met criteria for a manic episode or a major depressive episode. DSM-5 cyclothymic disorder is quite parallel to DSM-5 persistent depressive disorder in regard to both duration and intensity of symptoms.

Other patients have significant manic symptoms, but an adequate history is not elicited because of the situation (e.g., an emergency room visit); in such cases, the diag-nosis would be unspecified bipolar and related disorder. A variety of other patients are diagnosed with other specified bipolar and related disorder. These include people whose manic symptoms either persist for an inadequate duration (e.g., only 2–3 days rather than the required 4 days) or persist for greater than 4 days but do not meet the three of seven symptomatic criteria for hypomania. Still others meet criteria for hypo-mania but lack a history of major depressive disorder and therefore do not meet cri-teria for bipolar II disorder. Others have chronic hypomania and subthreshold depres-sive symptoms but do not meet the 24-month criterion for cyclothymia.

Bipolar spectrum diagnoses have generated significant controversy. One issue re-lates to duration. It is difficult to make a diagnosis in which the symptoms need be present for only a few days and do not necessarily cause significant distress. Another complication relates to symptom intensity. Distinguishing normal from abnormal is not always easy when the variables include such core human behaviors as talkative-ness, risk taking, need for sleep, and self-esteem.

To address this controversy, DSM-5 balances two competing interests. The first is to identify robust, discrete symptom clusters that occur within distressed patients. Accurate diagnosis is crucial for a cluster of disorders that cause significant dysfunc-tion and distress and are accompanied by a lifetime risk of suicide that is more than 20 times that in the general population. The second competing interest is to avoid pathologizing normal human experience. Absent reliable tests for "bipolar disorder," the onus is on the clinician to make use of these criteria and to follow available evi-dence in both the diagnosis and treatment of these challenging patients.

Suggested Readings

Cosgrove VE, Suppes T: Informing DSM-5: biological boundaries between bipolar I disorder, schizoaffective disorder, and schizophrenia. BMC Med 11:127, 2013

Kramer NE, Cosgrove VE, Dunlap K, et al: A clinical model for identifying an inflammatory phenotype in mood disorders. J Psychiatr Res 113:148–158, 2019

Strakowski SM (ed): The Bipolar Brain: Integrating Neuroimaging and Genetics, 2nd Edition. New York, Oxford University Press, 2022

CASE 3.1

Emotionally Disturbed

Donald M. Hilty, M.D., M.B.A.

An African American man who appeared to be in his 30s was brought to an urban emergency room (ER) by police after neighbors complained that he had been loudly knocking on many doors in the neighborhood. The referral form indicated that the man was "schizophrenic" and an "emotionally disturbed person." One of the police officers said that the man offered to pay them for sex while in the back seat of their patrol car. He referred to himself as the "New Jesus" and declined to offer another name. He refused to sit and instead ran through the ER. He was put into restraints and received intramuscularly administered lorazepam 2 mg and haloperidol 5 mg. Intravenous diphenhydramine (Benadryl) 50 mg was readied in case of extrapyramidal side effects. The admitting team wrote that he had "unspecified psychosis" and transferred him to the psychiatry team that worked in the ER.

Despite being restrained, the patient remained giddily agitated, talking about receiving messages from God. When asked when he had last slept, he said he no longer needed sleep, indicating that he had "been touched by Heaven." His speech was rapid, disorganized, and difficult to understand. A complete blood count, blood chemistries, and a toxicology screen were drawn. After an additional 45 minutes of agitation, he received another dose of lorazepam. This calmed him, but he still did not sleep. The restraints were removed.

An hour after receiving the initial haloperidol and lorazepam, the patient was interviewed while he sat in a chair in the ER. He was an overweight African American man who was disheveled and malodorous. He did not smell of alcohol. He made poor eye contact, instead looking at nearby people, a ticking clock, the examiner, a nearby nurse—at anything or anyone that moved. His speech was disorganized, rapid, and hard to follow. His leg bounced rapidly up and down, but he did not get out of his chair or threaten the interviewer. He described his mood as "not bad." His affect was labile. He often laughed for no particular reason but would get angrily frustrated when he felt misunderstood. His thought process was disorganized. He had grandiose delusions, and his perceptions were significant for "God talking to me." He denied other hallucinations and denied suicidal and homicidal ideation. When asked the date, he responded with an extended discussion about the underlying meaning of the day's date, which he missed by a single day. He remembered the names of the two police officers who had brought him to the hospital. He refused more cognitive testing. His insight and judgment appeared poor.

The patient's sister arrived an hour later, after having been called by a neighbor who had seen her brother, Mark Hill, being taken away in a police car. The sister said that her brother had seemed strange a week earlier, uncharacteristically arguing with relatives at a holiday gathering. He had claimed not to need sleep at that time and had been talking about his "gifts." She had tried to contact Mr. Hill since then, but he had not responded to phone, e-mail, or text messages. She said he did not like to talk about his issues, but she had twice seen a bottle of olanzapine in his house. She knew their father had been called "schizophrenic" and "bipolar," but she had not seen her father since she was a child. She said that Mr. Hill did not typically use drugs. She also said he was 34 years old and a middle school math teacher who had just finished a semester of teaching.

A review of Mr. Hill's electronic medical record indicated that he had experienced a similar episode 2 years earlier. At that time, a toxicology screen had been negative. He had been hospitalized for 2 weeks on the inpatient psychiatric service and was given a discharge diagnosis of "schizoaffective disorder"; he also was prescribed olanzapine and referred to an outpatient clinic for follow-up. The chart had additionally referred to two previous admissions to the county inpatient hospital, but records from that hospital were not available after hours.

Over the next 24 hours, Mr. Hill calmed significantly. He continued to believe that he was being misunderstood and that he did not need to be hospitalized. When asked, he agreed that he had a direct connection to God and "an important role on Earth," but he denied having a connection to anyone called the "New Jesus." His speech remained rapid and loud. The interviewer noted that he seemed easier to re-direct, though his thoughts continued to jump from idea to idea. He remained tense and jumpy but denied paranoia or fear.

Serial physical examinations revealed no abnormalities aside from blisters on his feet. The patient was not tremulous, and his deep tendon reflexes were symmetrical and graded 2 of 4. He showed no neurological asymmetry. His toxicology screen was negative and his blood alcohol level was zero. His initial lab results were pertinent for elevated blood urea nitrogen and a blood sugar level of 210 mg/dL. His mean corpuscular volume, aspartate aminotransferase/alanine aminotransferase ratio, and magnesium levels were normal. His BMI was 30.8.

Discussion

Safety was the primary initial goal for Mr. Hill. To that end, he was given sedating medications and was, for an hour, placed in restraints.

The team's attention quickly turned to diagnosis, and their understanding of the patient evolved over the 24 hours that he was in the ER. Upon admission, the team wrote that he had an "unspecified psychosis," which would be equivalent to DSM-5 "unspecified schizophrenia spectrum and other psychotic disorder," a diagnosis that is often used in emergency situations when patients present with psychotic symptoms without much collateral information. At that point, the critical diagnostic issue is between the diagnosis that appears most obvious (e.g., a psychosis) and diagnoses that are both common and potentially the most immediately dangerous (e.g., a psychosis or delirium induced by either substance intoxication or withdrawal).

The search in the electronic medical record was important in that it indicated that the patient had presented 2 years earlier with similar symptoms and a negative toxicology screen. Later on the day of the current admission, the evaluating team was further informed by a negative toxicology screen as well as labs suggesting that Mr. Hill was not a chronic, intense user of alcohol; these lab results included a blood alcohol level of zero and normal mean corpuscular volume, aspartate aminotransferase/alanine aminotransferase ratio, and magnesium levels. His sister's collateral information, in conjunction with Mr. Hill's normal reflexes, lack of tremor, and apparently intact cognition (good memory for the names of the police officers and orientation at least to the date), made alcohol withdrawal highly unlikely.

It was clear that Mr. Hill had some sort of psychosis, but the team did not seem to have developed a clear diagnosis. He had presented to the ER with a classic cluster of symptoms: an expansively irritable mood, grandiosity, a diminished need for sleep, pressured speech, racing thoughts, distractibility, agitation, and sexually inappropriate behavior. Blisters on his feet would be consistent with incessant walking, and elevated blood urea nitrogen and normal creatinine levels would be consistent with dehydration.

In other words, he met every DSM-5 criterion for a manic episode. His psychotic symptoms were loudly impressive, but they would be specifiers for the bipolar illness rather than an indication that the diagnosis belonged within the schizophrenia spectrum. Historical information—much of which became available only toward the end of Mr. Hill's day in the ER—indicated that he was a 34-year-old math teacher who had just finished his teaching semester. People with schizophrenia rarely are able to maintain a highly demanding job like teaching, whereas people with bipolar illness are often quite functional between episodes.

If Mr. Hill's presentation 2 years earlier was indeed similar to his presentation in the current episode, and there was no actual evidence for a history of intermorbid psychotic thinking, it is curious that the earlier team concluded that he had schizoaffective disorder. Cultural issues may have contributed to the earlier diagnosis of schizoaffective disorder. African Americans appear to be diagnosed with schizophrenia much more frequently than non-Latino white individuals, despite not having an elevated actual incidence of the disorder. It is unclear why. It is possible that clinicians from a different cultural subgroup fail to get an adequate history because of some sort of mutual misunderstanding. It is also possible that reduced access to mental health care—perhaps related to economic disparities or lower levels of trust in the medical and/or mental health care system—leads to systematic undertreatment of African Americans. This could lead to more persistent, severe, or bizarre psychotic symptoms, which might then be interpreted, mistakenly, as more likely to be associated with schizophrenia.

Misdiagnosis with a schizophrenia spectrum disorder would have consequences for Mr. Hill. By not having his bipolar disorder properly diagnosed, he would be less likely to receive a mood-stabilizing medication, which could lead to more episodes of both mania and depression. In addition, he might be treated chronically with an antipsychotic medication such as olanzapine, which is well known to cause large weight gains. Mr. Hill is noted to be obese (BMI 30.8) and to have a blood sugar level of 210 mg/dL. His treating team needs to aggressively clarify his diagnosis, both to mitigate the many negative effects of his likely bipolar illness and to avoid iatrogenic medication effects such as weight gain, diabetes, and metabolic syndrome.

Diagnosis

- Bipolar I disorder, current episode manic, severe, with mood-congruent psychotic features

Suggested Readings

Gara MA, Vega WA, Arndt S, et al: Influence of patient race and ethnicity on clinical assessment in patients with affective disorders. Arch Gen Psychiatry 69(6):593–600, 2012

Mazereel V, Detraux J, Vancampfort D, et al: Impact of psychotropic medication effects on obesity and the metabolic syndrome in people with serious mental illness. Front Endocrinol (Lausanne) 11:573479, 2020

Singh SP, Islam Z, Brown LJ, et al: Ethnicity, Detention and Early Intervention: Reducing Inequalities and Improving Outcomes for Black and Minority Ethnic Patients: The ENRICH Programme, A Mixed-Methods Study. Southampton, UK, NIHR Journals Library, 2013

Strakowski SM, Keck PE Jr, Arnold LM, et al: Ethnicity and diagnosis in patients with affective disorders. J Clin Psychiatry 64(7):747–754, 2003

CASE 3.2

Cycles of Depression

Michael Gitlin, M.D.

Nancy Ingram, a 33-year-old stock analyst and married mother of two children, was brought to the emergency room (ER) after 10 days of what her husband described as "another cycle of depression," marked by a hair-trigger temper, tearfulness, and almost no sleep. He noted that these "dark periods" had gone on as long as he had known her but that she had experienced at least a half dozen of these episodes in the prior year. He said they typically improved within a few weeks of restarting her fluoxetine. He added that he wondered whether alcohol and clonazepam worsened her symptoms, because she routinely ramped up their use when the dark periods began.

Ms. Ingram's husband said he had decided to bring her to the ER after he discovered that she had recently created a blog entitled Nancy Ingram's Best Stock Picks. Such an activity not only was out of character but also, given her job as a stock analyst for a large investment bank, was strictly against company policy. He said that she had been working on these stock picks around the clock, forgoing her own meals as well as her responsibilities at work and with her children. She countered that she was fine and that her blog would "make them as rich as Croesus."

The patient had first been diagnosed with depression in college, after the death of her father from suicide. He had been a wildly erratic, alcohol-abusing businessman whom the patient loved very much. Her paternal grandmother had several "nervous breakdowns," but her diagnosis and treatment history were unknown. Since college, her mood had generally been "down," interspersed with recurrent bouts of worsened dysphoria, insomnia, and uncharacteristically rapid speech and hyperalertness. She had tried psychotherapy sporadically and taken a series of antidepressant medications, but her husband noted that the baseline depression persisted and that the dark periods were increasing in frequency.

Her outpatient psychiatrist noted that Ms. Ingram appeared to have dysthymia (persistent depressive disorder) and recurrent major depressive disorder. He also said that he had never seen her during her periods of edginess and insomnia—she always refused to see him until the "really down" periods improved—and that she had refused him access to her husband or to any other source of collateral information.

On examination, the patient was pacing angrily in the exam room. She was dressed in jeans and a shirt that was carelessly unbuttoned. Her eyes appeared glazed and unfocused. She responded to the examiner's entrance by sitting down and explaining that this was all a miscommunication, that she was fine and needed to get home immediately to tend to her business. Her speech was rapid, pressured, and very difficult to interrupt. She admitted to not sleeping but denied that it was a problem. She denied hallucinations but admitted, with a smile, to a unique ability to predict the stock market. She refused cognitive testing, saying she would decline the opportunity to be "a trained seal, a guinea pig, Mr. Ed, and a barking dog, thank you very much, and may I leave now?" Her insight into her situation appeared poor, and her judgment was deemed to be impaired.

Discussion

Ms. Ingram presents with tearfulness, irritability, poor sleep, a sad mood, and increasingly unsuccessful treatments for recurrent major depressive disorder. When her symptoms are most intense and disabling, she refuses to see her outpatient psychiatrist. His evaluation has been limited, therefore, and the case report presents symptoms that do not seem to have been incorporated into the diagnostic evaluation. For example, Ms. Ingram presents with speech that is rapid and pressured. Depressed patients with marked anxiety may present with rapid, "pressured" speech, but it is more typical to find slow and nonspontaneous speech patterns in depression. She has also created a get-rich-quick investment blog that reflects poor judgment and could get her fired from her job.

These are classic manic symptoms, which should lead to a reformulation of her "depressive" symptoms. Diminished sleep is often found in depression but is generally accompanied by daytime fatigue. Ms. Ingram describes a diminished need for sleep without daytime fatigue; this combination is more typical of bipolar mania. Irritability can be part of depression, but it is especially typical of people who have mixed features of both depression and mania. Ms. Ingram's mocking, dismissive attitude during the interview further substantiates this diagnosis, as do her poor insight and judgment. The history indicates at least six of these episodes within the prior year, which meets DSM-5 criteria for the "with rapid cycling" specifier for bipolar manic episodes.

Although at least some of her prior "depressions" appear to have been marked by pressured irritability, the case report does not indicate whether the prior episodes were accompanied by the level of grandiosity, risk taking, and dysfunction that accompany the current episode. Nevertheless, it appears that Ms. Ingram does have a history of chronic depressive features, possibly persistent depressive disorder, and that these symptoms have been accompanied by hypomanic and, as of this presentation, clearly manic symptoms. This highlights the repeated observation that even though mania/hypomania is the defining feature of bipolar disorder, depression tends to be the dominant pole. On average, patients spend three times as much time depressed as manic/hypomanic. The combination of depressive and manic symptoms indicates that Ms. Ingram's rapid-cycling bipolar disorder qualifies for the "with mixed features" specifier.

The differential diagnosis also includes "mixed depressions," which consist of depressive episodes with an admixture of manic/hypomanic symptoms. However, Ms. Ingram manifests more of a full manic/hypomanic picture with some depressive symptoms, rather than a full depressive picture with a few hypomanic features. This suggests that manic episode with mixed features is the more accurate diagnosis and highlights the dimensional and fluid nature of depressive and manic/hypomanic symptoms within mood disorders.

Because Ms. Ingram never saw her psychiatrist during her past hypomanic episodes and refused to allow contact between him and others who know her, the psychiatrist was unaware of these hypomanic episodes and was treating her as if she had unipolar depression. This implies that she probably also had true depressive episodes (different from her recurrent mixed hypomanic periods), for which her psychiatrist prescribed fluoxetine.

Her past "response" to fluoxetine is not easily interpretable given the information presented. Possibilities include the following: that fluoxetine was effective for treating the depression that may have followed the mixed hypomanias (the classic mania-depression-interval sequence in bipolar disorder); that Ms. Ingram was cycling out of her episodes while taking fluoxetine, which had no positive effect; or that the use of the antidepressant, especially without a mood stabilizer, was inducing a more rapid cycling pattern, which would appear as rapid responses to an antidepressant with subsequent rapid relapsing into the next mood state.

Ms. Ingram's family history is consistent with major psychiatric illness, but it is not clear enough to specifically suggest bipolar disorder. A family history of suicide plus alcohol use disorder (in the patient's father) does not help distinguish between unipolar and bipolar depression. The description of Ms. Ingram's father as erratic could reflect the effect of the alcohol use, unrecognized bipolar disorder, or both. Similarly, the description of the patient's paternal grandmother as having had "nervous breakdowns" hints at a major psychiatric disorder but is diagnostically nonspecific.

The increased use of both clonazepam and alcohol during these manic states is very common. Bipolar disorders are associated with the highest rate of drug or alcohol use comorbidity among all psychiatric disorders, aside from other substance use disorders. In Ms. Ingram's case, use of clonazepam and alcohol could represent self-medication of her irritable dysphoria or the tendency of manic individuals to push any behavior to excess. Ms. Ingram's family history of alcohol use disorder elevates her risk even further.

Diagnosis

- Bipolar I disorder, current episode manic, with mixed features and rapid cycling

Suggested Readings

Baldessarini RJ, Salvatore P, Khalsa HM, et al: Morbidity in 303 first-episode bipolar I disorder patients. Bipolar Disord 12(3):264–270, 2010 20565433

Lee S, Tsang A, Kessler RC, et al: Rapid-cycling bipolar disorder: cross-national community study. Br J Psychiatry 196(3):217–225, 2010 20194545

Suppes T, Ostacher M: Mixed features in major depressive disorder: diagnoses and treatments. CNS Spectr 22(2):155–160, 2017 28462772

CASE 3.3

Suicidal Preoccupation

Maria A. Oquendo, M.D.

Olivia Jacobs, a 22-year-old graduate student in architecture, was referred for an urgent psychiatric consultation after she told her roommate that she was suicidal. Ms. Jacobs had a history of mood symptoms that had been under good control with lithium and sertraline, but her depressive symptoms had returned soon after she had arrived in a new city for school, 3 months earlier. She had become preoccupied with ways in which she might kill herself without inconveniencing others. Her dominant suicidal thoughts involved shooting herself in the head while leaning out the window, so as not to cause a mess in the dorm. Although she did not have access to a gun, she spent time searching the Web for places where she might purchase one.

Ms. Jacobs's psychiatric history began at age 15, when she began to regularly drink alcohol and smoke marijuana, usually when out at dance clubs with friends. Both of these substances calmed her, and she denied that either had become problematic. She had used neither alcohol nor marijuana since starting graduate school.

Around age 17, she began experiencing brief, intense depressive episodes, marked by tearfulness, feelings of guilt, anhedonia, hopelessness, low energy, and poor concentration. She would sleep more than 12 hours a day and neglect responsibilities at school and home.

These depressive episodes would generally shift after a few weeks into periods of increased energy, pressured speech, and unusual creativity. She would stay up most of the night working on projects and building architectural models. These revved-up episodes lasted about 5 days and were punctuated by feelings that her friends had turned against her and that they were not really friends at all. Worried especially about the paranoia, her family had brought her to a psychiatrist, who diagnosed her as having bipolar II disorder and prescribed lithium and sertraline. Although Ms. Jacobs's moods did not completely stabilize on this regimen, she did well enough at a local university to be accepted into a prestigious graduate program far from home. At that point the depression returned, and she became intensely suicidal for the first time.

Upon evaluation, the patient was visibly depressed and tearful, and had psychomotor slowing. She said it was very difficult to get out of bed and she was not attending class most days. She reported hopelessness, poor concentration, and guilt about spending family money for school when she was not able to perform. She stated that she thought about suicide most of the time and that she had found nothing to distract her. She denied recent drinking or smoking marijuana, stating she did not feel like "partying." She acknowledged profound feelings of emptiness and indicated that she had occasionally cut her arms superficially to "see what it would feel like." She stated that she knew that cutting herself in this way would not kill her. She reported depersonalization and occasional panic attacks. She denied having mood instability, derealization, problems with impulsivity, concerns about her identity, and fears of abandonment.

Discussion

Ms. Jacobs presents with a current depression marked by depressed mood, anhedonia, sleep problems, anergia, psychomotor retardation, excessive guilt, and recurrent, persistent thoughts about suicide. These symptoms cause significant distress and impairment and appear to have been present for 3 months, well beyond the 2 weeks required for a DSM-5 diagnosis of major depressive disorder.

In addition to the depressive symptoms, she has been treated for bipolar II disorder, which features symptoms of major depressive disorder and hypomania. According to her history, she has had multiple 5-day periods of increased energy, pressured speech, increased creativity and productivity, and diminished need for sleep. These conform to the definition of hypomania. In addition to those symptoms, however, the patient has transiently believed that her friends had turned against her and that they were not really friends at all. If these paranoid symptoms were considered psychotic, then she would warrant a diagnosis of bipolar I disorder. In this case, the paranoia appears closer to being an overvalued idea than a frank delusion, but careful assessment of the patient's ability to reality-test is important.

Ms. Jacobs's illness began when she was in her late teens. The average age at onset of bipolar disorder is about age 25, and symptoms typically start between ages 15 and 30 years. Early age at onset suggests a more severe form of illness, and although Ms.

Jacobs has often been very functional, she has already had multiple episodes of both depression and hypomania by age 22.

Ms. Jacobs also has a history of alcohol and marijuana use, which she identified as having a "calming effect." The extent of her substance use is not known, but half of those who meet criteria for bipolar disorder also have a comorbid alcohol and/or substance use disorder. Both of these substances can be a problem by themselves, of course, but either one might have also helped trigger some of her initial mood symptoms. She has not, however, used either of them during the 3 months of her most recent depression, and for her mood disorder to be considered "substance induced," her mood symptoms should not persist beyond 1 month after stopping both the alcohol and marijuana. In other words, regardless of the role of substances in initiating symptoms, Ms. Jacobs's bipolar II disorder has taken on a life of its own.

Anxiety disorders are also commonly comorbid with bipolar disorder. Ms. Jacobs described a "calming effect" from marijuana and alcohol, which is perhaps an indicator of unrecognized anxiety. She later experienced episodes of depersonalization and panic attacks, which she found extremely distressing. Pending further information, she may meet criteria for a specific anxiety disorder, but based on available data, she currently meets criteria for an unspecified anxiety disorder.

Borderline personality disorder is also frequently comorbid with early-onset bipolar disorder, especially type II. In Ms. Jacobs's case, the presence of depersonalization, feelings of emptiness, substance use, nonsuicidal self-injury, and preoccupation with suicidal thoughts could be considered symptoms of borderline personality disorder. At the same time, however, she denied problems with impulsivity (other than substance misuse), mood instability when not in episode, derealization, concerns about her identity, and fears of abandonment. Although the possibility of a personality disorder cannot be entirely dismissed, Ms. Jacobs does not currently meet criteria for borderline personality disorder. Instead, the overlapping symptoms are likely due to her anxiety and bipolar disorders.

Ms. Jacobs's suicidal ideation is worrisome. Bipolar disorder is associated with the highest suicide rates among all psychiatric conditions, accounting for 25% of all suicides. Roughly one-third of people with bipolar disorder report at least one suicide attempt, 8%–20% of bipolar patients die by suicide, and the lethality of attempts may be even higher in bipolar II than in bipolar I. It is difficult to predict which patients will act on their suicidal thoughts, although associations have been found with early age at onset, first episodes that are depressive, a family history of suicidal acts, and aggressive and impulsive behaviors. Given this patient's diagnosis and suicidal ideation, her current level of suicidal risk appears to be high.

Diagnoses

- Bipolar II disorder, current episode depressed; high level of concern about suicide
- Unspecified anxiety disorder

Suggested Readings

Chen YW, Dilsaver SC: Lifetime rates of suicide attempts among subjects with bipolar and unipolar disorders relative to subjects with other Axis I disorders. Biol Psychiatry 39(10):896–899, 1996

Oquendo MA, Currier D, Liu SM, et al: Increased risk for suicidal behavior in comorbid bipolar disorder and alcohol use disorders: results from the National Epidemiologic Survey on Alcohol and Related Conditions (NESARC). J Clin Psychiatry 71(7):902–909, 2010

Swartz HA, Suppes T (eds): Bipolar II Disorder: Recognition, Understanding, and Treatment. Washington, DC, American Psychiatric Association Publishing, 2019

CASE 3.4

Episodic Depressions

Victoria E. Cosgrove, Ph.D.
Trisha Suppes, M.D., Ph.D.

Pamela Kershaw was a 43-year-old married librarian who presented to an outpatient mental health clinic with a long history of episodic depressions. Most recently, she described depressed mood during the month since she began a new job. She said she was preoccupied with concerns that her new boss and colleagues thought her work was inadequate and slow and that she was unfriendly. She had no energy and enthusiasm at home, either, and instead of playing with her children or talking to her husband, she tended to watch television for hours, overeat, and sleep excessively. This had led to a 6-pound weight gain in just 3 weeks, which made her feel even worse about herself. She had begun to cry several times a week, which she reported as the sign that she "knew the depression had returned." She had also begun to think often of death, although she had never attempted suicide.

Ms. Kershaw said her memory about her history of depressions was a little fuzzy, so she brought in her husband, who had known her since college. They agreed that she had first become depressed in her teens and that she had experienced at least five discrete periods of depression as an adult. These episodes generally included depressed mood, anergia, amotivation, hypersomnia, hyperphagia, deep feelings of guilt, decreased libido, and mild to moderate suicidal ideation without plan. Her depressions were often punctuated by periods of "too much" energy, irritability, pressured speech, and flight of ideas. These episodes of excess energy could last hours, days, or a couple of weeks. The depressed mood would not lift during these periods, but she would "at least be able to do a few things."

When specifically asked, Ms. Kershaw's husband described distinctive times when Ms. Kershaw seemed unusually excited, happy, and self-confident, and like a "different person." She would talk fast, seem energized and optimistic, do the daily chores very efficiently, and start (and often finish) new projects. She would need little sleep and still be enthusiastic the next day. Ms. Kershaw recalled these periods but said they felt "normal." In response to a question about hypersexuality, Ms. Kershaw smiled for the only time during the interview, saying that although her husband seemed to be including her good periods as part of her illness, he had not been complaining when she had her longest such episode (about 6 days) when they first started dating in college. Since then, she reported that these episodes were "fairly frequent" and lasted 2 or 3 days.

Because of her periodic low mood and thoughts of death, she had seen various psychiatrists since her mid-teenage years. Psychotherapy tended to work "okay" until she had another depressive episode, when she would be unable to attend sessions and would then just quit. Three antidepressant trials of adequate dosage and duration (6 months to 3 years) were each associated with short-term relief of depression, followed by relapse. Both alone and in the presence of her husband, Ms. Kershaw denied any history of alcohol or substance misuse. A maternal aunt and maternal grandfather had been recurrently hospitalized for mania, although Ms. Kershaw was quick to point out that she was "not at all like them."

On examination, Ms. Kershaw was a well-groomed, overweight woman who often averted her eyes and tended to speak very softly. No abnormal motor movements were noted, but her movements were constrained, and she did not use hand gestures. Her mood was depressed. Her affect was sad and constricted. Her thought processes were fluid, though possibly slowed. Her thought content was notable for depressive content, including passive suicidal ideation without evidence of paranoia, hallucinations, or delusions. Her insight and judgment were intact.

Discussion

Ms. Kershaw's recurrent symptoms of depression have caused significant suffering as well as functional impairment. They are also the recurrent impetus for her to seek psychiatric treatment. It is, therefore, tempting to focus only on the depressive symptoms and arrive at a diagnosis of recurrent major depressive disorder.

It is generally useful to search broadly for diagnoses, however, and this is especially true in patients whose symptom course or specific symptoms are atypical or whose treatment response has been inadequate. Ms. Kershaw reports an aunt and a grandfather who were hospitalized with episodes of bipolar mania. Although family history is not part of DSM-5 criteria, a strong family history of bipolar disorder should prompt a careful investigation into diagnoses that fall into the bipolar spectrum. When specifically asked, Ms. Kershaw and her husband report that her depressions are often punctuated by episodes of irritability, pressured speech, and flight of ideas. In addition, they describe recurrent, multiday episodes that are not related to depression and in which she is noticeably different from her baseline: she sleeps less, functions more effectively, and seems uncharacteristically happy, excited, pressured, and optimistic.

Ms. Kershaw insists that her periods of pressured activity are not like those of her aunt and grandfather, and her symptoms do not, in fact, appear to reach the intensity and duration that are characteristic of bipolar mania. Instead, Ms. Kershaw's energized periods are best described by the term *hypomania*.

Both DSM-5 mania and hypomania require at least three of seven associated symptoms, but there are important differences. One difference is the effect of the symptoms: mania requires significant accompanying distress or dysfunction, whereas hypomania requires only that the symptoms be distinctly noticeable to an observer. The duration requirements are also different. Mania requires a week's persistence of symptoms, whereas hypomania requires 4 days. If an individual meets criteria for mania at any time, bipolar I disorder would be the primary mood-related diagnosis. If the criteria for hypomania have been met at any time without a lifetime history of mania, then diagnosis hinges on whether the individual has a history of major depressive disorder. If so, the individual would warrant a bipolar II disorder diagnosis. This is in contrast to bipolar I disorder, in which the depression history should be explored but is not integral to the DSM-5 diagnosis. As described in the introduction to this chapter, the so-called bipolar spectrum also includes categories for people who do not quite meet the criteria for number or duration of symptoms or whose symptoms developed in the context of a medical illness or the use of medications or substances of abuse.

Because individuals rarely ask psychiatrists to evaluate their "uncharacteristic energy and enthusiasm," the bipolar II diagnosis often hinges on a careful historical review. In Ms. Kershaw's case, she described times of needing less sleep and becoming unusually talkative, pressured, and productive; these would meet the symptomatic criteria for hypomania. Regarding the duration of symptoms, most of Ms. Kershaw's hypomanic episodes last only 2–3 days, which would not meet criteria for bipolar II disorder. She did, however, have one early episode lasting 6 days. Once a hypomanic episode has occurred in a patient with a history of at least one past depressive episode, bipolar II disorder becomes the diagnosis, even if future hypomanic episodes are below the 4-day threshold for a hypomanic episode.

As seen in Ms. Kershaw, hypomanic symptoms often intrude into depression in patients with bipolar II disorder. In other words, hypomania is not always associated with a "good" or "elevated" mood. It can be useful to ask, for example, about "energized depression."

Bipolar II disorder is not simply an attenuated version of bipolar I disorder. Most people with bipolar II disorder have comorbidities that range throughout DSM-5 and include eating disorders, personality disorders, and anxiety disorders. Suicide is an important risk and should be explicitly investigated. Ms. Kershaw's recurrent, debilitating episodes are typical. Furthermore, the diagnosis is often missed. As seen in Ms. Kershaw's situation, the hypomanic periods may not be troublesome and are often a welcome change from the depression. Nevertheless, accurate diagnosis is important for optimizing a treatment that is necessary to mitigate the pain and suffering that often accompany bipolar II disorder.

Diagnosis

- Bipolar II disorder, current episode depressed, of moderate severity

Suggested Readings

Miller S, Suppes T, Mintz J, et al: Mixed depression in bipolar disorder: prevalence rate and clinical correlates during naturalistic follow-up in the Stanley Bipolar Network. Am J Psychiatry 173(10):1015–1023, 2016

Nusslock R, Frank E: Subthreshold bipolarity: diagnostic issues and challenges. Bipolar Disord 13(7–8):587–603, 2011

Simon NM, Otto MW, Wisniewski SR, et al: Anxiety disorder comorbidity in bipolar disorder patients: data from the first 500 participants in the Systematic Treatment Enhancement Program for Bipolar Disorder (STEP-BD). Am J Psychiatry 161(12):2222–2229, 2004

Suppes T, Mintz J, McElroy SL, et al: Mixed hypomania in 908 patients with bipolar disorder evaluated prospectively in the Stanley Bipolar Treatment Network: a sex-specific phenomenon. Arch Gen Psychiatry 62(10):1089–1096, 2005

Wozniak J, Faraone SV, Martelon M, et al: Further evidence for robust familiality of pediatric bipolar I disorder: results from a very large controlled family study of pediatric bipolar I disorder and a meta-analysis. J Clin Psychiatry 73(10): 1328–1334, 2012

CASE 3.5

Irritability and Sadness

Robert L. Findling, M.D., M.B.A.

Rachel, a 15-year-old girl, was referred for a psychiatric evaluation because of worsening difficulties at home and at school over the prior year. The mother's chief concern was that "Rachel's meds aren't working." Rachel said she had no particular complaints.

In meetings with the patient and her mother, both together and separately, both reported that Rachel's grades had dropped from As and Bs to Cs and Ds, that she had lost many of her long-standing friends, and that conflicts at home had escalated to the point that her mother characterized her as "nasty and mean."

Rachel first saw a psychiatrist at age 7 years when she was evaluated for attention-deficit/hyperactivity disorder (ADHD) because of long-standing restlessness, impulsivity, and distractibility. After behavioral interventions were ineffective, the patient began treatment with a methylphenidate-based medication at age 8. Improvement was seen at school, in her social life, and at home. For the ensuing 6 years, Rachel had done well and was "pretty much like other kids as long as she took her medicine."

At around age 14, however, Rachel became "moody." Instead of being a "bubbly teenager," she would spend days by herself and hardly speak to anyone. During these periods of persistent sadness, she would sleep more than usual, complain that her friends didn't like her anymore, and not seem interested in anything. At other times, she would be a "holy terror" at home, frequently yelling at her sister and parents to the point that everyone was "walking on eggshells." At about that time, Rachel's grades plummeted, and her pediatrician increased the dosage of her ADHD medication.

Rachel's family history was pertinent for a father who "had real problems." Although her mother did not know his diagnosis, he had been treated with lithium. The father had left the family before Rachel was born, and the two had never met.

In exploring the periods of irritability, dysphoria, and social isolation, the clinician asked whether there had been times in which Rachel was in an especially good mood. The mother recalled multiple periods in which her daughter would be "giddy" for a week or two. She would "laugh at anything" and would enthusiastically help out with and even initiate household chores. Because these were the "good phases," the mother did not think these episodes were noteworthy.

Rachel had no general medical problems. She denied use of alcohol, illicit substances, and medications other than the prescribed ADHD medication.

On examination while alone, Rachel was a casually groomed teenager who was coherent and goal directed. She appeared wary and sad, with some affective constriction. She did not like how she had been feeling, saying she felt depressed for a week, then okay, then "hilarious" for a few days, then "murderous," like someone was "churning up my insides." She did not know why she felt like that, and she hated not knowing how she would be feeling the next day. She denied psychotic symptoms, confusion, and suicidal and homicidal thoughts. She was cognitively intact.

Discussion

Rachel presents with at least 1 year's history of diminished functioning at school, at home, and with friends. She appears to have several different moods, each of which seems to last at least 1 week. These include being irritable, withdrawn, and giddy, all of which seem to be significantly different from her baseline. The mother thinks these "might be a stage," but the persistence, recurrence, and intensity of these moods have begun to have repercussions in Rachel's life, and so the mother has become concerned.

In trying to formulate a diagnosis for Rachel, we notice that much of the case report appears to be filtered through the perspective of the mother. Although helpful, such a story is liable to emphasize behavior, because that is what is most readily observable to parents and teachers. When evaluating adolescents, it is important to explore the teenagers' own perspective on their mood states. Furthermore, it is useful to differentiate between mood swings that are reactive to an external event and mood episodes that tend to be spontaneous and episodic. In Rachel's case, the interview supplied some important information. For example, she clarified that she did not like these mood fluctuations and denied particular precipitants.

A complication of Rachel's history is the presence of relatively nonspecific symptoms. Irritability, dysphoria, and emotional lability are part of multiple psychiatric conditions, particularly during adolescence, when many major psychiatric disorders tend to begin. In addition, it is important to differentiate fluctuations in mood states that are developmentally expected from ones that are not. Nevertheless, from what is known of Rachel's history, a mood disorder is the most likely diagnosis.

Rachel's most striking clinical feature is the spontaneous fluctuation between different emotional states. She describes a week or two of hypomania followed by a week or two of sadness followed by a couple of weeks of irritability. These symptoms seem to fit DSM-5 cyclothymic disorder, which requires multiple hypomanic episodes and multiple subsyndromal depressive episodes over a 2-year period (1 year for adolescents like Rachel). To meet the criteria, she should have had symptoms for at least half that time and should have had no more than a 2-month stretch without symptoms. Furthermore, she should not ever have reached criteria for mania, major depressive disorder, or a schizophrenia spectrum disorder. Although cyclothymic disorder can be seen as a disorder that does not match the intensity of bipolar I disorder, it can cause significant distress and dysfunction and dramatically affect the trajectory of adolescence.

Although the potential differential diagnosis for Rachel is broad, several other diagnoses deserve specific mention. Further exploration could lead to a diagnosis of bipolar I or bipolar II disorder. Her father appears to have had a bipolar disorder (he had "real problems" and took lithium), and even if Rachel has cyclothymia, she is at risk for developing bipolar I or bipolar II disorder in the future.

As more of an alliance is developed with Rachel, it might be possible to more fully evaluate personality issues. For example, cyclothymia is often comorbid with borderline personality disorder. Sleep is not mentioned in the case report, but sleep-wake difficulties can fuel affective instability. Perhaps most likely in a 15-year-old girl is the possibility of substance misuse, because many drugs of abuse can induce mood symptoms via intoxication or withdrawal. Rachel might reveal substance misuse with time, but it might also be useful to get a toxicology screen that can be legitimately framed to Rachel as part of the routine evaluation. Even if the screen is positive only for her ADHD medication, her symptoms should lead to a consideration that she is taking excess amounts on some days and taking none on other days.

Diagnosis

• Cyclothymic disorder

Suggested Readings

Findling RL, Youngstrom EA, McNamara NK, et al: Early symptoms of mania and the role of parental risk. Bipolar Disord 7(6):623–634, 2005

Perugi G, Hantouche E, Vannucchi G, Pinto O: Cyclothymia reloaded: a reappraisal of the most misconceived affective disorder. J Affect Disord 183:119–133, 2015

Van Meter AR, Youngstrom EA, Findling RL: Cyclothymic disorder: a critical review. Clin Psychol Rev 32(4):229–243, 2012

Van Meter A, Youngstrom EA, Demeter C, Findling RL: Examining the validity of cyclothymic disorder in a youth sample: replication and extension. J Abnorm Child Psychol 41(3):367–378, 2013

Van Meter A, Youngstrom EA, Birmaher et al: Longitudinal course and characteristics of cyclothymic disorder in youth. J Affect Disord 215:314–322, 2017

CASE 3.6

God Has Cured Me!

Stephen J. Ferrando, M.D.

Sebastian Lopez, a 27-year-old Hispanic freelance editor, was brought to his long-time HIV clinic by his worried partner. As the patient entered the clinic waiting room, he announced, "God has cured me! I can stop my antivirals!"

While Mr. Lopez fidgeted on a chair, furiously writing on a yellow pad, his partner provided the recent history. He said that the patient had been doing well until approximately 1 month earlier. At that point, he began an unusually intense editing project. After about 10 days of little sleep, "boundless energy," and activity, Mr. Lopez seemed edgy, a little pressured, and "glassy-eyed." That night, the two of them went to a party to celebrate the completion of the work project. Despite several years of Narcotics Anonymous meetings and abstinence from illicit substances, Mr. Lopez took crystal methamphetamine, a stimulant. Acutely anxious and paranoid that they were being followed, Mr. Lopez drank three martinis but still did not sleep that night. Over the ensuing days the patient became less paranoid, but he appeared increasingly distracted and his speech was more pressured.

Mr. Lopez's work project was returned with multiple negative comments and requests for corrections. Instead of focusing on his editing, however, he stayed up late every night, intent on finding a cure for HIV. He made inappropriate, hypersexual advances toward other men at the gym, where he spent much of the day. He lost at least 5 pounds after deciding he should take vitamin supplements instead of food and his antiretroviral medication. He refused to go to the emergency room but finally agreed to come to his routine AIDS clinic appointment to show his doctors how well he had done despite not having taken his medications in over a month.

Mr. Lopez's psychiatric history was without a prior episode of clear-cut mania, but he had been depressed as a teenager during the early phase of his coming-out process. That episode was punctuated by a purposeful overdose and a 2-week psychiatric hospitalization and treatment with antidepressant medication and psychotherapy. Mr. Lopez had discontinued the medication because it made him "hyper and edgy," and he stopped the psychotherapy because "it was pointless." He used methamphetamine frequently for several years, which led to recurrent unprotected intercourse with strangers.

Mr. Lopez was diagnosed with HIV at age 22, at which point he went to an outpatient substance use disorder rehabilitation center and discontinued his use of stimulants and alcohol. His lowest CD4 lymphocyte count had been 216 cells/mm^3, when he was age 24, at which time his viral load was 1.6 million copies. He had been reportedly adherent to his antiretroviral medications since then. His most recent CD4 count, 6 months prior to this episode, had been 526 cells/mm^3. His viral load had been undetectable. He had suffered fatigue but had not had any AIDS-defining illnesses. A magnetic resonance imaging (MRI) scan of the brain revealed mild cortical atrophy and periventricular white matter disease in excess of what would be expected for his age. The partner was unsure when Mr. Lopez had discontinued his antiretrovirals but thought it might have been months earlier. He also wondered if Mr. Lopez had "lost a step" cognitively over the past year.

His family psychiatric history was significant for a maternal aunt who had received lithium and several courses of electroconvulsive therapy, but her diagnosis was unknown.

On examination, the patient was a sloppily dressed young man who told a pressured, disjointed story of events over the prior month. He was difficult to direct and was uncharacteristically irritable and devaluing. He was preoccupied with having discovered a cure for HIV through multivitamins and exercise. He denied hallucinations and suicidal and homicidal ideation. He refused cognitive testing, and his insight and judgment appeared poor.

Discussion

Mr. Lopez presents with many classic manic symptoms. He has had a distinct period of elevated, irritable mood with increased energy and goal-directed activity. These symptoms have been present every day, for all or almost all of the day, for several weeks. He demonstrates grandiosity, decreased need for sleep, pressure to keep talking, increased goal-directed activity, and impulsive hypersexuality. These behaviors easily meet the requirement of three of seven symptomatic criteria for a DSM-5 manic episode.

The diagnosis of bipolar mania also requires an assessment of etiology, with a particular focus on possible physiological effects of medications or a medical condition. This evaluation is complicated regarding Mr. Lopez.

In addition to a classic manic syndrome, Mr. Lopez has a personal history of depression, and during a course of antidepressant medication, he became "hyper and edgy." That response to medication suggests a manic or hypomanic response and an elevated risk for bipolar disorder. In addition, his aunt's use of lithium suggests a family history of bipolar disorder. Absent other comorbidities, this presentation would suggest the diagnosis of bipolar disorder, manic, single episode.

However, this case is complicated by two significant comorbidities: the use of crystal methamphetamine and his HIV infection. Amphetamines can induce paranoid psychosis and manic mood symptoms in the setting of both acute and chronic use. In this case, Mr. Lopez's symptoms appear to have begun before he apparently used the stimulant (he was edgy, hyperenergetic, pressured, and glassy-eyed), and they persisted for weeks after his only reported use of the crystal methamphetamine. Stimulant-induced mania typically resolves within days of abstinence, which would better fit Mr. Lopez's acute paranoid reaction to the crystal methamphetamine. In addition, he has a multiple-year history of crystal methamphetamine misuse without reported mania, which might further diminish the likelihood that amphetamine triggered this

DSM-5-TR™ Clinical Cases

episode. On the other hand, Mr. Lopez may have been hiding his use of crystal methamphetamine for weeks or months, or he may have used amphetamines to help him complete his recent editing project. Either stimulant would have contributed to sleep deprivation, which is both a precipitant and a symptom of mania.

HIV infection is also associated with bipolar disorder. Manic symptoms can occur at any stage of infection, but they are most closely associated with relatively late-stage HIV-associated neurocognitive disorder. Symptoms may be identical to a classic mania, but the neurocognitive disorder seems to contribute to unusually prominent irritability and cognitive difficulties. It is difficult to assess a noncompliant patient for cognitive decline, especially when he or she is manic, but Mr. Lopez has been said to have "lost a step" over the prior year, is irritable, and has an MRI scan that features the sort of nonspecific findings often found in patients with HIV infection and immune suppression. It appears that Mr. Lopez has been nonadherent to his antiretroviral medication for at least 1 month, possibly longer, and he has not had recent assessment of his T cells or viral load.

Tentatively, then, Mr. Lopez warrants a DSM-5 diagnosis of bipolar and related disorder due to HIV infection, with manic features. A toxicology screen might help clarify whether Mr. Lopez has continued to use amphetamines, whereas a T-cell count and viral load assessment can help determine the degree of immune suppression. After psychiatric stabilization and a resumption of antiretroviral medications, it would be useful to obtain a neuropsychological assessment to clarify the degree of neurocognitive impairment.

Diagnosis

• Bipolar and related disorder due to HIV infection, with manic features

Suggested Readings

Eggers C, Arendt G, Hahn K, et al; German Association of Neuro-AIDS und Neuro-Infectiology (DGNANI): HIV-1-associated neurocognitive disorder: epidemiology, pathogenesis, diagnosis, and treatment. J Neurol 264(8):1715–1727, 2017

Ferrando SJ, Nims C: HIV-associated mania treated with electroconvulsive therapy and highly-active antiretroviral therapy. Psychosomatics 47(2):170–174, 2006

Walter TJ, Iudicello J, Cookson DR, et al; on behalf of the Translational Methamphetamine AIDS Research Center (TMARC): The relationships between HIV-1 infection, history of methamphetamine use disorder, and soluble biomarkers in blood and cerebrospinal fluid. Viruses 13(7):1287, 2021

CASE 3.7

Bizarrely Silent

Jessica Daniels, M.D.

Taaj Mustafa, a 22-year-old recent college graduate, was brought to the emergency room (ER) by his friends after he appeared bizarrely silent after disappearing for 3 days. Mr. Mustafa's friends reported that he had recently undergone treatment for testicular cancer, but that he had been in a good mood when they had last seen him 4 nights earlier. He had not shown up for a planned get-together the following day and had then not responded to e-mails, texts, or phone calls. They had not known how to contact his parents or relatives and had no other history.

In the ER, Mr. Mustafa related to others in an odd manner, standing stiffly and not making eye contact or answering questions. After about 10 minutes, he suddenly grabbed a staff member by the arm. While he seemed to lack a purpose or intent to harm, he refused to let go, and the staff member was unable to extricate herself until a security guard intervened. At that point, he received intramuscular haloperidol and lorazepam. During the ensuing hour, his extremities became rigid, and while lying on a hospital bed, he held his arms above his head, with his elbows bent. He was admitted to the medical service. A head computed tomography (CT) scan, routine laboratory tests, and urine toxicology were noncontributory, except that his creatine phosphokinase (CPK) was elevated, at 906 IU/L. His heart rate was also elevated, at 110 beats per minute. He had no fever, and his blood pressure was within the normal range.

On examination, Mr. Mustafa was found to be a thin young man lying in bed, with his head held awkwardly off the pillow. He was stiffly raising his arms up and down. His hair was falling out in tufts. He stared straight ahead with infrequent blinks, making no eye contact. He was not diaphoretic and did not appear to be in pain. Physical examination revealed an initial resistance against any movement of his arms. When either arm was moved into a position by the examiner, it remained in that position. No myoclonus was evident. Speaking with a long latency and significantly decreased production, he expressed fear that he was dying. As he slowly expressed his anxiety, his body remained stiff and rigid. He denied auditory or visual hallucinations. He was fully awake and alert and was oriented to time and place but did not participate in other cognitive tests.

Mr. Mustafa was clinically unchanged for 3 days while he received intravenous fluids. No psychoactive medication was given. Laboratory tests, an electroencephalogram (EEG), and magnetic resonance imaging (MRI) of the brain were unrevealing, and his CPK trended downward after peaking at 1,100 IU/L. On the fourth hospital day, Mr. Mustafa was given a test dose of intravenous lorazepam 1 mg and then a repeat dose of 1 mg after 5 minutes. He did not become sedated. His mental status did not change, except that his speech was slightly more productive after the second dose. Intravenous lorazepam 1 mg every 4–6 hours was started. After 24 hours, his rigidity had resolved, his speech was fluent and pressured, and he became very active and agitated. He paced the hallways, followed the nurses around, and tried to leave the hospital. He told staff, other patients, and visitors that he was a great artist and that he had cured his cancer. His CPK normalized and tachycardia resolved. He remained afebrile.

Mr. Mustafa's parents arrived from out of town on the sixth hospital day. They reported that his only previous psychiatric history had been a depression that developed when he was diagnosed with testicular cancer 1 year earlier. Mr. Mustafa had been taking sertraline 50 mg/day and was doing well until 10 days prior to admission, when he learned that he had a recurrence of testicular cancer with metastasis to the retroperitoneum. He immediately underwent chemotherapy with cisplatin, etoposide, and dexamethasone. After receiving the chemotherapy, Mr. Mustafa had told his parents over the phone that he felt "excellent" but had then not returned their phone calls or e-mails. This was not entirely unusual behavior for their son, who was "a sketchy correspondent," but they had become increasingly worried and finally flew across the country when they had not heard from him in 10 days. The parents also mentioned that the only pertinent family history was a maternal uncle with severe bipolar disorder, which had been treated with electroconvulsive therapy.

Discussion

Mr. Mustafa presents with grossly disorganized and abnormal behavior. He manifests a rigid, bizarre posture with waxy flexibility. He lacks appropriate verbal and motor responses (mutism and stupor), maintains a rigid and fixed posture (catalepsy), and exhibits repetitive or ritualistic movements (stereotypy). Mr. Mustafa's symptoms easily meet the 3 of 12 psychomotor features required for a DSM-5 diagnosis of catatonia.

Catatonia has historically been linked to schizophrenia, and one-third of people with schizophrenia have an episode of catatonic symptoms at some point during their lives. It has become clear, however, that most patients with catatonia have a depressive or bipolar disorder. Still other patients have catatonic symptoms as part of a medical disorder (e.g., hepatic encephalitis), a reaction to a medication (e.g., neuroleptic malignant syndrome [NMS]), or a reaction to an illicit substance (e.g., cocaine). The breadth of potential etiologies is an important reason that DSM-5 generally uses the term *catatonia* as a modifying specifier rather than as the name of a specific type of disorder.

After catatonia is identified and the patient is stabilized, the next clinical focus is diagnosing the underlying cause. This search is urgent, because many of the causes of catatonia are medically dangerous. In addition, catatonia itself can cause severe morbidity and mortality due to dehydration, malnutrition, exhaustion, and profound immobility that can lead to thromboembolism and pressure ulcers. In addition, people with catatonia can hurt themselves or others. Regardless of etiology, catatonia can progress to malignant catatonia, which is marked by fever, autonomic instability, and high fatality rates.

Mr. Mustafa's normal neurological and physical examinations, head CT scan, brain MRI scan, and EEG appeared to rule out many of the acute neurological events that can mimic catatonia, such as a stroke (and akinetic mutism), central nervous system malignancy, and locked-in syndrome. Mr. Mustafa remained afebrile, which made it unlikely that his symptoms were caused by infectious encephalitis. A urine drug screen ruled out acute cocaine and phencyclidine intoxication. Other medical causes of catatonia were evaluated and ruled out through noncontributory assessments of thyroid, glucose, HIV, complete blood count, vitamin B_{12}, liver function, lupus antibodies, and a complete metabolic panel. Given his cancer history, a paraneoplastic panel was considered, but he recovered before a lumbar puncture was performed.

NMS is a serious concern. As described in the DSM-5 Section II chapter "Medication-Induced Movement Disorders and Other Adverse Effects of Medication," NMS is a psychiatric emergency characterized by muscle rigidity, fever, autonomic instability, cognitive changes, and an elevated CPK. Mr. Mustafa became "stiff" after receiving haloperidol in the ER, was confused, and had an elevated CPK. Mr. Mustafa was never febrile, however, and his vital signs remained stable except for mild tachycardia, which resolved with lorazepam treatment. His elevated CPK likely reflected recent agitation and rigidity and did not reach the greatly elevated range associated with NMS. Whereas NMS is associated with the use of antipsychotic medication, serotonin syndrome is associated with selective serotonin reuptake inhibitor (SSRI) antidepressants. Although Mr. Mustafa is taking sertraline and could have taken an overdose, he lacks the typical myoclonus and gastrointestinal symptoms.

With no obvious medical and neurological abnormalities, a psychiatric condition appears the most likely cause of the catatonia. While barely able to speak, Mr. Mustafa did say he was scared and worried that he was dying or dead. Extreme anxiety is the most common affective experience of catatonic patients, to the point that catatonia is sometimes viewed as an extreme "freeze" response. This affective experience does not point toward the underlying psychiatric condition, however, and, given the typical patient's inability to communicate, correct diagnosis is often delayed until the catatonia resolves.

Diagnosis and treatment often occur simultaneously with the use of low-dose intravenous lorazepam. Unlike most other patients, people with catatonia often appear more alert and engaged after administration of benzodiazepines. Mr. Mustafa's mutism and stupor seem to have shown subtle improvement immediately but then improved significantly after 24 hours. As his catatonia improved, his underlying mania became more evident. In addition, his parents provided invaluable collateral history that clarified that his manic episode was apparently triggered by a steroid-based chemotherapy regimen.

Diagnosis

- Steroid-induced bipolar and related disorder, with mania, severe, with mood-congruent psychotic features and catatonic features

Suggested Readings

Daniels J: Catatonia: clinical aspects and neurobiological correlates. J Neuropsychiatry Clin Neurosci 21(4):371–380, 2009

Fink M: Rediscovering catatonia: the biography of a treatable syndrome. Acta Psychiatr Scand Suppl (441):1–47, 2013

Smith JH, Smith VD, Philbrick KL, Kumar N: Catatonic disorder due to a general medical or psychiatric condition. J Neuropsychiatry Clin Neurosci 24(2):198–207, 2012

Walther S, Stegmayer K, Wilson JE, Heckers S: Structure and neural mechanisms of catatonia. Lancet Psychiatry 6(7):610–619, 2019

CASE 3.8

A Postpartum Change

Ian Jones, M.R.C.Psych., Ph.D.

Ursula Norman, a 32-year-old nurse, was brought to an emergency department 6 days after giving birth. Her husband stated that she had been behaving very strangely and that she had become convinced that she had smothered and killed her baby.

Her husband reported that after a normal pregnancy and uncomplicated delivery, Ms. Norman had happily gone home with their first child. On the third day after delivery, however, her mood and affect began to shift rapidly between elation and weepiness. She became irritable and anxious. She slept only an hour a night, even when her baby was asleep. Her behavior became increasingly bizarre, with overactivity and agitation. Her speech was rapid and digressive. Although not previously a religious person, she became convinced that God was speaking through her and that she had special powers that could solve the problems of the world. She told her husband that she could identify evil people by looking into their eyes and had begun to worry that she was surrounded by evil people, including her own mother. Most disturbing for her, whenever she was out of sight of her son, she became totally convinced that she had smothered him, and no one could convince her otherwise.

Ms. Norman had a history of three episodes of major depressive disorder in her teens and early 20s. These episodes resolved with psychotherapy and antidepressant medication. She also had a psychiatric admission for mania 3 years prior to the delivery of her child, after a flight from Asia to Europe. Following treatment with antipsychotic medication, she became depressed for several months. Although a diagnosis of bipolar disorder was discussed at this time, she was reluctant to accept this label, attributing the episode to stress and jet lag. She had discontinued the psychiatric medication in anticipation of getting pregnant.

Ms. Norman's own mother had been admitted to a psychiatric hospital shortly after the birth of her first child. This episode was not talked about in the family, and there were few other details. She had no other family history of note.

Until just before delivery of her child, Ms. Norman had been a highly functional nurse in a renal unit. Her husband was the head of a sales team, and they lived in comfortable social circumstances. She had no history of illicit drug use and, prior to pregnancy, drank only 2 or 3 units of alcohol a week.

On mental status examination, Ms. Norman wandered around the room, seemingly unable to sit for more than a few moments. She was distractible and overtalkative, and demonstrated flight of ideas, flitting from one subject to another. Her mood was labile. At times she appeared happily euphoric. At other times she was tearful, and she could become quickly irritable when she felt she was not being understood. It was clear that she had a number of delusional beliefs but was unwilling to discuss most of them with the examiner. She did insist that she had already killed her own child, which led to several minutes of tears, but she returned to an edgy euphoria within a few minutes. She denied intent to harm herself or anyone else. She appeared inattentive, with poor concentration, but would not participate in formal cognitive testing.

Physical examination and laboratory testing results were all within normal limits.

Discussion

Ms. Norman presents with flight of ideas, pressured speech, distractibility, agitation, lability, greatly diminished sleep, uncharacteristic hyperreligiosity, delusions about her friends and family, and the fixed, false belief that she has already killed her child. She has a history of multiple major depressive episodes and of one psychiatric hospitalization for mania. These qualify her for a DSM-5 diagnosis of bipolar I disorder, severe, with psychotic features.

Ms. Norman is also clearly experiencing an episode of what has traditionally been called postpartum psychosis—the abrupt onset of an affective psychosis in the early postpartum period. A number of features of her presentation are characteristic of postpartum psychosis. The onset is typically early in the postpartum period, generally in the first postpartum week. Episodes of postpartum psychosis commonly show a rapid onset and may deteriorate quickly to a florid and severe psychosis. As in Ms. Norman's case, episodes often manifest a "kaleidoscopic" presentation, with delusional thoughts, for example, changing frequently rather than becoming fixed and systematized. Because of these characteristics, postpartum psychosis is a true psychiatric emergency and admission is usually required. A comprehensive risk assessment is essential, both for suicidal ideation and for risk of harm to the baby.

Pregnancy leads to a severe postpartum episode in 1 in 1,000 pregnancies, but some women are at considerably higher risk. For example, women with bipolar disorder suffer severe postpartum episodes in approximately 1 in 4 deliveries. In women with a history of postpartum psychosis, the risk in subsequent pregnancies is greater than 1 in 2.

Women who are at high risk of a severe postpartum episode should be identified during the antenatal period. With her history of bipolar disorder and a probable family history of postpartum psychosis, Ms. Norman was at very high risk, despite having been well for several years. Given this history, she should have been under close monitoring throughout the pregnancy and postpartum period. After she recovers, it will become important to discuss plans with regard to future pregnancies with both her and her partner. Her case also illustrates that severe postpartum episodes can have a sudden onset in women who have been very well in pregnancy and who have no particular psychosocial predisposing factors.

Ms. Norman had a diagnosis of bipolar disorder prior to this pregnancy. In many cases, however, particularly when postpartum psychosis is the first episode, the diagnosis can be more uncertain. An early onset of a severe postpartum episode, even in the absence of a prior psychiatric history, should raise suspicion of a bipolar diagnosis.

The specific diagnosis of postpartum psychosis is not an option in DSM-5, but as is the case with postpartum depression, the term has remained in common usage by clinicians, women themselves, and user groups (e.g., Action on Postpartum Psychosis: www.app-network.org). Instead, DSM-5 suggests use of a descriptive specifier, "with peripartum onset."

There are a number of reasons why flagging the perinatal context of episodes is important. First, the new baby is an important consideration and may affect management decisions (e.g., hospitalization). Second, a severe postpartum episode has important implications for future pregnancies. Third, the close relationship of severe postpartum episodes to bipolar disorder should prompt careful assessments for a history of a bipolar disorder as well as inform future clinical psychiatric treatment.

Diagnosis

- Bipolar I disorder, current episode manic, severe, with psychotic features, with peripartum onset

Suggested Readings

Di Florio A, Forty L, Gordon-Smith K, et al: Perinatal episodes across the mood disorder spectrum. JAMA Psychiatry 70(2):168–175, 2013

Jones I, Heron J, Blackmore ER, et al: Puerperal psychosis, in Oxford Textbook of Women and Mental Health. Edited by Kohen D. Oxford, UK, Oxford University Press, 2010, pp 179–186

Munk-Olsen T, Laursen TM, Meltzer-Brody S, et al: Psychiatric disorders with postpartum onset: possible early manifestations of bipolar affective disorders. Arch Gen Psychiatry 69(4):428–434, 2012

Perry A, Gordon-Smith K, Di Florio A, et al: Mood episodes in pregnancy and risk of postpartum recurrence in bipolar disorder: The Bipolar Disorder Research Network Pregnancy Study. J Affect Disord 294:714–722, 2021

CASE 3.9

Depressed and Anxious

Holly A. Swartz, M.D.

Victoria Owens, a divorced 58-year-old event planner, scheduled an appointment with a psychiatrist for help with anxiety and depression. Ms. Owens arrived at the appointment well dressed and a little agitated. Speaking at a normal pace, she explained that her depressive symptoms had begun 2 years earlier in the setting of initiating divorce proceedings from her fourth husband. She described poor mood, incapacitating worry about her future, and poor concentration. These symptoms progressed to anhedonia, decreased energy, hypersomnia with interrupted sleep, passive suicidal ideation, and increased appetite with carbohydrate craving. She stopped going to work as an event planner and began spending most of the day in bed.

Ms. Owens initially sought treatment from a homeopath, who prescribed a variety of remedies that were not helpful. She eventually saw her internist, who prescribed alprazolam 0.25 mg three times a day as needed. This medication reduced her worry but had little effect on her mood. Her internist then initiated sertraline 50 mg/day, increasing the dosage (as tolerated) to 200 mg/day. Over the ensuing 2 months, Ms. Owens's sleep improved and she no longer experienced suicidal thoughts. However, she became more anxious, irritable, agitated, and energized and noted that her thoughts moved rapidly. She denied impulsivity and psychotic symptoms.

Ms. Owens had a long-standing history of similar depressive episodes. The first such episode occurred during college, lasted for several months, and was untreated.

When specifically asked, she described multiple periods in her life when she had moderately elevated mood, rapid thoughts, and increased energy. It seemed that many important life accomplishments occurred during these periods. For instance, as a young, recently divorced unemployed single mother, she agreed to throw a bridal shower for her best friend. She pored over bridal and craft magazines, determined to create a fabulous party on a shoestring budget. She became totally engrossed in the project, seeming to have abundant energy and ideas. The shower was a huge success and launched Ms. Owens's career as a party planner. She hid her mood swings from her clients and colleagues, leveraging her elevated mood states to project a high-energy "face," but then would retreat and avoid work when her mood became low. She also became more irritable during these high-energy episodes, and she believed that each of her marriages both began and ended because of her tendency to "get emotional" when she was in these elevated mood states. Although these periods could last for many weeks, she did not experience changes in sleep, engage in risky behaviors, speak quickly, or become grandiose, and she saw nothing problematic about them.

Ms. Owens also reported that she drank heavily when she was in her 40s but rarely did so now. She denied prior suicide attempts and psychiatric hospitalizations. Her mother had been treated for depression with sertraline, and her brother was treated with lithium for bipolar disorder.

Discussion

Ms. Owens has a history of recurrent depressive episodes accompanied by multiple high-energy, high-mood episodes that meet duration criteria (≥4 days) for hypomania but are not characterized by sufficient symptoms to meet full syndromal criteria for a hypomanic episode. She endorsed both elevated mood and energy during these episodes but only two of the seven Criterion B symptoms: racing thoughts and increased goal-directed activity. As is typical for individuals with subthreshold bipolar disorder, Ms. Owens experiences these episodes as ego-syntonic and does not report them spontaneously. Not surprisingly, subthreshold hypomanic episodes are easily missed unless the interviewer carefully probes for them.

Major depressive disorder would also be included in the differential diagnosis. Ms. Owens initially presented to her internist with classic symptoms of depression. Given her prior history of multiple depressive episodes and lack of spontaneous complaints about hypomania, her primary care physician likely assumed that Ms. Owens had major depressive disorder and treated her with an SSRI. The SSRI, however, precipitated a mixed state consisting of an irritable and anxious mood, rapid thoughts, and increased energy. When depressed patients such as Ms. Owens develop mixed, manic, or hypomanic symptoms following exposure to antidepressants, consideration should be given to a bipolar diagnosis. Ms. Owens's mixed state while taking an SSRI is not sufficient for a diagnosis of bipolar disorder but certainly raises a red flag. Her family history of bipolar disorder (in this case, a brother treated with lithium) further increases the likelihood that she has a form of bipolar disorder. Although the most common mood disorder among first-degree relatives of individuals with bipolar disorder is major depressive disorder, having a relative with bipolar disorder does increase the person's risk of having bipolar disorder as well.

Despite features consistent with bipolar disorder, Ms. Owens's clinical picture is complicated. In addition to subthreshold hypomanic symptoms, she also reported a history of unstable relationships, emotional lability, prior substance misuse, and anxiety. Bipolar disorder and personality disorders—especially borderline personality disorder—often co-occur and may be difficult to tease apart because they have clinical features in common. For instance, both bipolar disorder and borderline personality disorder are characterized by increased levels of impulsive behavior, affective lability, and irritability. In Ms. Owens's case, lability and irritability appear to be restricted to mood episodes, suggesting that they are secondary to a mood disorder rather than pervasive problems of affect regulation. However, comorbid mood disorder and personality disorder cannot be ruled out.

Up to one-third of patients with bipolar disorder are diagnosed with comorbid anxiety disorders, which are, in turn, associated with worse psychiatric outcomes. Bipolar disorder is often misdiagnosed as an anxiety disorder, perhaps because of the high rates of comorbidity. Similarly, substance use disorders and bipolar disorders often co-occur. Co-occurring anxiety and substance use disorder seem to follow the course of bipolar illness—that is, anxiety disorders tend to associate most with depressive symptoms, and substance use disorders are moderately associated with manic symptoms. Further exploration is needed to determine the presence of comorbidities, and there is a high probability that Ms. Owens suffers from more than one psychiatric disorder.

Diagnosis

• Unspecified bipolar and related disorder

Suggested Readings

Deltito J, Martin L, Riefkohl J, et al: Do patients with borderline personality disorder belong to the bipolar spectrum? J Affect Disord 67(1–3):221–228, 2001

Mantere O, Isometsä E, Ketokivi M, et al: A prospective latent analyses study of psychiatric comorbidity of DSM-IV bipolar I and II disorders. Bipolar Disord 12(3):271–284, 2010

Merikangas KR, Jin R, He JP, et al: Prevalence and correlates of bipolar spectrum disorder in the World Mental Health Survey Initiative. Arch Gen Psychiatry 68(3):241–251, 2011

Parker GB, Graham RK: Clinical characteristics associated with treatment-resistant bipolar disorder. J Nerv Ment Dis 205(3):188–191, 2017

Zimmerman M, Morgan TA: The relationship between borderline personality disorder and bipolar disorder. Dialogues Clin Neurosci 15:155–169, 2013

CHAPTER 4

Depressive Disorders

INTRODUCTION

John W. Barnhill, M.D.

Depression is one of the most commonly used words in psychiatry, and it is also one of the most ambiguous. As a symptom it can mean sadness, but as a diagnosis it can be applied to people who deny feeling sad. Depressed mood is a common, normal human experience, but it can also reflect a seriously debilitating, distressing, and potentially fatal condition. Depression can present in multiple ways, with many potential comorbidities, precipitants, and reliably associated symptoms.

It is important to recognize that depressive symptoms can be found in almost all disorders in DSM-5, and a chief complaint of "sadness" is only the beginning of the diagnostic inquiry. It is also useful to recall that essentially all of the major nonmood disorders in DSM-5 increase the likelihood of comorbid major depressive disorder. For example, although bipolar disorder has historically been viewed as "manic depression," and therefore as a subset of depression, it has become increasingly clear that while bipolar and depressive disorders have similarities, they also have substantive differences in regard to clinical presentation, family history, longitudinal course, and treatment. For these reasons, bipolar disorder was moved into its own chapter in DSM-5. The overlap persists, however, and the depressive and bipolar disorder chapters go into detail in an effort to distinguish the sometimes subtle differences between these diagnoses.

Major depressive disorder (MDD) remains the archetypal depressive disorder, and its diagnostic criteria are essentially unchanged in DSM-5. The diagnosis still hinges on the assessment of clinical presentation (presence of five of nine symptoms), history (persistence for longer than 2 weeks), and relevance (significant distress or impairment). To further subdivide this broad category, DSM-5 provides specifiers that distinguish the episode based on severity and recurrence as well as the presence of such factors as melancholia, psychotic features, and catatonia. A particularly useful change from DSM-IV is the delinkage of psychosis and severity, so the clinician can accurately describe people whose depressive symptoms are, say, moderate, but who have an associated psychosis.

The text within DSM-5-TR includes many different assessment tips. For example, many people with depression report insomnia or fatigue rather than depression per se, and a failure to look for depressive symptoms can lead to underdiagnosis. Psychomotor disturbance and guilt (whether delusional or near-delusional) are much less common in MDD than insomnia or fatigue but tend to be markers for greater severity.

Culture can affect the diagnosis of depression in multiple ways. Poverty, racism, and marginalization are examples of structural adversities that may contribute to the development of MDD. The prevalence, course, and symptomatology of depression vary among different cultures, but a depressive syndrome has been widely identified across cultures. Although such symptoms are not included in the official criteria, DSM-5-TR suggests being alert to depressive manifestations such as social isolation, anger, tearfulness, and diffuse pain. Somatic complaints are typical presenting complaints of depression in many cultures, and it can be helpful to tactfully explore the meaning of these symptoms as they relate to local social contexts.

Studies consistently indicate that women are significantly more likely than men to develop MDD. It has been hypothesized that these elevated rates are partly related to women's disproportionate exposure to interpersonal trauma over the life span. In addition, women may be at elevated risk because of their experiences in the reproductive life stages of the perimenstrual, peripartum, and perimenopausal periods.

The DSM-5 chapter on depressive disorders also included several changes from DSM-IV that have been the subject of significant scrutiny. The so-called bereavement exclusion has perhaps been the most discussed. It is widely understood that mourning the death of a loved one is a normal human reaction, and DSM-IV clarified that a 2-month period of bereavement was generally necessary before an MDD diagnosis could be made. Evidence indicated, however, that most grieving people do not develop the symptoms of MDD. In other words, MDD that occurs in the context of bereavement is not a "normal" reaction. The suffering of MDD tends to include more intense feelings of guilt, worthlessness, and suicidality, for example, and the functional decline is more severe. Furthermore, individuals who develop major depressive symptoms soon after the death of a loved one have elevated rates of depression in their personal and family histories, tend to have a worse prognosis, and tend to respond to antidepressant medications. In other words, individuals who develop all the characteristics of MDD following the death of a loved one are similar to people who develop MDD following any other serious stress and deserve the same level of clinical attention. DSM-5-TR extends this focus on grief by moving *prolonged grief disorder* from "Conditions for Further Study" (where it was called *persistent complex bereavement disorder* in DSM-5) into the main body of the text, where it is discussed in the chapter on trauma- and stressor-related disorders.

Just as most grief is a normal reaction to loss, temper tantrums are a normal part of childhood. There are, however, children whose low frustration tolerance and behavioral dyscontrol transcend those of normal human experience; their affective dysregulation not only is distressing to their parents, teachers, and classmates, but also is upsetting to the affected children and threatens to derail their normal development. In DSM-5, these children were categorized as having disruptive mood dysregulation disorder (DMDD). Controversies about DMDD fall into two camps. In the first, there is concern that the diagnosis might pathologize normal childhood experience. In the second, there is a view that such behavior is more accurately described within the bipolar spectrum of disorders. Evidence indicates, however, that DMDD does describe a cluster of prepubescent children who are significantly distressed and dysfunctional and who are at risk for a lifetime of difficulty. Furthermore, it appears that DMDD is not simply a childhood form of bipolar disorder. In fact, DMDD is much more likely to convert in adulthood to a depressive or an anxiety disorder than to a bipolar disorder.

Another change from DSM-IV was the shift of premenstrual dysphoric disorder (PMDD) from DSM-IV Appendix B ("Criteria Sets and Axes Provided for Further Study") into the main text of DSM-5. Just as DMDD does not refer to average expectable "temper tantrums," PMDD does not describe the transient, mild symptoms that are commonly described as "premenstrual syndrome." Instead, PMDD describes a robust cluster of symptoms that cause persistent, significant debility and distress.

Concerns have been raised that these changes could lead to the pathologizing of normal human experience and, secondarily, to the excess use of psychiatric medication. The field of psychiatry should indeed recognize both the limitations of current evidence and the external forces that might try to influence the field for their own reward. At the same time, evidence does indicate that these new diagnoses reflect clusters of people who are suffering and significantly dysfunctional. It is also true that people meeting these criteria are often already seeking psychiatric help, and that the development of rigorous diagnostic criteria allows for replicable research into effective biopsychosocial interventions.

Suggested Readings

Haroz EE, Ritchey M, Bass JK, et al: How is depression experienced around the world? A systematic review of qualitative literature. Soc Sci Med 183:151–162, 2017

Kirmayer LJ, Gomez-Carrillo A, Veissière S: Culture and depression in global mental health: an ecosocial approach to the phenomenology of psychiatric disorders. Soc Sci Med 183:163–168, 2017

Kramer P: Against Depression. New York, Penguin, 2006

Nemeroff CB, Schatzberg AF, Rasgon N, Strakowski SM (eds): The American Psychiatric Association Publishing Textbook of Mood Disorders, 2nd Edition. Washington, DC, American Psychiatric Association Publishing, 2022

Vines AI, Ward JB, Cordoba E, Black KZ: Perceived racial/ethnic discrimination and mental health: a review and future directions for social epidemiology. Curr Epidemiol Rep 4(2):156–165, 2017

CASE 4.1

Moody and Irritable

William C. Wood, M.D.

Wyatt was a 12-year-old-boy referred by his psychiatrist to an adolescent partial hospitalization program because of repeated conflicts that have frightened both class-mates and family members.

According to his parents, Wyatt was generally moody and irritable, with frequent episodes of being "a raging monster." It had become almost impossible to set limits. Most recently, Wyatt had smashed a closet door to gain access to a video game that had been withheld to encourage him to do homework. At school, Wyatt was noted to have a hair-trigger temper, and he had recently been suspended for punching another boy in the face after losing a chess match.

Wyatt had been an extremely active young boy, running "all the time." He was also a "sensitive kid" who constantly worried that things might go wrong. His tolerance for frustration had been less than that of his peers, and his parents quit taking him shopping because he would predictably become distraught whenever they did not buy him whatever toys he wanted.

Grade school reports indicated fidgetiness, wandering attention, and impulsivity. When Wyatt was 10 years old, a child psychiatrist diagnosed him as having attention-deficit/hyperactivity disorder (ADHD), combined type. Wyatt was referred to a be-havioral therapist and started taking methylphenidate, which led to an improvement in his symptoms. However, by fourth grade, his moodiness became more pronounced and persistent. He was generally surly, complaining that life was "unfair." Wyatt and his parents began their daily limit-setting battles at breakfast while he delayed getting ready for school, and then—by evening—continued their arguments about home-work, video games, and bedtime. These arguments often included Wyatt screaming and throwing nearby objects. By the time he reached sixth grade, his parents were tired and his siblings avoided him.

According to Wyatt's parents, he had no problems with appetite, and although they fought about when he would go to bed, he did not appear to have a sleep distur-bance. He appeared to find pleasure in his usual activities, maintained good energy, and had no history of elation, grandiosity, or decreased need for sleep lasting more than a day. Although they described him as "moody, isolated, and lonely," his parents did not see him as depressed. They denied any history of hallucinations, abuse, trauma, suicidality, homicidality, a wish to self-harm, or any premeditated wish to harm others. He and his parents denied he had ever used alcohol or drugs. His medical history was unremarkable. His family history was notable for anxiety and depression in the father, alcoholism in the paternal grandparents, and possible untreated ADHD in the mother.

On interview, Wyatt was mildly anxious yet easy to engage. His body twisted back and forth as he sat in the chair. In reviewing his temper outbursts and physical aggression, Wyatt said, "It's like I can't help myself. I don't mean to do these things. But when I get mad, I don't think about any of that. It's like my mind goes blank." When asked how he felt about his outbursts, Wyatt looked very sad and said earnestly, "I hate when I'm that way." If he could change three things in his life, Wyatt replied, "I would have more friends, I would do better in school, and I would stop getting mad so much."

Discussion

Wyatt's psychiatrist has referred him to an adolescent partial hospitalization program because of persistent irritability and severe recurrent temper outbursts.

In assessing this 12-year-old boy, it would be important to attend to the quality, severity, frequency, and duration of the outbursts. Are they outside the range of "developmentally normal" children? What are the provocations? Do the outbursts occur at home, at school, with peers, or in more than one setting? How are they affecting his life? What is this boy's general mood between the outbursts? Do the outbursts reflect a lack of control over his emotional reactions, or are they a behavior calculated to achieve an intended outcome? At what age did these emotional and/or behavioral outbursts begin? Are there corresponding neurovegetative depressive symptoms? Has he ever exhibited manic-like symptoms such as grandiosity, decreased need for sleep, pressured speech, or racing thoughts? If so, have these symptoms persisted long enough to meet criteria for a manic episode? Does he abuse substances? Has he ever experienced psychotic symptoms such as paranoia, delusions, or hallucinations of any kind?

In Wyatt's case, his intense irritability appears to be persistent, while his outbursts tend to be extreme and incongruent with his overall developmental level. They are clearly interfering with all aspects of his life. He does not appear to be in control of his behavior, and his irritability and outbursts are not bringing him anything positive; in fact, the three things he says he would most like to change are specifically related to either the symptom ("stop getting mad so much") or the consequences of his symptoms ("have more friends" and "do better in school"). These symptoms have been worsening since grade school. He lacks prominent neurovegetative symptoms of depression, and there is no history of mania, psychosis, or substance abuse.

In considering the differential diagnosis for age-incongruent "temper tantrums," it is useful to recognize that Wyatt does not manifest the decreased need for sleep, pressured speech, mood cycling, and racing thoughts that are found in bipolar disorder. In addition, his intense irritability persists between outbursts, which excludes oppositional defiant disorder, intermittent explosive disorder, and conduct disorder.

Wyatt does appear to meet criteria for disruptive mood dysregulation disorder (DMDD), a diagnosis introduced in DSM-5 that is listed among the depressive disorders. The core feature of DMDD is chronic, severe, persistent irritability that is incongruent with a child's developmental stage and is causing significant impairment. This core feature has two prominent clinical manifestations: frequent severe temper outbursts (verbal or behavioral) and chronic, persistently irritable or angry mood that is present between the severe temper outbursts.

By DSM-5 definition, DMDD cannot coexist with bipolar disorder or with either oppositional defiant disorder or intermittent explosive disorder. If the patient has ever had a manic episode, a diagnosis of bipolar disorder supersedes a DMDD diagnosis. If the patient meets criteria for intermittent explosive disorder or oppositional defiant disorder but also meets criteria for DMDD, the patient should only be diagnosed with DMDD.

DMDD can be comorbid with a variety of other diagnoses. For example, Wyatt presents with long-standing problems with attention and anxiety. When in grade school, he was diagnosed with ADHD, combined type, which indicates that he met most criteria in both ADHD categories: attention and hyperactivity/impulsivity. Wyatt is also noted to be a chronic worrier. Although this was not explored at length in the history, he may well qualify for an anxiety disorder.

It will be important to follow Wyatt longitudinally. The goal, of course, is to employ the most parsimonious diagnostic assessment and treatment plan, but these can change in the context of Wyatt's overall development. As an adolescent with a diagnosis of DMDD, he will continue to be at risk for a variety of comorbid psychiatric conditions, including other mood, anxiety, and substance use disorders.

Diagnoses

- Disruptive mood dysregulation disorder
- Attention-deficit/hyperactivity disorder, combined presentation

Suggested Readings

Bruno A, Celebre L, Torre G, et al: Focus on disruptive mood dysregulation disorder: a review of the literature. Psychiatry Res 279(Sep):323–330, 2019

Copeland WE, Angold A, Costello EJ, Egger H: Prevalence, comorbidity, and correlates of DSM-5 proposed disruptive mood dysregulation disorder. Am J Psychiatry 170(2):173–179, 2013

Mürner-Lavanchy I, Kaess M, Koenig J: Diagnostic instruments for the assessment of disruptive mood dysregulation disorder: a systematic review of the literature. Eur Child Adolesc Psychiatry Jul 7 2021 [online ahead of print]

Stringaris A, Vidal-Ribas P, Brotman MA, Leibenluft E: Practitioner review: definition, recognition, and treatment challenges of irritability in young people. J Child Psychol Psychiatry 59(7):721–739, 2018

CASE 4.2

Postpartum Sadness

Kimberly A. Yonkers, M.D.

Heather B. Howell, M.S.W.

Yvonne Perez was a 23-year-old woman who presented for an outpatient psychiatric evaluation 3 weeks after giving birth to her second child. She was referred by her breastfeeding nurse, who was concerned about the patient's depressed mood, flat affect, and fatigue.

Ms. Perez said she had been worried and unenthusiastic since finding out she was pregnant. She and her husband planned to wait a few years before having another child, and her husband made it clear that he would have preferred that she terminate the pregnancy, an option she would not consider because of her religion. He had also been upset that she was "too tired" to do paid work outside of the home during her pregnancy. She became increasingly dysphoric, hopeless, and overwhelmed after the delivery. Breastfeeding was not going well, and she began to believe her baby was "rejecting me" by refusing her breast, spitting up her milk, and crying. Her baby became very colicky, so she felt forced to hold him most of the day. She wondered whether she deserved this difficulty because she had not wanted the pregnancy.

Her husband was gone much of the time for work, and she found it very difficult to take care of the new baby and her lively and demanding 16-month-old daughter. Over the past several weeks she slept little, felt constantly tired, cried often, and worried about how she was going to get through the day. Her mother-in-law had just arrived to help her care for the children, and she thought Ms. Perez just had the typical postpartum blues that result from "hormones being out of whack."

Ms. Perez was an English-speaking Hispanic woman who had worked in a coffee shop until midway through her first pregnancy, almost 2 years earlier. She was raised in a supportive home by her parents and has a large extended family. She moved to a different region of the country when her husband was transferred for work, and she had no relatives nearby. Although no one in her family had seen a psychiatrist, several family members appeared to have been depressed. She had no prior psychiatric history or treatment. She denied illicit drug or alcohol use. She had smoked for several years but stopped when she was pregnant with her first child. Ms. Perez had a history of asthma. Aside from a multivitamin with iron, she took no medications.

On mental status examination, Ms. Perez was a casually dressed, cooperative young woman. She made some eye contact, but her eyes tended to drop to the floor when she spoke. Her speech was fluent but slow, with increased latency when answering questions. The tone of her speech was flat. She endorsed low mood, and her affect was constricted. She denied thoughts of suicide and homicide. She also denied any hallucinations and delusions, although she had considered whether the current situation was punishment for not wanting the child. She was fully oriented and could register three objects but only recalled one after 5 minutes. Her intelligence was average. Her insight and judgment were fair to good.

Discussion

Ms. Perez presents with low mood, poor energy and sleep, psychomotor retardation, guilt, and poor concentration. The case report does not address her appetite, her ability to find pleasure, or the presence of thoughts about death, but she clearly has more than the required five of nine symptoms to meet criteria for a DSM-5 diagnosis of a major depressive episode. Contributors include the recent delivery, a family history of depression, and multiple psychosocial stressors, including a lack of support from her husband, financial troubles, a colicky baby, and geographical distance from her family of origin.

The case report is not clear, but it appears that Ms. Perez had some depressive symptoms throughout the pregnancy; she was referred to a psychiatrist at this particular time not because she was dramatically more depressed but because she was seen by a health professional, the breastfeeding nurse. This may indicate either less severe symptoms or a lack of systematic screening for depression. If Ms. Perez had become depressed only a week or so after delivery, she may not have had symptoms for the 2 weeks that are required for a major depressive episode. In that case, adjustment disorder with depressed mood would be a more appropriate diagnosis. A postpartum onset might also increase her risk of having bipolar disorder rather than unipolar depressive disorder. Arguing against a diagnosis of bipolar disorder in this patient is the lack of any known manic or psychotic symptoms as well as the absence of a history of mood episodes or a family history of bipolar disorder. Still, the fact that she experienced precipitous worsening after delivery would increase the risk that she might develop bipolar disorder.

From the available history, it appears more likely that Ms. Perez had significant depressive symptoms throughout the pregnancy. She said she felt "worried and unenthusiastic" and had felt "too tired" to work. This would not be an unusual depression trajectory, because half of women who are found to be depressed after delivery were already depressed during pregnancy. DSM-5 now includes a specifier, "with peripartum onset," for women who develop a mood disorder during or soon after a pregnancy. Ms. Perez also worries that her infant is rejecting her and that her current situation is a punishment. These appear to be overvalued ideas rather than delusions, but it would be reasonable to conduct ongoing assessments for psychotic thinking.

It is also important to do a suicide risk assessment for everyone with symptoms of major depressive disorder. Ms. Perez denies such symptoms, but it would be potentially useful to explore any thoughts she might have of death, of her family being better off without her, and of her children being better off dead.

The depressive subtype is important to clarify because many women with postpartum subsyndromal depressive symptoms improve spontaneously within weeks of delivery. This can occur even in the absence of formal treatment. For this reason, and because many women wish to continue breastfeeding, an initial treatment approach may be psychotherapeutic rather than pharmacological.

Diagnosis

- Major depressive disorder, single episode, moderate severity, without psychotic features, with peripartum onset

Suggested Readings

Gastaldon C, Solmi M, Correll CU, et al: Risk factors of postpartum depression and depressive symptoms: umbrella review of current evidence from systematic reviews and meta-analyses of observational studies. Br J Psychiatry 27:1–12, 2022

Sharma V, Doobay M, Baczynski C: Bipolar postpartum depression: an update and recommendations. J Affect Disord 219:105–111, 2017

Yonkers KA: Treatment of psychiatric conditions in pregnancy starts with planning. Am J Psychiatry 178(3):213–214, 2021

CASE 4.3

Grief and Depression

Richard A. Friedman, M.D.

Andrew Quinn, a 60-year-old businessman, returned to see his longtime psychiatrist 2 weeks after the death of his 24-year-old son. The young man, who had struggled with major depressive disorder and substance use disorder, had been found surrounded by several emptied pill bottles and an incoherent suicide note.

Mr. Quinn had been very close to his troubled son, and he immediately felt crushed, like his life had lost its meaning. In the ensuing 2 weeks, he had constant images of his son and was "obsessed" with how he might have prevented the substance abuse and suicide. He worried that he had been a bad father and that he had spent too much time on his own career and too little time with his son. He felt constantly sad, withdrew from his usual social life, and was unable to concentrate on his work. Although he had never previously drunk more than a few glasses of wine per week, he increased his alcohol intake to half a bottle of wine each night. At that time, his psychiatrist told him that he was struggling with grief and that such a reaction was normal. They agreed to meet for support and to assess the ongoing clinical situation.

Mr. Quinn returned to see his psychiatrist weekly. By the sixth week after the suicide, his symptoms had worsened. Instead of thinking about what he might have done differently, he became preoccupied that he should have been the one to die, not his young son. He continued to have trouble falling asleep, but he also tended to awake at 4:30 A.M. and just stare at the ceiling, feeling overwhelmed with fatigue, sadness, and feelings of worthlessness. These symptoms improved during the day, but he also felt a persistent and uncharacteristic loss of self-confidence, sexual interest, and enthusiasm. He asked his psychiatrist whether he still had normal grief or had major depressive disorder.

Mr. Quinn had a history of two prior major depressive episodes that improved with psychotherapy and antidepressant medication, but no significant depressive episodes since his 30s. He denied a history of alcohol or substance use disorders. Both of his parents had been "depressive" but without treatment. No one in the family had previously committed suicide.

Discussion

In the weeks after his son's suicide, Mr. Quinn developed sadness, insomnia, social withdrawal, diminished pleasure in activities, and poor concentration. This symptom cluster is typical of grief, recognized by both the lay public and medical professionals as a normal human reaction to the death of a loved one.

At the first meeting with the psychiatrist, Mr. Quinn demonstrated multiple symptoms that are typically found in major depressive disorder (MDD), but his symptoms at that point appeared to be better conceptualized as normal bereavement. Such a view is supported by the fact that grief—despite causing distress and dysfunction—typically runs its course within 2–6 months without specific clinical attention. Grief can also evolve into a full-blown episode of MDD, especially in a patient like Mr. Quinn, who has a history of recurrent MDD.

A prior version of DSM (DSM-IV) specifically acknowledged the normalcy of grief by mandating that a diagnosis of MDD be deferred for 2 months unless the clinical presentation was characterized by unusually severe symptoms such as suicidal ideation or psychosis. This so-called bereavement exclusion was included in DSM-IV for a good reason: although uncomplicated grief can be painful, it is short-lived and benign, and does not severely impair function or increase the risk of suicide as does MDD.

Some people, however, do develop an autonomous mood disorder after the death of a loved one, as well as after other traumas, such as financial ruin, losses from a natural disaster, or a serious medical illness or disability. Severely distressing and causing serious impairment, such mood syndromes warrant clinical attention prior to reaching DSM-IV's 2-month cutoff.

Because of the significant symptomatic overlap between bereavement and MDD, the difficulty in predicting which symptoms will persist or intensify and which will improve on their own, and the uncertainty over what is psychologically different between the loss of a loved one and, for example, the loss of a home due to a natural disaster, there has been significant attention paid to fine-tuning the differences between MDD and bereavement.

Attempting to distinguish between depression and normal grief raises a core concern in psychiatry, both from within and outside the field: what is normal? Various DSM-5 drafts were debated, and many people (including myself) worried that removal of the bereavement exclusion would medicalize normal grief and erroneously assign a psychiatric diagnosis to healthy people.

In assessing depressive symptoms in the context of grief, DSM-5 suggests that Mr. Quinn's psychiatrist use her clinical judgment in differentiating between the emptiness and loss that are typical of grief and the persistently depressed mood, anhedonia, and pessimistic ruminations that are more typical of MDD. In grief, the dysphoria should gradually attenuate over weeks, though interrupted perhaps by pangs of grief that tend to focus on the deceased. The depressive symptoms of MDD are less exclusively connected to the deceased, less likely to be interrupted by positive emotions and humor, and more likely to be accompanied by self-criticism and feelings of worthlessness.

When Mr. Quinn was seen 2 weeks after his son's suicide, his psychiatrist rightly viewed his reaction as within the bounds of a normal grief reaction. At the same time, Mr. Quinn had risk factors for MDD that are often not present in people who are grieving. He has a personal history of two prior major depressive episodes, his family history is positive for depression in both parents, and his son may also have been depressed. All of these factors increase Mr. Quinn's likelihood of developing MDD in the context of the death of his son.

While deferring a diagnosis of MDD, the psychiatrist continued to meet weekly with Mr. Quinn. After about 6 weeks, his symptoms had worsened, both in terms of intensity and the development of cognitive and neurovegetative symptoms, making the diagnosis of MDD clear. The DSM-IV 2-month bereavement exclusion might have encouraged Mr. Quinn's psychiatrist to delay a diagnosis of MDD for another several weeks, until the 2-month mark had been reached. DSM-5, by contrast, did not specifically limit the use of an MDD diagnosis during the time frame between 2 weeks and 2 months. For Mr. Quinn, this shift likely means that he would more quickly receive a diagnosis of MDD under DSM-5.

Experts in favor of the removal of the 2-month bereavement exclusion might be reassured by Mr. Quinn's clinical assessment. With worsening symptoms and a strong personal and family history of depression, Mr. Quinn probably warrants specific clinical attention.

For most grieving people, however, their depressive symptoms do not indicate MDD. For example, a study using data from the National Epidemiologic Survey on Alcohol and Related Conditions showed that subjects who had a bereavement-related depressive syndrome at baseline were no more likely over a 3-year follow-up period to have a major depressive episode than were those who had no lifetime history of MDD at baseline. These data confirm the widely held view that for most people, grief resolves on its own.

Nevertheless, 10%–20% of bereaved individuals go on to experience a more chronic and debilitating syndrome. DSM-5-TR addresses this complexity by adding *prolonged grief disorder* to the main body of the DSM text. Called *persistent complex bereavement disorder* in DSM-5, where it was included in Section III's "Conditions for Further Study," DSM-5-TR's prolonged grief disorder is characterized by a cluster of dysfunctional reactions to the death of a loved one at least 12 months earlier. The reaction is characterized by an intense longing for the loved one and/or a disturbing preoccupation with the deceased. In addition, the patient should manifest at least three of eight symptom clusters that are referable to the death: identity disruption, a sense of disbelief about the death, avoidance of reminders of the death, intense emotional pain, difficulty reintegrating into relationships, emotional numbness, a sense of meaninglessness, and loneliness. In addition, this cluster of reactions must have occurred more days than not since the loved one's death and almost every day for the month leading up to the evaluation. The clinician must also link the symptoms with the loss of the loved one, so that the symptoms (such as identity disruption or loneliness) are not better explained by a different disorder, such as MDD.

Whether one is evaluating someone who is suffering acutely, like Mr. Quinn, or someone who is still suffering a year or more after a loss, DSM-5-TR urges clinicians to use their judgment when trying to distinguish between clinical depression and grief. A reasonable argument could be made for treating the patient for MDD in equivocal cases, especially if the patient appears to fulfill requirements for MDD. It remains to be seen whether these changes will help identify patients who warrant clinical attention—or will encourage the medicalization of grief. In the meantime, clinicians should continue to recognize that although grief can sometimes trigger MDD, grief itself is an entirely normal emotional response to loss that requires no psychiatric intervention.

Diagnosis

• Major depressive disorder

Suggested Readings

Friedman RA: Grief, depression and the DSM-5. N Engl J Med 366(20):1855–1857, 2012

De Stefano R, Muscatello MRA, Bruno A, et al: Complicated grief: a systematic review of the last 20 years. Int J Soc Psychiatry 67(5):492–499, 2021

McCabe PJ, Bor W: Bereavement is different: a multinational bereavement symptom model validation. Psychiatry Res 300:113926, 2021

Mojtabai R: Bereavement-related depressive episodes: characteristics, 3-year course, and implications for the DSM-5. Arch Gen Psychiatry 68(9):920–928, 2011

Zetumer S, Young I, Shear MK, et al: The impact of losing a child on the clinical presentation of complicated grief. J Affect Disord 170:15–21, 2015

CASE 4.4

Lost Interest in Life

Anthony J. Rothschild, M.D.

Barbara Reiss was a 51-year-old white woman who was brought to the emergency room by her husband with the chief complaint "I feel like killing myself."

Ms. Reiss had begun to "lose interest in life" about 4 months earlier. During that time, she reported depression every day for most of the day. Symptoms had been worsening for months. She had lost 9 lb (current weight 105 lb) without dieting because she did not feel like eating. She had trouble falling asleep almost every night and woke at 3:00 A.M. several mornings per week (she normally woke at 6:30 A.M.). She had diminished energy, concentration, and ability to perform her administrative job at a dog food processing plant. She was convinced that she had made a mistake that would lead to the deaths of thousands of dogs. She expected that she would soon be arrested, and would rather kill herself than go to prison.

Her primary care physician had recognized the patient's depressed mood 1 week earlier and had prescribed sertraline and referred her for a psychiatric evaluation.

Ms. Reiss denied a previous psychiatric history. One sister suffered from depression. Ms. Reiss denied any history of hypomania or mania. She typically drank a glass of wine with dinner and had started drinking a second glass before bed in hopes of getting a night's sleep. She had been married to her husband for 20 years, and they had three school-age children. She had been employed with her current company for 13 years. She denied illicit drug use.

The physical examination performed by the primary care physician 1 week earlier was noncontributory. All laboratory testing was normal, including complete blood count, electrolytes, blood urea nitrogen, creatinine, calcium, glucose, thyroid function tests, folate, and vitamin B_{12}.

On mental status examination, Ms. Reiss was cooperative and exhibited psychomotor agitation. She answered most questions with short answers, often simply saying "yes" or "no." Speech was of a normal rate and tone, without tangentiality or circumstantiality. She denied having hallucinations or unusual thoughts. She described the mistakes she believed she had made at work and insisted that she would soon be arrested for the deaths of dogs, but she insisted this was all true and not "a delusion." Recent and remote memory were grossly intact.

Discussion

Ms. Reiss exhibits all nine of the symptomatic criteria for major depressive disorder (MDD): depressed mood, loss of interest or pleasure, weight loss, insomnia, psychomotor agitation, loss of energy, excessive guilt, trouble concentrating, and thoughts of death. Only five are necessary for a DSM-5 MDD diagnosis.

Before a depressive disorder diagnosis is made, a medical cause should be ruled out. A recent medical examination was noncontributory, and there is no indication that Ms. Reiss even has a medical comorbidity, much less one that could cause a depression. It is also important to explore the possibility of bipolar disorder. The case report makes no mention of such symptoms as pressured speech or risk taking, but manic symptoms can sometimes be missed, and a bipolar disorder diagnosis would significantly affect treatment. The patient reports two nightly glasses of wine, which is unlikely to be contributory. If she is significantly underestimating her alcohol intake, however, she would be at risk for alcohol-induced depressive disorder. Multiple medications and substances of abuse can also cause serious depression and psychosis. Collateral history might be helpful, as would a toxicology screen.

Ms. Reiss also exhibits psychotic symptoms (delusions) in the context of MDD. New to DSM-5 was the separation of psychotic features from the MDD severity rating. In other words, MDD with psychotic features is not inevitably considered "severe." This has not changed in DSM-5-TR. Ms. Reiss's psychotic symptoms would be classified as mood congruent because the content of her delusions is consistent with the typical depressive themes of inadequacy, guilt, disease, death, nihilism, or deserved punishment.

Psychotic features often can be missed in MDD. Although Ms. Reiss's delusions about killing dogs appear to have been spontaneously reported and are unlikely to be true, many patients are more guarded and will not easily give up such information. Furthermore, fixed, false beliefs that are not bizarre can sound reasonable to the clinician. One way to approach this issue with patients is to avoid the use of words such as *psychosis* or *delusional* and instead to ask patients about their "irrational worries." Clinicians may also find the Psychotic Depression Assessment Scale (PDAS; https://psychoticdepressionassessmentscale.com) to be a useful tool for the assessment of patients with MDD with psychotic features.

Diagnosis

- Major depressive disorder, single episode, moderate, with psychotic features

Suggested Readings

Dubovsky SL, Ghosh BM, Serotte JC, Cranwell V: Psychotic depression: diagnosis, differential diagnosis, and treatment. Psychother Psychosom 90(3):160–177, 2021

Østergaard SD, Meyers BS, Flint AJ, et al: Measuring psychotic depression. Acta Psychiatr Scand 129(3):211–220, 2014

Rothschild AJ: Challenges in the treatment of major depressive disorder with psychotic features. Schizophr Bull 39(4):787–796, 2013

Rothschild AJ, Winer J, Flint AJ, et al: Missed diagnosis of psychotic depression at 4 academic medical centers. J Clin Psychiatry 69(8):1293–1296, 2008

CASE 4.5

Despair*

Cheryl C. Munday, Ph.D.
Jamie Miller Abelson, M.S.W.

Crystal Smith, a 33-year-old African American homemaker, came to an outpatient clinic seeking "someone to talk to" about feelings of despair that had intensified over the previous 8–10 months. She was particularly upset about marital conflict and an uncharacteristic irritability with her mother-in-law.

Ms. Smith said she had begun to wake before dawn, feeling down and tearful. She had difficulty getting out of bed and completing her usual household activities. At times, she felt guilty for not being her "usual self." At other times, she became easily irritated with her husband and impatient with her mother-in-law for minor transgressions. She relied on her mother-in-law for assistance with her children, but recently her mother-in-law appeared to be less available. Ms. Smith worries that she has become a burden to her mother-in-law. Her related guilt, in combination with her insomnia and fatigue, have made it very difficult for Ms. Smith to get her children to school on time. In the past few months, she had lost 13 pounds without dieting. She denied current suicidal ideation, saying she "would never do something like that," but acknowledged having thought that she "should just give up" and that she "would be better off dead." She decided to make an appointment after she attended her good friend's wedding and found she did not enjoy any of it.

Two months previously, Ms. Smith had seen a psychiatrist for several weeks and received fluoxetine. She reluctantly gave it a try, discontinuing it quickly because it made her feel even more tired. She had also dropped out of therapy, indicating that the psychiatrist did not seem to understand her.

Ms. Smith lived with her husband of 13 years and two school-age children. Her husband's parents lived next door. She said her marriage was good, although her husband suggested she "go see someone" so that she would not be "pacing and yelling at everyone all the time." While historically sociable, she now rarely talked to her own mother and sisters, much less her friends. Previously a regular churchgoer, she had quit attending because she felt her faith was "weak." Her pastor had always been

---

*This case is dedicated to the memory of James S. Jackson, Ph.D., in recognition of his leadership of research on the mental health of Black Americans.

supportive, but she had not contacted him with her problems because "he wouldn't want to hear about these kinds of issues."

Ms. Smith described herself as having been an outgoing, friendly child. She grew up with her parents and three siblings. She recalled feeling quite upset at age 10–11 when her parents divorced and her mom remarried. Because of fights with other kids at school, she met with a school counselor with whom she felt a bond. Unlike the psychiatrist she had recently consulted, Ms. Smith felt the counselor did not "get into my business" and helped her recover. She said she became quieter as she entered junior high school, with fewer friends and little interest in studying. She married her husband at age 20 and worked in retail sales until the birth of their first child when she was 23 years old.

Ms. Smith had not used alcohol since her first pregnancy, and she denied any use of illicit substances. She also denied past and current use of prescribed medications, other than the brief trial of the antidepressant medication. She reported generally good health.

On mental status examination, Ms. Smith was a casually groomed young woman who was coherent and goal directed. She had difficulty making eye contact with the white middle-aged therapist. She was cooperative but mildly guarded and slow to respond. She needed encouragement to elaborate her thinking. She was periodically tearful and generally appeared sad. She denied confusion, psychosis, hallucinations, current suicidal ideation, and homicidality. Cognition, insight, and judgment were all considered normal.

Discussion

Ms. Smith presents with 8–10 months of a persistently depressed mood, anhedonia, poor sleep, diminished appetite with weight loss, anergia, psychomotor agitation, and thoughts of death. She easily meets the requirement of five of nine symptom criteria for major depressive disorder (MDD). There is no evidence that the symptoms are caused by a substance or another medical condition. She is distressed and dysfunctional to an extent that warrants clinical attention. She therefore meets criteria for DSM-5 MDD. In addition, Ms. Smith has classic melancholic features: she reports loss of pleasure in almost all activities, describes a distinct quality of depressed mood (characterized by profound despondency or despair), is regularly worse in the morning, has had significant weight loss, and is reportedly motorically agitated.

Ms. Smith's irritability is prominent. Irritability may be more readily endorsed than sadness, especially by African Americans, among whom psychiatric stigma is high. Although a complaint of irritability can be part of mania or hypomania, Ms. Smith lacks other symptoms of mania. Further exploration of her guilty feelings would help determine whether they are excessive. Many African American women expect to function as a steadfast maternal figure with strong religious faith, a culturally normative gender role, and they might be more likely to present with excessive fatigue rather than a complaint of depression.

An important depression specifier is whether the MDD is a single episode or recurrent. It is not clear whether Ms. Smith had MDD after her parents' divorce when she was a child. To clarify, the clinician should explore further those long-ago symptoms. She was referred to a school counselor at that time because of irritability and fights with classmates, but underlying depressive thoughts and feelings associated with her parents' divorce would be consistent with a mood disorder. Knowledge of her parents' divorce might have helped teachers recognize that she was experiencing depressive symptoms, but it would not have been unusual for her to have been labeled "impulsive and disruptive" rather than seen as a depressed young girl who needed help.

Although she had been willing to seek professional help, Ms. Smith has had a mixed experience with mental health care professionals. She felt a bond with her school counselor, noting that the therapist did not "get into her business" but did help her recover. More recently, she had quickly dropped out of mental health care treatment because the psychiatrist "did not understand her," and the antidepressant medication made her "tired." At the time of the evaluation, Ms. Smith is noted (by the self-described middle-aged white therapist) as guarded and having difficulty making eye contact. More information would be needed, and it is common for people with depression to not feel an alliance or to discontinue recommended medication.

Nevertheless, Ms. Smith's evaluation and treatment may be getting derailed by cultural issues. Race, ethnicity, socioeconomic status, and gender are increasingly being realized as affecting the development of a therapeutic alliance, an accurate diagnosis, and a workable therapeutic plan. Furthermore, lower use of mental health care services by African Americans and delays in seeking treatment may contribute to illness persistence. Use of the revised DSM-5-TR Core Cultural Formulation Interview might facilitate more sensitive communication between clinician and patient and enhance the clinician's understanding of the patient's personal narrative. Ms. Smith's outcome may depend on her therapist's ability and willingness to tactfully address the cultural issues that are likely to be affecting Ms. Smith's depression and her course of treatment.

Diagnosis

• Major depressive disorder, moderate, with melancholic features

Suggested Readings

Aggarwal NK, Cedeno K, Lewis-Fernandez R: Patient and clinician communication practices during the DSM-5 cultural formulation interview field trial. Anthropol Med 27(2):192–211, 2020

Fava M, Hwang I, Rush AJ, et al: The importance of irritability as a symptom of major depressive disorder: results from the National Comorbidity Survey Replication. Mol Psychiatry 15(8):856–867, 2010

Hays K, Gilreath T: Profiles of depression help seeking among Black Americans: a latent class approach. J Nerv Ment Dis 205(8):627–633, 2017

Lewis-Fernández R, Aggarwal NK, Lam PC, et al: Feasibility, acceptability and clinical utility of the Cultural Formulation Interview: mixed-methods results from the DSM-5 international field trial. Br J Psychiatry 210(4):290–297, 2017

Neighbors HW, Caldwell C, Williams DR, et al: Race, ethnicity, and the use of services for mental disorders: results from the National Survey of American Life. Arch Gen Psychiatry 64(4):485–494, 2007

Walton QL, Shepard Payne J: Missing the mark: cultural expressions of depressive symptoms among African-American women and men. Social Work in Mental Health 14(6):637–657, 2016

CASE 4.6

Feeling Low for Years

Benjamin Brody, M.D.

Diane Taylor, a 35-year-old laboratory technician, was referred to the outpatient psychiatry department of an academic medical center by the employee assistance program (EAP) of her employer, a major pharmaceutical company. Her supervisor had referred Ms. Taylor to the EAP after she had become tearful while being mildly criticized during an otherwise positive annual performance review. Somewhat embarrassed, she told the consulting psychiatrist that she had been "feeling low for years" and that hearing criticism of her work had been "just too much."

A native of western Canada, Ms. Taylor came to the United States to pursue graduate studies in chemistry. She left graduate school before completing her doctorate and began work as a laboratory technician. She reported feeling frustrated with her job, which she saw as a "dead end," yet feared that she lacked the talent to find more satisfying work. As a result, she struggled with guilty feelings that she "hadn't done much" with her life.

Despite her troubles at work, Ms. Taylor felt that she could concentrate without difficulty. She denied ever having active suicidal thoughts, yet sometimes wondered, "What is the point of life?" When asked, she reported that she occasionally had trouble falling asleep. However, she denied any change in her weight or appetite. Although she occasionally would go out with coworkers, she said that she felt shy and awkward in social situations unless she knew the people well. She did enjoy jogging and the outdoors. Although her romantic relationships tended to "not last long," she felt that her sex drive was normal. She noted that her symptoms waxed and waned but had remained consistent over the past 3 years. She had no symptoms suggestive of mania or hypomania.

Ms. Taylor was an only child. Growing up, she had a close relationship with her father, a pharmacist who owned a drugstore. She described him as a "normal guy who liked to hunt and fish" and liked to take her hiking. Her mother, a nurse, stopped working shortly after giving birth and had seemed emotionally distant and depressed.

Ms. Taylor became depressed for the first time in high school when her father was repeatedly hospitalized after developing leukemia. At that time she was treated with psychotherapy and responded well. She had no other psychiatric or medical history, and her medications were a multivitamin and oral contraceptives. When offered several different treatments, she expressed a preference for a combination of medication and psychotherapy. She started taking citalopram and began a course of supportive psychotherapy. After several months of treatment, she revealed that she had been sexually abused by a family friend during her childhood. It also emerged that she had few women friends and a persistent pattern of dysfunctional and occasionally abusive relationships with men.

Discussion

It has long been recognized that depressive illnesses are not always episodic, and a significant minority of patients suffer from chronic forms of depression with varying degrees of severity. Early versions of DSM characterized mild, chronic depression as a personality disorder. In DSM-III, however, the milder form of chronic depression was introduced as an affective illness called dysthymic disorder. That move reflected a growing body of research suggesting that the condition can respond to antidepressant medication, but the move was controversial. Do these patients feel dysphoric *because* of their chronic social dysfunction, occupational difficulties, and negative cognitive styles? Alternatively, does their chronic underlying depression lead to an atrophy of their relationships and interpersonal skills and a selective attentional bias to negative life events? Debate about the nature and validity of the diagnosis persists.

When first conceptualized in DSM-III, dysthymia was described as being a less severe but more chronic variant of acute major depressive disorder (MDD). Evidence accumulated, however, that "pure" dysthymia (i.e., persistent mild depression without episodes of MDD) was uncommon. This led to the description of a spectrum of chronic depressive syndromes, of which dysthymia was the most mild. Slightly more severe was "double depression," or a major depressive episode superimposed on a baseline dysthymic state. The next most severe involved two or more major depressive episodes bridged by periods of incomplete improvement. Two years of symptoms severe enough to meet full criteria for MDD represented the most severe form. In practice, many patients found it difficult to recall their symptom fluctuations well enough to make these distinctions meaningful. DSM-5-TR now aggregates contemporary descriptions of these patterns as specifiers under the diagnosis persistent depressive disorder.

Does Ms. Taylor meet the criteria for this DSM-5-TR diagnosis? She has certainly had chronic symptoms. Despite significant occupational and interpersonal impairment, she endorses psychological but not neurovegetative symptoms of depression, which fall below the threshold for MDD. However, whether that has consistently been the case over the past 2 years is difficult to tell. It is possible, for example, that although Ms. Taylor denied difficulty concentrating at the time of evaluation, her employers may have felt otherwise at times in the past. The criteria allow for the possibility that although she may have slipped into MDD at times, the current diagnosis is still persistent depressive disorder.

The interplay of affective illness, childhood trauma history, and personality also emerges from Ms. Taylor's story. She manifests personality traits (withdrawal, restricted affectivity, intimacy avoidance, and sensitivity to criticism) that shape how she sees the world. These traits can perpetuate her depressive symptoms and offer important clues for treatment. Her history of childhood abuse, for example, suggests a need for combination therapy that will likely be more effective than psychotherapy or antidepressant medication alone. Regardless of whether Ms. Taylor meets criteria for a comorbid avoidant personality disorder, her avoidant personality traits are liable to complicate treatment and portend a poor outcome. Alternatively, these dysfunctional personality traits may improve with resolution of her persistent depressive symptoms.

Diagnosis

- Persistent depressive disorder

Suggested Readings

Nübel J, Guhn A, Müllender S, et al: Persistent depressive disorder across the adult lifespan: results from clinical and population-based surveys in Germany. BMC Psychiatry 20(1):58, 2020

Rhebergen D, Graham R: The re-labelling of dysthymic disorder to persistent depressive disorder in DSM-5: old wine in new bottles? Curr Opin Psychiatry 27(1):27–31, 2014

Schramm E, Klein DN, Elsaesser M, et al: Review of dysthymia and persistent depressive disorder: history, correlates, and clinical implications. Lancet Psychiatry 7(9):801–812, 2020

CASE 4.7

Mood Swings

Margaret Altemus, M.D.

Emma Wang, a 26-year-old investment banker, referred herself to an outpatient psychiatrist because of "mood swings" that were ruining her relationship with her boyfriend.

She said their latest argument was triggered by his being slightly late for a date. She had yelled at him and then, out of the blue, ended the relationship. She felt despondent afterward, guilty and self-critical. When she called him to make up, he had refused, saying he was tired of her "PMS [premenstrual syndrome] explosions." She had then cut herself superficially on her left forearm, which she had found to be a reliable method to reduce anxiety since she was a young teenager.

She said these mood swings came out of the blue every month and that they featured tension, argumentativeness, anxiety, sadness, and regret. Sometimes she yelled at her boyfriend, but she also got upset with friends, work, and her family. During the week in which she was "Mr. Hyde," she avoided socializing or talking on the phone; she wouldn't be her "usual fun self," she said, and would alienate her friends. She was able to work when she felt "miserable," but she did have relatively poor energy and concentration. She was also edgy and "self-pitying" and regretful that she had chosen to "waste" her youth working so hard for an uncaring financial institution.

When she was feeling "desperate," she would be determined to seek treatment. Soon after the onset of her period, however, she would improve dramatically, return to her old self, and not find the time to see a psychiatrist. During the several weeks after her period, she said she felt "fine, terrific, the usual."

She said the mood swings always started 7–10 days before the start of her menstrual period, "like terrible PMS." Her periods were regular. She had premenstrual breast tenderness, bloating, increased appetite, and weight gain. Almost as soon as her period began, she felt "suddenly good." She denied alcohol or illicit substance use and had no history of psychotic, manic, or obsessional symptoms. She denied any suicidal thoughts and any prior suicide attempts and psychiatric hospitalizations. She denied allergies and medical problems. She took one medication, her birth control pill. Her family history was pertinent for a mother with possible depression. Ms. Wang was born in Taiwan and came to the United States at age 14 to attend boarding school. After graduating from an elite business school, she had moved in with her older sister.

On mental status examination, Ms. Wang was a fashionably dressed East Asian woman wearing tasteful jewelry and carrying a designer bag. Her hair was slightly askew. She maintained good eye contact and was pleasant and cooperative throughout the interview. Her speech was normal in rate, rhythm, and volume. She described her mood as "generally good," and her affect was full, reactive, and mildly irritable. Her thought process was linear, and she showed no evidence of delusions, obsessions, or hallucinations. She denied suicidal and homicidal ideation. Her insight, judgment, and impulse control were intact, although she noted a history of perimenstrual impairment in these areas.

Discussion

Ms. Wang presents with mood swings, irritability, nonsuicidal self-injury (cutting), interpersonal instability, anxiety, sadness, social withdrawal, diminished concentration and energy, and anhedonia. She also describes physical symptoms such as increased appetite, clumsiness, fatigue, and bloating. These symptoms are severe enough to impair her social relationships and her function at work.

This history could fit a number of psychiatric disorders, but Ms. Wang also indicates that these symptoms occur only during a circumscribed time before the onset of her menses. At other times of the month, she is upbeat, energetic, and optimistic. Disappearance of symptoms after onset of menses is key to the diagnosis of premenstrual dysphoric disorder (PMDD).

Ms. Wang reports 7–10 days of symptoms premenstrually, which is on the longer end of the spectrum of symptom duration for PMDD. Some women have symptoms starting at ovulation and lasting for 2 weeks, but a shorter duration of symptoms is more common. Among women with premenstrual symptoms, the most symptomatic days, averaging across all women, are the 4 days preceding and the 2 days following onset of menses.

Ms. Wang's cutting behavior is not typical of PMDD. Impaired impulse control suggests borderline traits in addition to PMDD symptoms. Comorbid disorders do not exclude the diagnosis of PMDD. Many psychiatric disorders have exacerbations during the premenstrual period, but in such cases the patient does not return to her normal self after the menstrual period begins. Ms. Wang suggests that she has "PMS," or premenstrual syndrome, which is a medical condition but not a DSM-5 diagnosis. Criteria for PMS tend to be less rigorous than for PMDD and do not require an affective component.

PMDD is not associated with abnormalities in circulating levels of estrogen or progesterone. Instead, women with PMDD seem to be more sensitive to normal luteal hormone fluctuations. Hormone blood levels are, therefore, not part of the diagnostic evaluation. Although hormonal contraceptives might be expected to help with symptoms, women taking oral contraceptives often continue to have premenstrual mood symptoms (as seen in Ms. Wang).

One component that is crucial in making the PMDD diagnosis is an accurate longitudinal history. Retrospective symptom reports are often inaccurate throughout psychiatry, and that is true for premenstrual symptoms. Validated scales are available for assessing PMDD, such as the Daily Record of Severity of Problems. At this early stage of evaluation, DSM-5 would indicate that Ms. Wang has a provisional diagnosis of PMDD. Only after she has recorded symptoms over two menstrual cycles could she be said to have DSM-5 PMDD.

Diagnosis

• Premenstrual dysphoric disorder (provisional)

Suggested Readings

Bezerra de Carvalho A, de Azevedo Cardoso T, Mondin TC, et al: Prevalence and factors associated with premenstrual dysphoric disorder: a community sample of young adult women. Psychiatry Res 268:42–45, 2018

Hartlage SA, Freels S, Gotman N, Yonkers K: Criteria for premenstrual dysphoric disorder: secondary analyses of relevant data sets. Arch Gen Psychiatry 69(3): 300–305, 2012

Yonkers KA, Simoni MK: Premenstrual disorders. Am J Obstet Gynecol 218(1):68–74, 2018

CASE 4.8

Stress, Drugs, and Unhappiness

Edward V. Nunes, M.D.

Frank Young, a 40-year-old business executive, was brought for a psychiatric consultation by his wife. While Mr. Young sat quietly beside her, she reported that a change had come over him during the last 6 months. He was either quiet and withdrawn or uncharacteristically irritable. He had begun to drink alcohol to excess in social situations, sometimes embarrassing her. He often came home late, or not at all, claiming to have been at the office. When away from home, he rarely answered phone calls and text messages. She wondered if he was having an affair. Mr. Young denied seeing anyone else and indicated he had just been having a hard time.

After his wife left the psychiatrist's office, Mr. Young reported a great deal of stress at work over the last year as he tried to deal with industry-wide setbacks and personal financial losses. He said he felt down and depressed most of the time. He reported difficulty sleeping most nights, loss of interest in his wife and children, low energy, and feelings of failure and self-criticism. He had frequent thoughts of wanting to be dead and of suicide, but he denied any suicidal intent or plans.

When asked about the alcohol, he acknowledged that he had been drinking heavily for at least 6 months. When asked about other substances, he asked about therapeutic confidentiality and then acknowledged that he had been using cocaine several times per week for about 9 months. He kept his cocaine use from his wife because he knew she would be judgmental. In the beginning, cocaine put him in a reliably positive, optimistic mood, and he found that he could more successfully churn through large volumes of otherwise tedious and discouraging work. Although his work required some socializing in the evening, he also began to regularly go to bars in the evening just so that he would have a place to comfortably combine cocaine with alcohol. He craved the high from cocaine, went out of his way to obtain it, and spent a lot of time getting high that he would previously have been spending with his family.

When asked to clarify the sequence of work stress, cocaine use, and depression symptoms, he reported that he had felt worried and discouraged about work for a year, but the feelings of depression, loss of interest, irritability, insomnia, and low self-esteem had not begun until about 6 months earlier, 3 months after he had begun to use cocaine regularly. He experienced those depressive symptoms most of the day every day, whether or not he had taken cocaine within the last several days.

Mr. Young denied any previous episodes of depression, other mood or anxiety disorders, or suicide attempts. He drank socially. He had experimented with cannabis and cocaine as a teenager but had never developed a pattern of regular use or impairment until the past year.

Discussion

Mr. Young has significant depression. He meets criteria for cocaine use disorder of at least moderate severity and may also have an alcohol use disorder. He also has significant work stress and appears to be in a tense marriage. The relationships between his mood, his substance use, and his stress are complicated but crucial to the development of an effective treatment strategy.

The first difficulty in evaluating substance use disorders is getting an accurate history about behaviors that are often embarrassing and illegal. Mr. Young was quite forthcoming about his cocaine use, but only after he was specifically asked about alcohol and substance use. Waiting for patients to spontaneously report illicit substance use is likely to lead to not getting the information. This is problematic given that substance use is widespread and frequently co-occurs with other psychiatric disorders. An empathic, nonjudgmental interviewing style will usually help the patient open up. In other words, asking about alcohol and common drugs of abuse with a matter-of-fact attitude indicates to the patient that his or her answers will not be surprising and will provide information that can improve the treatment. As seen with Mr. Young, family members are often the ones to bring a substance use disorder patient to consultation. They can be important allies in clarifying the symptoms and implementing a treatment plan. Mr. Young needed time alone with the clinician to tell his story, but it was very useful to hear his wife's observations.

A careful exploration of the history can help differentiate between diagnoses that are associated with similar symptoms. Cocaine withdrawal typically causes depressive symptoms, for example, as do major depressive disorder (MDD) and cocaine-induced depressive disorder. One important differentiating factor is the temporal relationship between symptoms and the use of the substances.

According to DSM-5, an independent MDD would be diagnosed if the depression began before the onset of substance use disorder or persisted for a substantial period of time beyond cessation of substance use. The amount of time is left to the clinician's judgment, but about 1 month is suggested. MDD would also be diagnosed if the involved substance was deemed unlikely to cause a depressive syndrome or if the patient had previously experienced recurrent non-substance-induced major depressive episodes. Mr. Young had never had a major depressive episode until after he started using cocaine, and there has not been a substantial abstinent period since; thus, independent MDD cannot be diagnosed.

It is also important to consider the possibility that Mr. Young's symptoms are the direct result of intoxication and/or withdrawal. Intoxication with and withdrawal from cocaine and alcohol can cause depressed mood and sleep disturbance, but symptoms would be expected to resolve within a day or two of the last use. Mr. Young's depression and insomnia persist, regardless of the timing of his last use. In addition, other depressive symptoms such as suicidal ideation are not typically part of intoxication or withdrawal.

Mr. Young, therefore, is diagnosed with a substance-induced depressive disorder, which is linked to depressions that appear to have been induced by the ongoing use of a substance and that seem to have taken on a life of their own. If Mr. Young's depression persists after a month of abstinence, his diagnosis would shift to MDD, although the clinician would likely consider the cocaine to have triggered the depression.

It is useful to identify substance-induced depressive disorder. Compared with independent MDD, substance-induced depressive disorder is associated with an increased suicide risk. Furthermore, the additional depression diagnosis reduces the likelihood that someone with a substance use disorder will achieve abstinence. Substance-induced depressive disorder should be kept on a patient's list of diagnoses and followed carefully.

Diagnoses

- Cocaine use disorder, moderate
- Substance (cocaine)-induced depressive disorder

Suggested Readings

Dakwar E, Nunes EV, Bisaga A, et al: A comparison of independent depression and substance-induced depression in cannabis-, cocaine-, and opioid-dependent treatment seekers. Am J Addict 20(5):441–446, 2011

Nunes EV, Liu X, Samet S, et al: Independent versus substance-induced major depressive disorder in substance-dependent patients: observational study of course during follow-up. J Clin Psychiatry 67(10):1561–1567, 2006

Wai JM, Shulman M, Nunes E: Mood disorders, in The American Psychiatric Association Publishing Textbook of Substance Use Disorders, 6th Edition. Edited by Brady KT, Levin FR, Galanter M, Kleber HD. Washington, DC, American Psychiatric Association Publishing, 2021

CASE 4.9

Anhedonia and Restless Sleep

Thomas W. Meeks, M.D.

George Anderson, a 73-year-old married man, was referred to a psychiatrist for an evaluation of depression after screening positive on the Geriatric Depression Scale during a neurology appointment. For most of the 2 years since his diagnosis with Parkinson's disease, Mr. Anderson had coped well and continued to engage in many of his usual activities. His wife of 49 years noted that 1–2 years before developing Parkinson's disease, Mr. Anderson had become somewhat less enthusiastic and motivated compared with his baseline personality, but not to the point of causing any concern or impairment. The only other neuropsychiatric symptom preceding his Parkinson's diagnosis was his wife's report that during the past 5 years he frequently "thrashed about" while asleep.

Three months prior to the referral, however, Mr. Anderson began to decline social invitations from family and friends. He reported that he had withdrawn socially because he had lost pleasure in things that used to excite him, although he denied persistent feelings of sadness or worry. He recognized that he was not his "usual self" and tried, to no avail, to give himself "pep talks." He had worked as a high school science teacher until retirement at age 67, and reported having learned "the power of seeing the glass half full" from his students. He felt frustrated that he could not "snap out of it" for the first time in his life but was hopeful about getting professional help. He denied wishing for death, explaining that although he was not afraid of death, he wanted to enjoy life as long as possible. He added, "God does not give me more than I can handle. I can't ask for a better family, and I have had a full life."

Other new symptoms over the prior few months included increasing fatigue, impaired concentration and memory, unintentional weight loss, and sleep-onset insomnia. Further history on his more chronic sleep symptoms revealed that, around 3:00 A.M. or 4:00 A.M. on most nights, Mr. Anderson began violently moving his extremities and moaning as though in distress, all while still seemingly asleep in bed. He often awakened his wife with these movements and occasionally struck her in his sleep. She sometimes used a different bedroom because of this. When he awoke from such an incident, he was coherent and briefly anxious, often reporting that he had been dreaming of swimming or running from something.

His wife took over driving shortly after his Parkinson's disease diagnosis, but Mr. Anderson was otherwise independent in activities of daily living such as paying bills and managing his medications. His wife described him as "maybe a little more forgetful" over the past few years, but neither of them was concerned about this mild memory loss.

Past medical history included prostate cancer (in remission), glaucoma, and gout. Labs from his recent neurology visit were unremarkable, including blood counts, serum chemistries, thyroid function, and vitamin B_{12} levels. Family psychiatric history was positive only for a granddaughter with ADHD. He denied past problematic substance use and all current substance use except two or three glasses of wine monthly. He denied any previous depressive episodes, psychiatric treatment, or psychiatric evaluations.

On mental status examination, Mr. Anderson was pleasant, cooperative, and interpersonally engaging. Resting tremor, shuffling gait, hypophonia, and bradykinesia all were evident at mild to moderate levels. He occasionally smiled, but his affect was difficult to fully gauge because of masked facies. He reported his mood as "blah." There was no evidence of psychosis.

On cognitive testing, he had some difficulty on the Trail Making Test part B, figure copying, and word-list recall, the latter being helped by category prompts. On a standardized brief cognitive assessment, he scored 25 out of 30 points, which was in the normal range.

Discussion

Although Mr. Anderson denies sad mood, he does have evidence of anhedonia along with five other depressive symptoms (weight loss, insomnia, fatigue, poor concentration, and psychomotor retardation), all for longer than 2 weeks. These symptoms are distressing to him and are significantly impacting his social functioning. This could indicate major depressive disorder (MDD). However, Mr. Anderson has no personal or family history of depression, an atypically late age at symptom onset, and symptom development exclusively during the course of Parkinson's disease.

When depressive symptoms are temporally associated with the onset or progression of another medical condition, and are not explained by delirium, the DSM-5 diagnosis "depressive disorder due to another medical condition" should be considered. This diagnosis is intended for situations in which the direct *physiological* effects of another medical condition (e.g., effects of insufficient thyroid hormones on the brain) cause depressive symptoms. This diagnosis is *not* intended to describe individuals whose symptoms arise from a psychological reaction to illness. In Mr. Anderson's case, adjustment disorder with depressed mood may be a more appropriate diagnosis. These two possible etiologies of depressive symptoms (physiological vs. psychological) among persons with another medical condition are difficult to fully delineate from one another and may coexist. There are, however, many cases in which the evidence suggests one condition substantially more than the other.

Clinically significant depressive symptoms occur in up to half of persons with Parkinson's disease and may occur throughout the disease course. Depressive symptoms have been linked with neurobiological changes observed in Parkinson's disease, such as dysregulation and neuronal loss in monoamine pathways that are implicated in development of MDD. Yet Parkinson's-associated depression also appears distinct from MDD, with differing patterns of treatment response to antidepressants. In addition, Parkinson's disease tends to feature more prominent apathy/anhedonia than is seen in MDD, which may reflect the dopamine depletion that is the principal pathology of Parkinson's disease.

Depressive symptoms in Parkinson's disease do not consistently correlate with the severity of motor impairment or disability and often somewhat predate awareness of motor symptoms. These findings, together with Mr. Anderson's historical resiliency and positive coping style, suggest that a physiological explanation is more likely than a psychological one. In other words, depressive disorder due to another medical condition is a more appropriate diagnosis than adjustment disorder.

If the criteria for symptom duration and number are met for MDD, the specifier "with major depressive–like episode" should be added to the diagnosis. Because symptoms from a nonpsychiatric medical illness can overlap with depressive symptoms, diagnostic ambiguity may arise. For instance, persons with Parkinson's disease may experience symptoms such as fatigue, psychomotor retardation, sleep disturbance, cognitive impairment, and weight loss independent of depressed mood or anhedonia. However, in Mr. Anderson's case, these symptoms developed or worsened in conjunction with his newly disabling anhedonia, which suggests that criteria for a major depressive episode are met, except for the probable causation by another medical condition.

As often occurs in Parkinson's disease, Mr. Anderson has a sleep disturbance consistent with rapid eye movement (REM) sleep behavior disorder. This sleep disorder is characterized by "repeated episodes of arousal during sleep associated with vocalization and/or complex motor behaviors" that may result in "injury to self or the bed partner." Upon awakening, affected persons typically have a clear sensorium and a sense of having "acted out" their dreams. Polysomnography would reveal absence of atonia during REM sleep but would not be required in order to make the diagnosis in the context of a synucleinopathy such as Parkinson's disease. Symptoms typically occur 90 minutes or more into sleep and more often in the second half of the night, when REM sleep density increases. Although Mr. Anderson's history (including onset of sleep disturbance prior to Parkinson's disease symptoms) is consistent with REM sleep behavior disorder, his new initial insomnia is not explained by this diagnosis and is more likely related to his depressive disorder.

Cognitive changes, particularly impairments of visuospatial, executive, and memory retrieval functions, often develop and gradually progress in Parkinson's disease. Mr. Anderson's cognitive test results are typical of such cognitive changes, but his new-onset subjective difficulty with concentration is more likely secondary to depression. His cognitive problems are mild and not overtly impairing. Available information does not clearly indicate that a neurocognitive disorder is present, although neuropsychological testing and prospective monitoring of cognition should be considered, given that at least 30% of persons with Parkinson's disease develop an associated major neurocognitive disorder.

In addition to meeting criteria for two DSM-5 disorders, Mr. Anderson displays evidence of resilience, wisdom, and other signs of psychological health. He demonstrates positive coping skills (e.g., cognitive reframing, use of social supports) and long-term supportive relationships, spirituality, gratitude, optimism, and developmentally appropriate ego integrity, including a realistic yet nonmorbid perspective about personal mortality. Unfortunately, even individuals with few risk factors for depression and evidence of lifelong healthy psychological functioning are not immune to the neuropsychiatric effects of certain medical conditions.

Diagnoses

• Depressive disorder due to another medical condition (Parkinson's disease), with major depressive–like episode
• Rapid eye movement sleep behavior disorder

Suggested Readings

Boeve BF: Idiopathic REM sleep behaviour disorder in the development of Parkinson's disease. Lancet Neurol 12(5):469–482, 2013

Borgonovo J, Allende-Castro C, Izquierdo AL, et al: Changes in neural circuitry associated with depression at pre-clinical, pre-motor and early motor phases of Parkinson's disease. Parkinsonism Relat Disord 35:17–24, 2017

Jeste DV, Savla GN, Thompson WK, et al: Association between older age and more successful aging: critical role of resilience and depression. Am J Psychiatry 170(2):188–196, 2013

Marsh L: Depression and Parkinson's disease: current knowledge. Curr Neurol NeuroSci Rep 13(12):409, 2013

Pfeiffer RF: Non-motor symptoms in Parkinson's disease. Parkinsonism Relat Disord 22 (suppl 1):S119–S122, 2016

CASE 4.10

Mixed Features, but Not Bipolar

Joseph F. Goldberg, M.D.

Helena Bates was a 27-year-old single administrative assistant who presented for a psychiatric evaluation and treatment for depression. She had recently begun an intensive outpatient program after a first lifetime hospitalization for an impulsive overdose following the breakup of a 2-year relationship. She said she had been feeling increasingly sad and hopeless for 1–2 months prior to the breakup. About a month before her admission, she began seeing a new psychotherapist who told her she had "borderline traits" and "situational mood swings."

During these 4–8 weeks, Ms. Bates's mood had been moderately depressed throughout the day most days, with no diurnal variation and intact mood reactivity. She had recently gained about 10 pounds from "overeating comfort food and junk." She denied prominent irritability or argumentativeness. She described her self-esteem as "none" and had found it hard to feel motivation or to concentrate on routine tasks. By contrast, sometimes she would have "bursts" of nonstop thinking about her estranged boyfriend and devising ways to "get him back," alternating with "grieving his loss." She described times of being flooded with strategies to regain his interest (including purchasing a full-page newspaper "open letter" to him) and recently found herself awake until 5:00 or 6:00 A.M. journaling or calling friends in the middle of the night "for support." She would then "trudge through the day" without fatigue after only 2–3 hours of sleep. These symptoms began prior to her hospitalization. She denied drug or alcohol misuse and self-injurious behavior. Until this particular breakup, she denied a history of particularly intense or chaotic relationships, as well as a history of suicidal thoughts or gestures. Indeed, Ms. Bates seemed horrified by her own impulsive overdose.

Previously, Ms. Bates had seen a counselor in high school for "moodiness" and poor grades. She became "depressed" in college. At that time, she began escitalopram and psychotherapy, but improved quickly and stopped both after a few weeks. While in the hospital following her suicide attempt, she started taking vilazodone and quetiapine at bedtime "for sleep."

Ms. Bates was the youngest of three children who grew up in a middle-class suburban home. She attended public school and a state college as "mostly a B student" and hoped to someday go to law school. She described herself as having been a "quiet, anxious" child and "not a troublemaker." Her older brother abused multiple substances, although Ms. Bates said she herself had never used illicit substances. Her older sister was treated for "panic attacks and depression," and Ms. Bates knew of several aunts and cousins whom she thought were "depressed."

On examination, Ms. Bates was a pleasant, well-related, casually but appropriately dressed, moderately overweight woman, appearing her stated age, who made good eye contact. Her speech was somewhat rapid and verbose but interruptible and non-pressured. She had no abnormal motor movements, but she gestured dramatically and with excessive animation. Her mood was depressed, and her affect was tense and dysphoric but with full range and normal responsivity. Ms. Bates's thought processes were somewhat circumstantial but generally coherent, linear, and logical. Her thought content was notable for passive thoughts that she might be better off dead, but without intent or plan; she had no delusions, hallucinations, or homicidal thoughts. Her higher integrative functioning was grossly intact, as were her insight and judgment.

Discussion

Ms. Bates meets DSM-5 criteria for a major depressive episode, manifesting pervasive depressed mood with at least five associated features (suicidal thoughts, poor concentration, low self-esteem, hyperphagia, and psychomotor agitation). She also describes several symptoms consistent with mania or hypomania: a decreased need for sleep with nocturnal hyperactivity and no consequent next-day fatigue, probable racing thoughts, and rapid, verbose speech (as noted on interview). Although the examiner deemed Ms. Bates's insight and judgment globally intact at the time of the interview, some of her recent thoughts (e.g., posting an open letter in a newspaper) and actions (calling friends in the middle of the night) suggest impaired judgment involving behaviors with the potential for painful consequences.

Although Ms. Bates does have some manic symptoms, she does not meet DSM-5 requirements for a diagnosis of mania or hypomania. She would be said to have subsyndromal hypomania along with the syndromal depression. This combination qualifies her for the DSM-5-TR diagnosis of major depressive disorder with mixed features (MDD-MF). Previously, "mixed features" applied only to bipolar I disorder, whereas the term can now modify major depressive disorder and both bipolar I and bipolar II disorders.

For practicing clinicians, MDD-MF can pose a nosological conundrum. Clinical investigators who enroll subjects in mood disorder trials often agonize over the precision with which DSM-5-TR symptoms are present in sufficient number and duration to constitute or meet criteria for a distinct diagnostic entity, such as a bipolar II disorder hypomanic episode. Fundamentally, the construct of MDD-MF pertains to instances in which 1) MDD is present but concomitant manic or hypomanic symptoms are too few in number or duration to "qualify" as a formal syndrome of mania or hypomania, and 2) there is no previous history of a full manic or hypomanic episode that would merit a lifetime diagnosis of bipolar I or II disorder. Herein lies a potential difference between the clinical approach adopted by most real-world practitioners and that adopted by investigators in clinical trials: the latter may be fastidious in determining whether diagnostic symptom and duration criteria for a specific entity are evident, whereas the former more often take a global, less finicky approach to gauging the presence of a salient diagnostic entity, such as hypomania.

The spirit of the diagnosis reflects the observation that many unipolar depressed patients display subthreshold signs of hypomania. Concrete application of the DSM-5 construct of MDD-MF requires following the "rules" for counting symptoms. DSM-5 disallows the counting of four potential manic/hypomanic symptoms—namely, *insomnia* (as opposed to decreased need for sleep), *distractibility, indecisiveness,* and *irritability*—because they can also reflect MDD. DSM-5 identifies "abnormally and persistently increased activity or energy" as a mandatory criterion for diagnosing bipolar II hypomania, but this feature is not necessary to define MDD-MF. In the current case, if Ms. Bates had irritable mood in addition to her racing thoughts, rapid speech, and decreased need for sleep, she would meet DSM-5 criteria for bipolar II hypomania, and the mixed features specifier would then apply by virtue of her concomitant depressive symptoms.

The DSM-5-TR mixed features specifier requires that symptoms of the opposite polarity (in this case, mania/hypomania) be present "the majority of days during the episode." This latter criterion means that if Ms. Bates's manic/hypomanic symptoms had been present for fewer than 4 days (the minimum duration criterion for diagnosing bipolar II hypomania), her subthreshold hypomania symptoms would not count toward either a "mixed" or a "manic/hypomanic" designation and her diagnosis would simply be MDD. Some authors criticized DSM-5's stringency of discounting subthreshold hypomania symptoms if they involved only *two* manic/hypomanic symptoms or if they failed to persist for the full duration of an episode, because such presentations (referred to in the literature as "depressive mixed states") have been observed when as few as two mania/hypomania symptoms coexist with syndromal unipolar depression for as few as 2–4 days, and represent a construct that more closely resembles bipolar than unipolar disorder in family history, age at onset, and suicide risk.

One might speculate that Ms. Bates's psychomotor activation and subthreshold hypomania could have arisen as a consequence of the recent introduction of the novel serotonergic drug vilazodone. However, in this case, the history indicates that her subthreshold hypomanic symptoms predated her hospitalization and SSRI introduction; it would be important for the examiner to determine that this chronology is accurate (which would suggest that her mixed symptoms are not iatrogenic), because the mixed features specifier requires that symptoms be "not attributable to the physiological effects of a substance." Note that this qualifying statement is in contrast to the DSM-5 criteria for a manic/mixed/hypomanic episode, insofar as the emergence of mania/hypomania symptoms associated with recent antidepressant exposure is now classified as a bipolar disorder (similar to the viewpoint in DSM-III-R) and no longer as a substance-induced mood disorder (as in DSM-IV-TR).

Follow-up studies of MDD patients with subthreshold hypomania indicate an approximately 25% chance of eventually developing a full mania or hypomania. Therefore, although not all MDD patients who display subthreshold mixed features will develop syndromal mania or hypomania, such patients warrant particularly careful evaluation, treatment, and longitudinal monitoring.

Ms. Bates's symptoms of impulsivity and hyperactivity may have contributed to her acute presentation being wrongly identified as borderline personality disorder. Her longitudinal history does not support a pattern of symptoms suggestive of borderline personality disorder, and her suicide attempt and affective instability are readily accounted for by a current full affective syndrome.

Since the emergence of MDD-MF as a new entity in DSM-5, few dedicated clinical trials have examined its effective treatment. Notably, one large randomized trial with lurasidone for MDD-MF found improvement in both depressive and subthreshold manic symptoms. Additionally, in bipolar disorder, antidepressant use in the setting of even subthreshold mania symptoms has been shown to destabilize mood, prompting some experts, by extrapolation, to advise avoiding monoaminergic antidepressants in MDD-MF. Further studies are needed to help identify optimally safe and effective pharmacotherapies for MDD with mixed features in patients who do not meet diagnostic criteria for a lifetime categorical diagnosis of bipolar disorder.

Diagnosis

• Major depressive disorder with mixed features

Suggested Readings

Angst J, Cui L, Swendsen J, et al: Major depressive disorder with subthreshold bipolarity in the National Comorbidity Survey Replication. Am J Psychiatry 167(10):1194–1201, 2010
Fiedorowicz JG, Endicott J, Leon AC, et al: Subthreshold hypomanic symptoms in progression from unipolar major depression to bipolar disorder. Arch Gen Psychiatry 168(1):40–48, 2011
Serretti A, De Ronchi D, Olgiati P: Irritable mood and subthreshold hypomanic episodes correlate with more severe major depression. Neuropsychobiology 80(5):425–436, 2021
Suppes T, Silva R, Cucchiaro J, et al: Lurasidone for the treatment of major depressive disorder with mixed features: a randomized, double-blind, placebo-controlled study. Am J Psychiatry 173(4):400–407, 2016

CASE 4.11

Floundering

Peter D. Kramer, M.D.

Ian Campbell was a 32-year-old architect who presented for psychiatric consultation because he was floundering at work. His boss had expressed concern after he failed to make progress on a simple project. When Mr. Campbell explained that he had been distracted by problems at home, his boss suggested that more seemed wrong. Mr.

Campbell called his internist, who sent him to a neurologist, who referred him for psychiatric evaluation.

Mr. Campbell had encountered this problem, difficulty concentrating, before. In college, after his father died of a chronic illness, Mr. Campbell had been unable to study and had taken time off. Twice at his prior job, he experienced episodes lasting months in which he had difficulty making decisions. One of these intervals followed a romantic setback.

The patient's mother and sister had been diagnosed with major depressive disorder and treated successfully with medication. A maternal uncle had committed suicide.

The current impairment's onset accompanied the breakdown of Mr. Campbell's marriage of 6 years. Two months earlier, his wife had filed for divorce, announcing that she would live in the distant city her work had taken her to. Mr. Campbell had expected to feel relief; he said his wife had been hostile throughout the marriage. He had begun to entertain fond thoughts of a coworker. Nevertheless, he felt "flat"—unable to imagine a future.

Closer questioning revealed that Mr. Campbell's problems went beyond impaired cognition. He described apathy and diminished energy. Jazz was a passion, but he no longer attended recitals—although impaired concentration probably played a role as well. Listening, the psychiatrist noted probable retardation of speech. Mr. Campbell said that his employer had mentioned that he was "moving in slow motion." The problems were worse in the mornings. In the evenings, Mr. Campbell noticed a spark of energy. He put on music and reviewed reports that he had ignored during the workday.

Mr. Campbell declined to characterize himself as sad. He was pleased that the marriage was ending. But the psychiatrist was struck by her own affect in Mr. Campbell's presence; she felt glum, pessimistic, even weepy.

She questioned Mr. Campbell at length about depressed mood, changed sleep and appetite, feelings of guilt or worthlessness, and thoughts of death. None of these attributions, he said, applied. Nor had he had indicators of disorders that can be confused with depression. Between episodes of impairment, he felt and functioned well.

The psychiatrist decided that the problem at hand was close enough to depression to warrant treatment. Factors that influenced her decision included the partial syndromal presentation, diurnal variation, periodic recurrence, lack of future orientation, and her own empathic experience. She proposed psychotherapy centered on Mr. Campbell's decompensation in the face of loss. He insisted that he did not see the impending divorce in that light. The two agreed on brief psychotherapy supplemented by antidepressants. Within weeks, Mr. Campbell was functioning at full capacity. During the treatment, the psychiatrist was unable to elicit evidence of depressive symptoms beyond those noted in the initial history. All the same, she was convinced that the impaired concentration was a sign and symptom of something very much like major depressive disorder.

Discussion

The operational definition of major depressive disorder (MDD), which reached official standing in the third edition of DSM, is one of the great inventions in modern medicine. The approach has catalyzed productive research in fields ranging from cell biology to social psychiatry. Most of what is known about mood disorder, from the abnormalities it represents in the brain to the harm it does in lives, arises from the delineation of depression out of the inchoate domain of neurosis and psychosis.

That said, the definition is arbitrary. Historians have traced the DSM criteria to a 1957 *Journal of the American Medical Association* article whose lead author, a Boston psychiatrist, Walter Cassidy, had tried to systematize the study of a condition similar to today's MDD. For diagnosis, Cassidy required that patients have six of 10 symptoms from a list that included slow thinking, poor appetite, loss of concentration, and others that remain current. Later asked how he chose six, Cassidy said, "It sounded about right."

Operational approaches to depression, from DSM to the Hamilton Rating Scale for Depression, are attempts to create reliability in the face of an inherently ill-defined phenomenon—that is, clinicians' working diagnoses. Psychiatrists identified depressed patients using prevailing methods—sometimes with attention to their own empathic resonance with the patient; the symptom- and severity-based definitions translated the impressionistic into reproducible form.

Depression, however, has no known natural boundary. Behavioral geneticists find the DSM criteria arbitrary. Number, severity, and duration of symptoms each represent a continuum of disability. Patients who suffer four severe symptoms of depression for 2 weeks tend to do badly down the road. Five moderately disabling symptoms for 10 days confer a poor prognosis. Five mild symptoms, if they persist, predict substantial risk.

In this case, Mr. Campbell appears not to have had the five of nine criteria necessary for a diagnosis of MDD, but he would likely qualify for a DSM-5 diagnosis of other specified depressive disorder (depressive episode with insufficient symptoms). It is important to recognize that depression's harm—suffering, future full episodes, work and social problems, suicide—is only slightly less in people who narrowly miss full criteria. In one analysis, later MDD was as common in those who reported three or four symptoms as in those who reported five. Estimates of heritability are similar, too; "minor" depression in one sibling predicts full depression in an identical twin. One form of other specified depressive disorder appears especially dangerous: recurrent brief depression is associated with high rates of attempted suicide.

These other specified forms of depression are probably less prevalent than MDD. Studies that find lifetime rates for MDD on the order of well over 25% find the lifetime risk for these less severe syndromes to be on the order of 8%–9%. Patients with fewer symptoms tend also to have fewer accompanying mental illnesses. They are, for instance, less likely than patients with MDD to become dependent on drugs of abuse or on alcohol.

The DSM-5 categories unspecified depressive disorder and other specified depressive disorder acknowledge an important clinical reality: effectively, the near penumbra of depression *is* depression. Low-level episodes can appear as precursors of MDD and as sequelae, even in the absence of persistent depressive disorder; on its own, low-level depression represents suffering and confers risk.

Mr. Campbell's doctor will want to take his complaints seriously. Mr. Campbell may have entered a "depressive episode with insufficient symptoms," but the insufficiency relates to the symptom count for a major depressive episode, not to the level of illness needed to trigger clinical concern. Especially when peripheral factors—such as, in this case, the diurnal variation typical of classic depression—suggest mood disorder, the clinician will suspect that effectively the condition *is* depression and will approach the situation with the corresponding urgency and thoroughness.

Diagnosis

- Other specified depressive disorder (depressive episode with insufficient symptoms)

Suggested Readings

Cassidy WL, Flanagan NB, Spellman M, Cohen ME: Clinical observations in manic-depressive disease: a quantitative study of one hundred manic-depressive patients and fifty medically sick controls. J Am Med Assoc 164(14):1535–1546, 1957

Havens L: A Safe Place: Laying the Groundwork of Psychotherapy. Cambridge, MA, Harvard University Press, 1989

Kendler KS, Muñoz RA, Murphy G: The development of the Feighner criteria: a historical perspective. Am J Psychiatry 167(2):134–142, 2010

Kramer P: Against Depression. New York, Viking, 2005

Vandeleur CL, Fassassi S, Castelao E, et al: Prevalence and correlates of DSM-5 major depressive and related disorders in the community. Psychiatry Res 250:50–58, 2017

CASE 4.12

Insomnia and Physical Complaints

Russell F. Lim, M.D.

Ka Fang, a 59-year-old widowed Hmong woman, was referred to a mental health care clinic after she recurrently complained to her primary care physician of fatigue, chronic back pain, and insomnia. Over the preceding 11 months, the internist had prescribed clonazepam for sleep and Vicodin (hydrocodone/acetaminophen) for pain. Her sleep had improved and her pain decreased, but she continued to feel tired all day. At that point, the internist referred her for the psychiatric evaluation.

Ms. Fang had immigrated to the United States from Thailand a decade earlier. Natives of Laos, she and her family had spent almost two decades in a Thai refugee camp following the Vietnam War. Her family had resettled in the Sacramento area with the assistance of a local church group.

When questioned through a Hmong interpreter, Ms. Fang denied depressed mood. When asked if she enjoyed things, she said that she felt privileged to be in America and had no right to complain. She said she felt she was not doing enough to help her family. She was embarrassed by her fatigue because she did not "do anything all day." She denied any intention to harm herself.

She said she was very proud of all her children, especially her son, who had been an excellent student in Thailand and spoke good English. Nevertheless, her son, his wife, and their two young children followed many of the cultural practices that they had followed in Laos and Thailand, and often prepared Hmong food for dinner. He and his wife had bought a small farm outside Sacramento and were doing well, cultivating Asian vegetables. Her son had employed her two daughters on the farm until both had moved back to live in the Hmong community in Sacramento.

Ms. Fang indicated that the transition to California had gone better than she had expected. The biggest disappointments for her had been her husband's unexpected death from a heart attack 1 year earlier and the fact that most of her extended family had remained in Thailand.

On mental status examination, the patient was short and heavyset. She wore a floral short-sleeve blouse, black polyester slacks, black flip-flops, and no makeup. She had white strings tied around her wrists. Her eyes were generally downcast, but she seemed alert. She appeared sad and constricted but denied feeling depressed. Her speech was slow and careful. She denied all hallucinations, suicidality, and homicidality. Cognitive testing revealed normal attention and concentration. She had little formal education and appeared to be functionally illiterate. Her insight into her illness appeared limited.

When asked about the strings around her wrists, Ms. Fang explained that she had recently sought out a Hmong shaman, who had organized several soul-calling ceremonies to reunite with distant relatives.

Discussion

Ms. Fang presents for an evaluation of psychiatric contributions to her fatigue, insomnia, and pain. She endorses symptoms of insomnia, feelings of worthlessness, and fatigue, but she denies a depressed mood, anhedonia, agitation, weight loss, poor concentration, or thoughts of suicide. She fulfills only three of nine DSM-5-TR major depressive disorder criteria; five are needed to make the diagnosis.

Ms. Fang reports a number of pertinent cultural issues. She lives in a Hmong-speaking household with her son and his family on their farm outside of Sacramento. They raise vegetables, their apparent occupation when they lived in Laos and Thailand. In Hmong culture, the young married couple generally lives with the family of the husband, making the mother-in-law especially prominent. Although Ms. Fang expresses her appreciation for her situation, she may still feel marginalized and lonely, especially in the context of her husband's death 1 year earlier and her daughters having moved back to the Hmong community in Sacramento. Being functionally illiterate—not uncommon in societies in which the limited educational resources are primarily channeled to boys—Ms. Fang is not able to avail herself of tools to maintain connections, such as e-mail and newspapers. Her feelings of isolation are likely connected to the strings that the interviewer noticed on her wrists. Shamanistic soul-calling ceremonies are intended to reunite families, and she may be especially in need given her distance from her daughters, her Southeast Asian home, her Hmong culture, her extended family, and her ancestors.

In assessing whether Ms. Fang has a mood disorder, it is useful to know that there is no word in the Hmong language for depression. Like many people from other cultures, Ms. Fang describes somatic symptoms such as insomnia, anergia, and bodily aches to express depressed feelings. These probably are not adequate to meet symptomatic criteria for a DSM-5 major depressive disorder, and, by report, her symptoms have not yet persisted for the 2 years required for persistent depressive disorder. It would be useful to get collateral information from one of her children, who might be able to provide information that could solidify the diagnosis. As it stands, she best fits the diagnosis of other specified depressive disorder (depressive episode with insufficient symptoms).

Diagnosis

• Other specified depressive disorder (depressive episode with insufficient symptoms)

Suggested Readings

Culhane-Pera KA, Vawter DE, Xiong P, et al: Healing by Heart: Clinical and Ethical Case Stories of Hmong Families and Western Providers. Nashville, TN, Vanderbilt University Press, 2003

Lim RF (ed): Clinical Manual of Cultural Psychiatry. Washington, DC, American Psychiatric Publishing, 2006

Llorente M: Culture, Heritage, and Diversity in Older Adult Mental Health Care. Washington, DC, American Psychiatric Association Publishing, 2019

Parekh R, Al-Mateen CS, Lisotto MJ, Carter RD (eds): Cultural Psychiatry With Children, Adolescents, and Families. Washington, DC, American Psychiatric Association Publishing, 2021

CHAPTER 5

Anxiety Disorders

INTRODUCTION

John W. Barnhill, M.D.

The DSM-5 chapter on anxiety disorders brings together a cluster of presentations in which anxiety, fear, and avoidance are prominent. Among the most prevalent psychiatric diagnoses, anxiety disorders can also be among the most difficult to definitively diagnose. One complicating factor is that anxiety, fear, and avoidance are normal and adaptive responses, leading to some inevitable ambiguity in evaluations of people with mild symptoms.

Another complicating factor is that anxiety-related emotions can be experienced as physical symptoms. Fear—a normal response to a real or perceived imminent threat—is almost always associated with autonomic hyperarousal; such hyperarousal can be difficult for patients to identify or describe, especially if it is chronic. Similarly, anxiety—the emotional experience of fear unaccompanied by a clear threat—may be experienced as muscle tension and vigilance, which can blend imperceptibly into background noise for someone with chronically elevated anxiety levels.

A third complication is that anxiety disorders are often comorbid with one another and with mood, substance, and personality disorders, which can make it difficult to adequately attend to the manifestations of each diagnosis.

Finally, definitions of anxiety disorders are descriptive of phenomena with unknown pathophysiologies, and despite many advances, the field of psychiatry is not yet close to definitively identifying nosological categories based on underlying etiology.

DSM-5-TR maintains several changes that were initially made in DSM-5. For example, panic continues to be described in two different ways. Panic attacks are often comorbid, and they can now be identified as a specifier for all DSM-5-TR anxiety disorders, as well as for some other psychiatric disorders. When persistent panic attacks induce an ongoing, significant fear of further panic attacks, the more likely diagnosis is panic disorder.

Historically linked to panic disorder, agoraphobia continues to be identified as a distinct diagnosis that can develop in the context of a variety of stressors and psychiatric syndromes. As with specific phobia and social anxiety disorder, agoraphobia no longer requires that individuals over age 18 perceive the anxiety as unreasonable. Instead, the clinician can make a judgment as to whether the anxiety is out of proportion to the actual danger or threat. To reduce the likelihood of overdiagnosing transient fears, these disorders must persist for at least 6 months for all individuals rather than just for those under age 18.

All of the DSM-5 structural changes were maintained in DSM-5-TR. For example, separation anxiety disorder was moved into the chapter on anxiety disorders from the chapter on neurodevelopmental disorders. The diagnosis still requires an onset before age 18, but the chapter move is intended to encourage clinicians to recognize the 6% of adults who meet criteria for this childhood-onset disorder.

DSM-5 also created two new chapters for conditions that had largely been conceptualized as anxiety disorders: disorders related to OCD (i.e., OCD as well as conditions such as body dysmorphic disorder) and disorders related to trauma and stress (i.e., PTSD as well as adjustment disorders). These new chapters include clusters of disorders in which anxiety may play a prominent role but which also have other features (e.g., obsessions/compulsions or a significant trauma history).

DSM-5-TR describes temperamental traits often implicated in the development of anxiety symptoms. These include *negative affectivity* (or neuroticism), which refers to the disposition to experience negative emotions, and *anxiety sensitivity*, which refers to the disposition to believe that symptoms of anxiety are harmful. Also relevant to the anxiety disorders are such traits as behavioral inhibition, harm avoidance, and an attentional bias to threat.

Cultural awareness is emphasized throughout DSM-5-TR. In addition to describing recent evidence regarding rates of anxiety disorders within subgroups based on gender, ethnicity, home country, and so on, DSM-5-TR encourages clinicians to maintain a broad sensitivity to culture, including a recognition that not all patients believe in a Western medical model of disease. Clinician curiosity into alternative explanatory models can improve the therapeutic alliance and patient adherence. For example, within Cambodian culture, *khyâl* (wind) attacks involve dizziness, tinnitus, and neck soreness. Catastrophic cognitions and panic attacks can be triggered by the perceived dangerousness of a symptom, such as neck soreness, that may be understood to reflect disorder of *khyâl*. The clinician would not be expected to know all culturally mediated disorders from all regions of the world, but a successful medical interaction might depend on listening for clues that the patient (or a respected parent or grandparent) has theories about medicine and health that do not conform to a Western medical model. Tactful interviewing can often lead to a more precise diagnosis and a more culturally sensitive treatment plan.

Although anxiety is pervasive, and anxiety disorders are perhaps the most common psychiatric disorder, DSM-5 emphasizes that underdiagnosis of anxiety disorders can have serious consequences. Frequently misdiagnosed and undertreated,

DSM-5-TR™ Clinical Cases

anxiety disorders are commonly associated with decreased work performance and life satisfaction and with increases in suicidality, disability days, medical and psychiatric comorbidities, and medical resource use.

The various anxiety-related disorders can often be clearly differentiated but are frequently comorbid with each other and with other psychiatric diagnoses, including major depressive disorder, personality disorders, and substance use disorders. A chief complaint of "anxiety" does not make the diagnosis but is instead the beginning of a clinical thought process that can range throughout DSM-5.

Suggested Readings

Hofmann SG Hinton DE: Cross-cultural aspects of anxiety disorders. Curr Psychiatry Rep 16(6):450, 2014

Horwitz AV, Wakefield JC: All We Have to Fear: Psychiatry's Transformation of Natural Anxieties Into Mental Disorders. New York, Oxford University Press, 2012

Milrod B: The Gordian knot of clinical research in anxiety disorders: some answers, more questions. Am J Psychiatry 170(7):703–706, 2013

Simon NM, Hollander E, Rothman BO, Stein DJ (eds): The American Psychiatric Association Publishing Textbook of Anxiety, Trauma, and OCD-Related Disorders, 3rd Edition. Washington, DC, American Psychiatric Association Publishing, 2020

CASE 5.1

Fears and Worries

Loes Jongerden, M.A.

Susan Bögels, Ph.D.

Logan was a 12-year-old boy who was referred to mental health care for long-standing anxiety about losing his parents and relatively recent fears about getting a severe disease.

Although his parents described a long history of anxiety, Logan's acute problem began 5 weeks prior to the consultation, when he watched a television show about rare and fatal diseases. Afterward, he became scared that he might have a hidden disease. His parents reported three "panic attacks" in the prior month, marked by anxiety, dizziness, sweats, and shortness of breath. About that same time, Logan began to complain of frequent headaches and stomachaches. Logan's own theory was that his bodily aches were caused by his fears about being ill and about his parents going away, but the pain was still uncomfortable. He insisted he was not scared about having more panic attacks but was petrified about being left sick and alone. These illness fears developed several times a week, usually when Logan was in bed, when he "felt something" in his body, or when he heard about diseases.

Logan had begun to suffer from anxieties as a young child. Kindergarten was notable for intense separation difficulties. He was briefly bullied in third grade, which led to his first panic attacks and worsening anxiety. According to his parents, "there always seemed to be a new anxiety." These included fear of the toilet, the dark, sleeping alone, being alone, and being pestered.

Logan's most persistent fear revolved around his parents' safety. He was generally fine when both were at work or at home, but when they were in transit, or anywhere else, he was generally afraid that they would die in an accident. When the parents were late from work or when they tried to go out together or on an errand without him, Logan became frantic, calling and texting incessantly. Logan was predominantly concerned about his mother's safety, and she had gradually reduced her solo activities to a minimum. As she said, it felt like "he would like to follow me into the toilet." Logan was less demanding toward his father, who believed his wife had been too soft and overprotective.

Logan and his family underwent several months of psychotherapy when Logan was age 10. The father said therapy helped his wife become less overprotective, and Logan's anxiety seemed to improve. Logan's mother agreed with this assessment, although she said she was not sure what she was supposed to do when her son was panicking whenever she tried to leave the house or whenever he worried about getting a disease.

Logan's developmental history was otherwise unremarkable. His grades were generally good. His teachers agreed that he was quiet but had several friends and collaborated well with other children. He was quick, however, to negatively interpret the intentions of other children. For example, he tended to be very sensitive to any indication that he was being picked on.

Logan's family history was pertinent for panic disorder, agoraphobia, and social anxiety disorder in the mother. The maternal grandmother was described as "at least as" anxious as Logan's mother. The father denied psychiatric illness in his family.

On examination, Logan was a friendly, articulate boy who was cooperative and goal directed. He was generally in a "good mood" but cried when talking about his fears of dying and getting sick. He denied suicidality and hopelessness but indicated he was desperate to get over his problems before starting high school. His cognition was good. His insight and judgment appeared intact except as related to his anxiety issues.

Discussion

Logan has had separation fears since he was a young child. To qualify for separation anxiety disorder, DSM-5 requires three of eight symptoms. Logan has at least five, including long-standing, excessive, and disturbing fears of anticipated separations; of harm to his parents; of events that could lead to separations; and of being left alone. He also had physical complaints that could be traced to fears of dying and separation.

Logan also has panic attacks. He does not meet criteria for a panic disorder, however, because he is not afraid of having an attack. Instead, his panic seems related to fears of separation or getting a disease. Panic attacks would, therefore, be listed as a specifier of separation anxiety disorder.

Although Logan is anxious about having an illness, his symptoms do not appear to meet criteria for illness anxiety disorder: the duration of his fear of diseases is not 6 months, he does not visit doctors, and he seeks reassurance not about his health but about being left alone by his attachment figures. His symptoms do not meet criteria for generalized anxiety disorder because his predominant concern is specifically about separation from his parents. He may have met criteria for social anxiety disorder in the past (fear of being pestered), but social fears do not appear to dominate the current clinical picture.

Anxiety disorders have been present in the mother and grandmother, which may indicate a genetic predisposition. Multigenerational anxiety may also be transmitted via learning, modeling, and overprotective parenting. In Logan's case, the mother is noted to have panic disorder, agoraphobia, and social anxiety disorder, and both parents agree that her own anxieties have influenced her parenting style. In particular, Logan's fears appear to be rewarded: the parents stay home, rarely leave Logan alone, and respond quickly to all his calls and text messages. They appear to have frequent conversations about his fears but may not spend enough time discussing compensatory strategies. The father does seem to try to encourage Logan's autonomy, but the parents appear to not agree on the correct overall strategy. Unsupportive coparenting may have contributed to the maintenance of Logan's problems.

One potentially important change in DSM-5 was the relocation of separation anxiety disorder into the anxiety disorders chapter. In DSM-III and DSM-IV, it was discussed in the chapter aimed at disorders that begin in infancy, childhood, and adolescence. Separation anxiety disorder can extend into adulthood, however, and Logan's mother may herself have had adult separation anxiety disorder (as well as other anxiety disorders). Her own fears of separation may well be affecting how she is raising her son and be contributing to his ongoing anxiety.

Diagnosis

- Separation anxiety disorder with panic attacks

Suggested Readings

Aktar E, Van Bockstaele B, Pérez-Edgar K, et al: Intergenerational transmission of attentional bias and anxiety. Dev Sci 22:e12772, 2019

Baartmans JMD, van Steensel FJA, Mobach L, et al: Social anxiety and perceptions of likeability by peers in children. Br J Dev Psychol 38(2):319–336, 2020

Majdandzic M, de Vente W, Feinberg ME, et al: Bidirectional associations between coparenting relations and family member anxiety: a review and conceptual model. Clin Child Fam Psychol Rev 15(1):28–42, 2012

Patel AK, Bryant B: Separation anxiety disorder. JAMA 326(18):188, 2021

CASE 5.2

Panic

Carlo Faravelli, M.D.

Maria Greco was a 23-year-old single woman who was referred for psychiatric evaluation by her cardiologist. In the prior 2 months, she had presented to the emergency room four times for acute complaints of palpitations, shortness of breath, sweats, trembling, and the fear that she was about to die. Each of these events had a rapid onset. The symptoms peaked within minutes, leaving her scared, exhausted, and fully convinced that she had just experienced a heart attack. Medical evaluations done right after these episodes yielded normal physical exam findings, vital signs, lab results, toxicology screens, and electrocardiograms.

The patient reported a total of five such attacks in the prior 3 months, with the panic occurring at work, at home, and while driving a car. She had developed a persistent fear of having other attacks, which led her to take many days off work and to avoid exercise, driving, and coffee. Her sleep quality declined, as did her mood. She avoided social relationships. She did not accept the reassurance offered to her by friends and physicians, believing that the medical workups were negative because they were performed after the resolution of the symptoms. She continued to suspect that something was wrong with her heart and that without an accurate diagnosis, she was going to die. When she had a panic attack while asleep in the middle of the night, she finally agreed to see a psychiatrist.

Ms. Greco denied a history of previous psychiatric disorders except for a history of anxiety during childhood that had been diagnosed as a "school phobia."

The patient's mother had committed suicide by overdose 4 years earlier in the context of recurrent major depressive disorder. At the time of the evaluation, the patient was living with her father and two younger siblings. The patient had graduated from high school, was working as a telephone operator, and was not dating anyone. Her family and social histories were otherwise noncontributory.

On examination, the patient was an anxious-appearing, cooperative, coherent young woman. She denied depression but did appear worried and was preoccupied with ideas of having heart disease. She denied psychotic symptoms, confusion, and all suicidality. Her cognition was intact, insight was limited, and judgment was fair.

Discussion

Ms. Greco has panic attacks, which are abrupt surges of fear and/or discomfort that peak within minutes and are accompanied by physical and/or cognitive symptoms.

In DSM-5, panic attacks are seen as a particular kind of fear response and are not found only in anxiety disorders. Therefore, panic is conceptualized in two ways within DSM-5. The first is as a "panic attack" specifier that can accompany any DSM-5 diagnosis. The second is as a panic disorder when the individual meets the more restrictive criteria for the disorder.

Ms. Greco appears to satisfy the multiple criteria required for panic disorder. First, her panic attacks are recurrent, and she more than meets the requirement for four of 13 panic symptoms: palpitations, sweating, trembling, smothering, chest pain, and a persistent fear of dying. The diagnosis also requires that the panic attacks affect the person between episodes. Not only does she constantly worry about having a heart attack (despite medical workups and frequent reassurance), she avoids situations and activities that might trigger another panic attack. These symptoms should also last at least 1 month, and Ms. Greco has been symptomatic for 2 months.

The diagnosis of panic disorder also requires an evaluation for the many other causes of panic. These include medications, medical illness, substances of abuse, and other mental disorders. According to the history, this 23-year-old woman takes no medications, has no medical illness, and denies use of substances of abuse. Her physical examinations, electrocardiograms, routine lab results, and toxicology screens are either normal or negative. It might be useful to ask Ms. Greco specifically about herbal and complementary medications, but it appears that her symptoms are psychiatric in origin.

Many psychiatric disorders are associated with panic, and Ms. Greco may have been primed for panic attacks by another condition. She reports a childhood history of anxiety and "social phobia" (DSM-5-TR social anxiety disorder), although those symptoms appear to have remitted. Her mother killed herself 4 years earlier in the context of recurrent major depressive disorder. Details are unknown. Such a traumatic event would undoubtedly have had an effect on Ms. Greco. In fact, there would likely be two different traumas: the abrupt effects of the suicide and the more long-standing effects of having a chronically or recurrently depressed mother. Further exploration might focus on the psychosocial events leading up to these panic attacks.

For example, Ms. Greco's "school phobia" may have been a manifestation of undiagnosed separation anxiety disorder, and her recent panic may have developed in the setting of dating, sexual exploration, and/or a move away from her father and younger siblings. She does not present a pattern of panic in response to social anxiety or a specific phobia, but she also denies that her symptoms are psychiatric, so she may not recognize the link between her panic symptoms and another set of symptoms. It might be useful to assess Ms. Greco for anxiety sensitivity, which is the tendency to view anxiety as harmful, and for "negative affectivity," which is the proneness to experience negative emotions. Both of these personality traits may be associated with the development of panic.

Because certain symptom clusters are often not recognized spontaneously by patients as either symptoms or clusters of symptoms, it would be useful to look more specifically for disorders such as posttraumatic stress disorder and obsessive-compulsive disorder. In addition, it might be helpful to explore the sequence of symptoms. For example, the patient's panic seems to have led to her worries about heart disease. If the illness worries *preceded* the panic, she might also have an illness anxiety disorder or somatic symptom disorder.

Frequently comorbid with panic are depressive and bipolar disorders. Ms. Greco does have depressive symptoms, including insomnia and a preoccupation with death, but otherwise her symptoms do not appear to meet the criteria for a depression diagnosis. Her symptoms would, however, need to be observed longitudinally. Not only does her mother's history of depression increase her risk for depression, but Ms. Greco may not be especially insightful into her own emotional states. It would also be useful to specifically look for symptoms of bipolar disorder. Mania and hypomania are often forgotten by patients or are not perceived as problematic, and a missed diagnosis could lead to inappropriate treatment and an exacerbation of bipolar symptoms. If possible, a tactful review of her mother's symptoms may be useful, because both suicidality and suicide are more common in bipolar disorders than in depressive disorders. Furthermore, the development of panic appears to increase the risk of suicidal thoughts.

Although more should be explored, Ms. Greco does appear to have a panic disorder. DSM-5 suggests the assessment of whether the panic is expected or unexpected. It appears that Ms. Greco's initial panic attacks occurred in situations that might have been seen as stressful, such as while driving and at work, and so may or may not have been expected. Her last episode happened while she was asleep, however, so her panic attacks would be classified as unexpected.

DSM-5 delinked agoraphobia from panic disorder. They can be comorbid, but agoraphobia is now recognized as developing in situations besides panic. In Ms. Greco's case, her active avoidance of driving, exercise, and caffeine is better conceptualized as a behavioral complication of panic disorder rather than a symptom of agoraphobia. Accurate diagnosis and treatment are important to prevent her symptoms from becoming more severe and chronic.

Diagnosis

- Panic disorder

Suggested Readings

Bentley KH, Franklin JC, Ribeiro JD, et al: Anxiety and its disorders as risk factors for suicidal thoughts and behaviors: a meta-analytic review. Clin Psychol Rev 43:30–46, 2016

Faravelli C, Gorini Amedei S, Scarpato MA, Faravelli L: Bipolar disorder: an impossible diagnosis. Clin Pract Epidemiol Ment Health 5:13, 2009

MacKinnon DF, Zandi PP, Cooper J, et al: Comorbid bipolar disorder and panic disorder in families with a high prevalence of bipolar disorder. Am J Psychiatry 159(1):30–35, 2002

CASE 5.3

Adolescent Shyness

Barbara L. Milrod, M.D.

Nadine was a 15-year-old girl whose mother brought her for a psychiatric evaluation to help with her long-standing shyness.

Although Nadine was initially reluctant to say much about herself, she said she felt constantly tense. She added that the anxiety had been "really bad" for several years and was often accompanied by episodes of dizziness and crying. She was generally unable to speak in any situation outside of her home or school classes. She refused to leave her house alone for fear of being forced to interact with someone. She was especially anxious around other teenagers, but she had also become "too nervous" to speak to adult neighbors she had known for years. She said it felt impossible to walk into a restaurant and order from "a stranger at the counter" for fear of being humiliated. She also felt constantly on her guard, needing to avoid the possibility of getting attacked, a strategy that really only worked when she was alone in her home.

Nadine tried to conceal her crippling anxiety from her parents, typically telling them that she "just didn't feel like" going out. Feeling trapped and incompetent, Nadine said she contemplated suicide "all the time." In the month before her mother finally brought her in for a psychiatric evaluation, Nadine had begun to cut herself on her thighs to "feel pain and relieve stress." No one in the family was aware of this development.

Nadine had always been "shy" and had been teased at recess since she started kindergarten. The teasing had escalated to outright bullying by the time she was in seventh grade. The bullying took on a cultural/racially motivated undertone; Nadine and her family were of a different ethnicity than the vast majority of her schoolmates. For 2 years, day after difficult day, Nadine's peers turned on her "like a snarling wolf pack," calling her "stupid," "ugly," and "crazy." Not infrequently, one of them would stare at her and tell she would be better off committing suicide. One girl (the ringleader, as well as a former elementary school chum) hit Nadine on one occasion, giving her a black eye. Nadine did not fight back. This event was witnessed by an adult neighbor, who told Nadine's mother. When Nadine's mother asked her about the incident, Nadine denied it, saying she had "fallen" on the street. She did, however, mention to her mother "in passing" that she wanted to switch schools, but her delivery was so offhand that at the time, her mother casually advised against the switch. Nadine suffered on, sobbing herself to sleep most nights and wishing that she would not wake up.

Full of hope and ideas of escape from the bullies and their narrowness, Nadine transferred to a specialty arts high school for ninth grade. Although the bullying ceased, her anxiety symptoms paradoxically worsened. She felt even more unable to venture into public spaces and felt increasingly embarrassed by her inability to develop the sort of independence typical of a 15-year-old. She said she had begun to spend whole weekends "trapped" in her home and had become scared to even read by herself in the local park. Nadine's social anxiety had evolved into true agoraphobia. She had nightly nightmares about the bullies in her old school. Her preoccupation with suicide grew.

Her parents had thought she would outgrow being shy and sought psychiatric help for her only after a teacher remarked that her anxiety and social isolation were keeping her from making the sort of grades and doing the sort of extracurricular activities that were necessary to get into a good college.

Nadine described her mother as loud, excitable, aggressive, and "a little frightening." Her father was a successful tax attorney who worked long hours. Nadine described him as shy in social situations ("He's more like me"). Nadine said she and her father sometimes joked that the goal of any evening was to avoid tipping the mother into a rage. Nadine added that she "never wanted to be anything like her mother."

Discussion

Nadine appears to have an underlying shy temperament. Unfortunately, with sandbox logic, shy children are often picked on. If they never learn adequate ways to defend themselves, bullying can escalate, particularly during their middle and high school years. This pattern can lead these anxiety-prone and already high-risk adolescents to be traumatized by their peers. In Nadine's case, the added element of cross-cultural discrimination and intimidation heightened her sense of helplessness and shame. The intensity of her anxiety symptoms, her increasing social isolation, and her sense of having no one to whom she could turn combined to increase her risk of suicidal thoughts and behaviors.

By the time Nadine saw a psychiatrist, her distress had persisted for years and she appears to have developed a cluster of three DSM-5 diagnoses that are frequently comorbid. First, she has marked and excessive anxiety about multiple social situations, including those with her peers. These situations always invoke fears of embarrassment and a sense of her incompetence, again partially fueled by the culturally loaded bullying. Nadine tries to avoid these situations as best she can. She therefore meets the symptomatic criteria for DSM-5-TR social anxiety disorder, which is her primary diagnosis.

As is common among children and adolescents, Nadine's fears took on a life of their own after the bullying experience. She initially avoided anxiety-provoking social situations, which is an aspect of her social anxiety disorder. That anxiety gradually expanded and exploded, however, and she began to have panic attacks if she even tried to leave her house by herself. When she became persistently unable to even go alone to a nearby park, she would be said to have a second DSM-5 diagnosis, agoraphobia. Such expansion is so common among children and adolescents that contemporary treatment studies tend to focus interventions on a range of DSM-defined anxiety disorders rather than on a single disorder.

Nadine should also be considered for a third diagnosis: DSM-5-TR posttraumatic stress disorder (PTSD). She has experienced intense and prolonged bullying, which constitutes trauma according to DSM-5-TR Criterion A, especially when a child is socially isolated and going through a vulnerable period of development. To meet DSM-5-TR criteria for PTSD, Nadine would need to manifest clinically significant symptoms for at least 1 month in four different areas: intrusion (the nightmares, which she reported nightly), avoidance (of peers), negative alterations of cognitions and mood (exaggerated and negative views about herself, panic attacks when she fears reexposure to her trauma, i.e., bullying by her neighborhood peers), and alterations in arousal and reactivity (being always on her guard). Because some of these symptoms can also refer to Nadine's social anxiety disorder, clinical judgment is required to avoid overdiagnosing PTSD. Nevertheless, it does appear that these two conditions are comorbid in Nadine. It is also important to explore the possibility that these anxiety symptoms might be attributable to a nonpsychiatric medical condition or to the use of medications or substances, but none of these appear to be involved in Nadine's case.

When evaluating adolescent trauma, it is useful to recall that although other children are generally the bullies, teachers and administrators can contribute to the problem by paying inadequate attention to schoolyard dynamics or by tacitly tolerating them. This appears to be true in Nadine's case. As she reported, "There is no way that my teachers did not know what was happening to me." In addition, Nadine's parents seem to have been able to ignore her desperate situation until they became concerned about her college admissions.

It is also useful to recognize that Nadine's mother is a loud, explosive woman whom Nadine has avoided "upsetting" since very early childhood. This tenuous mother–child relationship (or dysregulated attachment relationship) likely played a formative role in Nadine's shyness. Fear of her mother's explosions might have contributed to Nadine's persistent sense that she was not safe, for example, and might have prevented her from developing the tools that she needed to be successfully assertive. As the psychiatric evaluation evolves, it might be reasonable to discuss with Nadine the possibility that her failure to defend herself against the bullying might be related to her intense desire not to be anything like her loud and frightening mother.

Diagnoses

- Social anxiety disorder, severe
- Posttraumatic stress disorder, moderate
- Agoraphobia, severe

Suggested Reading

Busch F, Milrod B, Chen C, Singer M: Trauma-Focused Psychodynamic Psychotherapy: Bringing Evidence-Based Psychodynamic Treatment to Patients With PTSD. New York, Oxford University Press, 2021

Milrod B: Separation anxiety disorder and other anxiety disorders, in Separation Anxiety Disorder: A Guide to the Clinical Syndrome. Edited by Pini S, Milrod B. Berlin, Springer, in press

Schneier F, Milrod B (section eds): Part IV (Anxiety Disorders and Obsessive-Compulsive and Related Disorders), in Gabbard's Treatments of Psychiatric Disorders, 5th Edition. Edited by Gabbard GO. Arlington, VA, American Psychiatric Association Publishing, 2014, pp 341–456

CASE 5.4

Flying Fears

Katharina Meyerbröker, Ph.D.

Olaf Hendricks, a 51-year-old married businessman, presented to an outpatient psychiatrist with problems relating to periodically feeling helpless and lacking confidence. He reported that he usually feels fine except when he is confronted with his inability to travel by airplane. His only daughter had delivered a baby in the prior year, and although he desperately wanted to meet his first granddaughter, he felt unable to fly across the Atlantic Ocean to where his daughter lived.

The patient's anxiety about flying had begun 3 years earlier when he was on an airplane that landed during an ice storm. He had last flown a year earlier but had cried during both takeoff and landing; he had then found himself unable to return from that trip by airplane and instead took a train from Rome to Amsterdam. He had gone with his wife to an airport one additional time, 1 year prior to the evaluation, to fly to his daughter's wedding in the United States. Despite having drunk a significant amount of alcohol, Mr. Hendricks felt unable to board the airplane. After that failed effort, he tended to feel intense anxiety when he even considered the possibility of flying. Anxiety about business trips had led him to decline a promotion as well as an external job offer. Mr. Hendricks sees himself as a "family man" and feels terrible that he failed to attend his daughter's wedding and has not yet been able to meet his granddaughter.

Aside from guilt and regret related to his inability to fly, Mr. Hendricks denied other symptoms of depression and anxiety. He had increased his alcohol consumption to three glasses of wine nightly in order to "unwind," but denied any history of alcohol complications or withdrawal symptoms. He also denied a family history of psychiatric problems.

He denied experiencing anxiety in other situations, indicating that his colleagues saw him as a forceful and successful businessman who could "easily" deliver speeches in front of hundreds of people. When specifically asked, he reported that as a child, he had been "petrified" that he might get attacked by a wild animal. This fear had led him to refuse to go on family camping trips or even on long hikes in the country. As an adult, he said that he had no worries about being attacked by wild animals because he lived in a large city and took vacations by train to other large urban areas.

Discussion

Mr. Hendricks has such intense anxiety about flying that he will not get on airplanes despite being intensely motivated to do so. Even the thought of airplanes and airports causes significant distress. This fear is persistent and has caused significant functional impairment. He meets diagnostic criteria, therefore, for specific phobia. DSM-5 also includes specifiers to describe the phobia. In Mr. Hendricks's case, the phobic stimulus is flying, which would be coded as a "situational" specifier. (Other common situational stimuli include elevators and enclosed spaces.)

Most people with specific phobia fear more than one object or situation. Although Mr. Hendricks initially denies other anxieties, he does describe having had a highly distressing fear of being attacked by wild animals when he was younger. This fear led him to skip camping trips and hikes. He now lives in an urban environment where he is highly unlikely to come across a wild animal, but DSM-5 allows for a diagnosis of a specific phobia even when the phobic stimulus is not likely to be encountered. From a clinical perspective, uncovering such phobias is important because avoidance can not only cause fairly obvious distress and dysfunction (an inability to fly leading to an inability to visit family or optimally perform at work) but can also lead to life decisions that may not be completely conscious (a fear of wild animals leading to systematic avoidance of non-urban areas).

In addition to animals and situations, there are a number of other categories of phobic stimuli. These include the natural environment (e.g., heights, storms), blood-injection-injury (e.g., needles, invasive medical procedures), and other stimuli (e.g., loud sounds or costumed characters).

Specific phobia is most often comorbid with other anxiety disorders as well as depressive, substance use, somatic symptom, and personality disorders. Mr. Hendricks denies that his alcohol use is causing distress or dysfunction, so it does not appear to meet criteria for a DSM-5 disorder, but further exploration might indicate that his nightly drinking is causing problems with some aspects of his life. Similarly, further exploration of his depressive moods might identify a mood disorder that may be a focus for clinical attention. If it turns out that the flying phobia is a symptom of another disorder (e.g., a manifestation of agoraphobia), then the other disorder (the agoraphobia) would be the more accurate diagnosis. As it stands now, however, Mr. Hendricks appears to have fairly classic specific phobia.

Diagnoses

- Specific phobia, situational (flying on airplanes)
- Specific phobia, animals

Suggested Readings

Böhnlein J, Altegoer L, Muck NK, et al: Factors influencing the success of exposure therapy for specific phobia: a systematic review. Neurosci Biobehav Rev 108:796–820, 2020

Eaton WW, Bienvenu OJ, Miloyan B: Specific phobias. Lancet Psychiatry 5(8):678–686, 2018

Emmelkamp PMG: Specific and social phobias in ICD-11. World Psychiatry 11 (suppl 1):93–98, 2012

Zimmerman M, Dalrymple K, Chelminski I, et al: Recognition of irrationality of fear and the diagnosis of social anxiety disorder and specific phobia in adults: implications for criteria revision in DSM-5. Depress Anxiety 27(11):1044–1049, 2010

CASE 5.5

Always on Edge

Ryan E. Lawrence, M.D.
Deborah L. Cabaniss, M.D.

Peggy Isaac was a 41-year-old administrative assistant who was referred for an outpatient evaluation by her primary care physician with a chief complaint of "I'm always on edge." She lived alone and had never married or had children. She had never before seen a psychiatrist.

Ms. Isaac had lived with her longtime boyfriend until 8 months earlier, at which time he had abruptly ended the relationship to date a younger woman. Soon thereafter, Ms. Isaac began to agonize about routine tasks and the possibility of making mistakes at work. She felt uncharacteristically tense and fatigued. She had difficulty focusing. She also started to worry excessively about money and, to economize, she moved into a cheaper apartment in a less desirable neighborhood. She repeatedly sought reassurance from her office mates and her mother. No one seemed able to help, and she worried about being "too much of a burden."

During the 3 months prior to the evaluation, Ms. Isaac began to avoid going out at night, fearing that something bad would happen and she would be unable to summon help. More recently, she avoided going out in the daytime as well. She also felt "exposed and vulnerable" walking to the grocery store three blocks away, so she avoided shopping. After describing that she had figured out how to get her food delivered, she added, "It's ridiculous. I honestly feel something terrible is going to happen in one of the aisles and no one will help me, so I won't even go in." When in her apartment, she could often relax and enjoy a good book or movie.

Ms. Isaac said she had "always been a little nervous." Through much of kindergarten, she had cried inconsolably when her mother tried to drop her off. She reported seeing a counselor at age 10, during her parents' divorce, because "my mother thought I was too clingy." She added that she had never liked being alone, having had boyfriends constantly (occasionally overlapping) since age 16. She explained, "I hated being single, and I was always pretty, so I was never single for very long." Nevertheless, until the recent breakup, she said she had always thought of herself as "fine." She had been successful at work, jogged daily, maintained a solid network of friends, and had "no real complaints."

On initial interview, Ms. Isaac said she had been sad for a few weeks after her boyfriend left, but denied ever having felt worthless, guilty, hopeless, anhedonic, or suicidal. She said her weight was unchanged and her sleep was fine. The patient denied psychomotor changes. She did describe significant anxiety, with a Generalized Anxiety Disorder–7 score of 18, indicating severe anxiety.

Discussion

Ms. Isaac has become edgy, easily fatigued, and excessively worried during the 8 months since her boyfriend broke up with her. She has difficulty focusing. Her worries cause distress and dysfunction and lead her to repeatedly seek out reassurance. Although some of these symptoms could also be attributable to a depressive disorder, she lacks most other symptoms of major depressive disorder. Instead, Ms. Isaac meets criteria for DSM-5 generalized anxiety disorder (GAD).

More acutely, Ms. Isaac has developed intense anxiety about leaving her apartment and entering the local supermarket. These symptoms suggest that Ms. Isaac may meet DSM-5 criteria for agoraphobia, which requires fears and avoidance of at least two different situations. Her agoraphobia symptoms have persisted only a few months, however, which is less than the 6-month DSM-5 requirement. Depending on whether the clinician thought the agoraphobia symptoms warranted clinical attention, Ms. Isaac could receive an additional diagnosis of "unspecified anxiety disorder (agoraphobia with inadequate duration of symptoms)."

GAD is common, with a lifetime prevalence of 5.7% in the community and approximately 8% in primary care settings, where patients may present with physical symptoms (e.g., headaches, gastrointestinal issues, musculoskeletal pain).

Cognitive-behavioral therapy and/or medication (e.g., a selective serotonin reuptake inhibitor or serotonin-norepinephrine reuptake inhibitor) will likely improve Ms. Isaac's symptoms. She may also wish to explore what might have precipitated her GAD. Although it is not possible to be certain why someone develops a mood or anxiety disorder, consideration of psychosocial stressors that are coincident with the onset of symptoms can help with formulation, goal setting, and treatment.

In this case, Ms. Isaac developed acute anxiety symptoms after her live-in boyfriend broke up with her and she moved into another apartment. Both of these events were acutely upsetting. The next part of answering "Why now?" involves thinking about how the stressors relate to long-standing issues in Ms. Isaac's life. She noted that she had "never [been] single for very long," and gave a history of difficulties with separation that began in childhood. Anxiety that is triggered by separation may suggest problems with attachment, and adult attachment styles are thought to be linked to a person's earliest relationships. Those with secure attachments are able to form intimate relationships with others but are also able to soothe and regulate themselves when alone.

Individuals with insecure attachments, on the other hand, may cling to loved ones, be unable to self-regulate when alone, and have ambivalent feelings about those upon whom they are dependent. Thinking in this way, one can hypothesize that Ms. Isaac may have become symptomatic because of an insecure attachment style linked to her earliest relationship with her mother.

Clues that this may be the case include her mother's feeling that Ms. Isaac was "too clingy" during the divorce and Ms. Isaac's ambivalent feelings about her mother's efforts to be supportive. It would be helpful to understand more about Ms. Isaac's earliest relationships and the sorts of problematic attachment patterns that have developed during her romantic relationships. Such patterns would likely be recapitulated in the therapeutic relationship, where they could become a focus of treatment.

Diagnosis

• Generalized anxiety disorder

Suggested Readings

Newman MG, Shin KE, Zuellig AR: Developmental risk factors in generalized anxiety disorder and panic disorder. J Affect Disord 206:94–102, 2016

Orvati Aziz M, Mehrinejad SA, Hashemian K, Paivastegar M: Integrative therapy (short-term psychodynamic psychotherapy and cognitive-behavioral therapy) and cognitive-behavioral therapy in the treatment of generalized anxiety disorder: a randomized controlled trial. Complement Ther Clin Pract 39:101122, 2020

Stein MB, Sareen J: Generalized anxiety disorder. N Engl J Med 373:2059–2068, 2015

CASE 5.6

Anxiety and Cirrhosis

Andrea DiMartini, M.D.
Catherine Crone, M.D.

A psychiatric transplant liaison service was called to evaluate Robert Jennings, a 50-year-old married white man, for a liver transplant in the context of an alcohol use disorder, advanced cirrhosis, and no other prior psychiatric history. Several weeks earlier, he had been hospitalized with acute alcohol-associated hepatitis and diagnosed with end-stage liver disease. Prednisolone 40 mg/day was prescribed for treatment of the hepatitis. Prior to that hospitalization, he had been unaware that his alcohol consumption was seriously damaging his health and was shocked to learn that he would eventually require a liver transplant. Upon discharge, he began an addiction treatment program that was mandatory for him to be listed for possible transplantation.

Outpatient psychiatric consultation was requested by the transplant team after the patient's family expressed concern that he had recently become increasingly irritable and anxious and seemed to be having difficulty coping with the requirements for transplantation. Mr. Jennings's primary care physician had recently prescribed alprazolam 0.5 mg as needed for his anxiety. This was initially helpful, but after several days his family noticed he seemed more irritable, lethargic, and forgetful.

When interviewed, the patient said that he had been tired for months prior to the diagnosis and that the fatigue had hampered his ability to work (his job required making deliveries for a shipping firm). Although the diagnosis had been a shock, he said he had left the hospital feeling "great, better than I'd felt in years." For about a week after discharge, he described having enhanced energy and a sense of well-being, but he then began to feel anxious and restless. He slept poorly, unable to concentrate, and worried constantly about his health, finances, and family. He became less engaged with his family and stopped watching movies, normally his favorite pastime.

He denied having nightmares, flashbacks, avoidant behaviors, or racing thoughts. He also denied low mood, tearfulness, appetite changes, anhedonia, helplessness, hopelessness, or suicidality. He reported that he had started drinking daily 10 years earlier, stating that he enjoyed the taste of beer and liked socializing with friends after work. He developed tolerance to alcohol, needing to consume six to eight drinks per night to achieve the same effect. He described some withdrawal symptoms in the morning but did not drink during work hours; he underwent random testing due to his job as a truck driver. He did miss some family activities, preferring to drink, and this had been a source of marital conflict. He admitted feeling guilty about his alcohol use and its impact on him and his family. He denied using any alcohol since his hospitalization. He admitted to anger over having to undergo addiction counseling and had argued with the transplant team about this requirement. He denied having been an anxious person and considered himself able to handle most of life's challenges without being overwhelmed. His family confirmed his description of himself and viewed his recent behavior as uncharacteristic.

On mental status examination, Mr. Jennings was a thin, jaundiced, tired-appearing man. His gait was normal, but he was fidgety while seated. He maintained eye contact and responded appropriately, although he repeatedly made comments like, "Something isn't right" and "It's not all in my head." His affect was anxious and irritable, and his speech was terse. He appeared distracted but denied confusion and disorientation. He had no delusions or hallucinations. His thoughts were logical and coherent, without disorganization, and there was no latency to his responses. He scored 26 out of 30 on the Montreal Cognitive Assessment, missing points for recall and serial 7s. He scored in the normal range for Trail Making Test A and B but asked to have the instructions repeated for Trails B.

Discussion

Mr. Jennings has been fatigued for several months. Diagnosis and treatment of his hepatic cirrhosis were followed by a weeklong burst of euphoria, followed by anxiety, irritability, cognitive disturbances, and insomnia. The evaluating team would look broadly for causes of Mr. Jennings's psychiatric complaints, but the initial search would focus on medical causes. Liver disease rarely induces anxiety directly, but he did receive prednisolone while in the hospital, and steroid therapy frequently induces an initial sense of well-being, followed within 1–2 weeks by more negative or unpleasant symptoms of mood or anxiety disturbance.

Other diagnoses should also be considered. Fatigue, difficulty concentrating, and a reduction in pleasurable activities point to the possibility of major depressive disorder, for example, although some of these symptoms could be attributable to progressive physical limitations from his advanced liver disease. Utilizing a broad or "inclusive" approach to the diagnosis of depression in medically ill patients might suggest that these symptoms be counted under the DSM-5 diagnostic criteria for major depressive disorder despite their potential physical origin. However, further review of Mr. Jennings's presentation indicated that although he complained of feeling irritable, he had no problems with persistent low mood, tearfulness, or other associated depressive symptoms (e.g., anhedonia, appetite changes, inappropriate thoughts of guilt, or recurrent thoughts of death or suicide). Major depressive disorder would seem unlikely.

Anxiety disorders such as generalized anxiety disorder and panic disorder should also be considered. It could be that the discontinuation of his alcohol use has led to the unmasking of an underlying anxiety disorder. However, Mr. Jennings denied having past symptoms of anxiety and reported drinking for pleasure and to socialize; he did not appear to be drinking to manage anxiety or stress. In addition, his symptoms seem directly related to the steroids and lack the duration to qualify for one of the other anxiety disorders.

Illness, treatments, and potentially life-threatening circumstances can lead to acute stress disorder, adjustment disorder, and PTSD. Although he does have symptoms of heightened arousal and reactivity, Mr. Jennings denies intrusive recollections or avoidance behaviors. He does not, therefore, meet criteria for a trauma-related disorder. Furthermore, it is notable that he initially felt well despite his diagnosis and only later developed changes in his mood and behavior. This pattern would not rule out a trauma diagnosis but does reduce its likelihood.

An additionally important diagnostic area to consider is Mr. Jennings's dependence on alcohol. Early in abstinence, patients often experience symptoms of anxiety, irritability, and depression. These symptoms contribute to the high rates of relapse following alcohol rehabilitation. Even in the context of life-threatening illness and the need for transplantation, a significant number of individuals relapse. Although it may be tempting to prescribe benzodiazepines to treat anxiety symptoms, these medications can produce cravings and precipitate relapse, and should be avoided. This patient is denying alcohol use, but he is on a transplant list, and a relapse could lead to a delisting. To monitor unrevealed alcohol use, it would be warranted to monitor him by ongoing interviews and random toxicology screenings.

Mr. Jennings's current presentation could also be related to a neurocognitive disorder. Patients with advanced liver disease frequently have problems with minimal hepatic encephalopathy, a phenomenon that is characterized by subtle but important changes in both physical and mental functioning. Compared with hepatic encephalopathy (DSM-5 delirium due to another medical condition), minimal hepatic encephalopathy does not present with disturbance of consciousness or with overt behavioral or cognitive functioning changes. Rather, patients may present with mild personality or behavioral changes such as irritability, excessive fatigue, or sleepiness, along with subtle subcortical cognitive impairment or slowing. Impairments in psychomotor speed, visual attention, and perception are typically not evident with basic screening such as the Montreal Cognitive Assessment but require specific psychometric testing that would elicit these deficits (e.g., Trail Making Test A and B, Digit Span, finger-tapping speed).

Identifying minimal hepatic encephalopathy is important because patients with this diagnosis typically do not improve with the use of antidepressants or anxiolytics but instead require treatment with ammonia-reducing agents. The combination of minimal hepatic encephalopathy and slower hepatic metabolism makes patients more sensitive to adverse drug side effects (e.g., cognitive slowing from benzodiazepines, sedatives, pain medications, or anticholinergic medications). In Mr. Jennings's case, the worsening of symptoms may have resulted from the use of a benzodiazepine. These patients need to avoid medications that may worsen cognitive functioning, and they should also be monitored for development of overt hepatic encephalopathy. Because cognitive difficulties that accompany minimal hepatic encephalopathy are known to impair daily functioning and skills such as driving, this patient may need to be counseled on whether he can or should continue to drive (which would have significant implications for his work as a deliveryman). After discontinuing the alprazolam and receiving treatment for high ammonia levels (if present), he could be retested to establish his cognitive baseline.

Diagnoses

- Alcohol use disorder, moderate, in early remission
- Medication-induced anxiety disorder (steroids)

Suggested Readings

Kruckenberg KM, Shenai N, Dew MA, et al: Transplant-related trauma, personal growth and alcohol use outcomes in a cohort of patients receiving transplants for alcohol associated liver disease. Gen Hosp Psychiatry 72:73–80, 2021

Rogal S, Shenai N, Kruckenberg K, et al: Post-transplant outcomes of persons receiving a liver graft for alcoholic liver disease. Alcohol Alcohol 53(2):157–165, 2018

Obsessive-Compulsive and Related Disorders

INTRODUCTION

John W. Barnhill, M.D.

When evaluating a patient whose preoccupations and rituals have become persistent, excessive, and impairing, clinicians are encouraged to consider each of the disorders within the chapter on obsessive-compulsive and related disorders. These include obsessive-compulsive disorder, body dysmorphic disorder, hoarding disorder, trichotillomania (hair-pulling disorder), and excoriation (skin-picking) disorder.

Obsessive-compulsive disorder (OCD) is characterized by the presence of obsessions and/or compulsions. Obsessions are unwanted and repetitive thoughts that often involve such concerns as pathological doubt, fear of contamination, somatic concerns, and a need for symmetry. Compulsions are the repetitive behaviors that are performed in response to the distress of the obsessions. Common compulsive behaviors include checking, ordering, cleaning, and mental rituals.

Body dysmorphic disorder (BDD) is characterized by a preoccupation with one or more physical flaws that are not readily apparent to others. In addition, a diagnosis of BDD requires repetitive behaviors (such as excessive grooming or reassurance seeking) and significant distress or dysfunction. If the preoccupation is primarily about weight, however, then that patient would receive an eating disorder diagnosis if diagnostic criteria for an eating disorder are met.

Once a diagnosis is made, DSM-5 includes multiple specifiers for many of its diagnoses. OCD, BDD, and hoarding disorder are unusual in having an "insight" specifier. The insight specifier characterizes patients as having good or fair insight, poor insight, or absent insight/delusional beliefs. For example, people who are delusionally convinced that their BDD beliefs are true would not be coded as having a comorbid psychotic disorder (e.g., delusional disorder) but would instead be noted to have BDD with absent insight.

Trichotillomania (hair-pulling), and excoriation (skin-picking) are the most common body-focused, repetitive behavior disorders. Hair-pulling disorder was previously listed among the impulse-control disorders not elsewhere classified, along with such disorders as pyromania and intermittent explosive disorder. Skin-picking disorder was new in DSM-5. Both disorders involve the sort of persistent, repetitive dysfunctional behaviors that characterize all of the obsessive-compulsive and related disorders.

Hoarding disorder was also new in DSM-5. It was previously listed as a possible criterion for obsessive-compulsive personality disorder or considered a symptom of OCD. In some cases, hoarding-type behavior is a symptom of OCD (e.g., if trash accumulates because of fears of becoming contaminated by touching it), but evidence indicates that dysfunctional hoarding often exists without an accompanying OCD diagnosis.

As continues to be true throughout much of DSM-5, this chapter includes categories for patients whose symptoms are assessed to be secondary to medications, substances, or another medical condition. DSM-5 also allows clinicians to identify clinically relevant conditions that do not meet full criteria for a disorder. For example, a presentation that meets criteria for body dysmorphic disorder in a person who has significant physical flaws—a circumstance that would preclude the use of that diagnosis (which requires that any physical flaws be no more than "slight")—could be recorded as "other specified obsessive-compulsive and related disorder (body dysmorphic–like disorder with actual flaws)." The "other specified" diagnosis might also be used to refer to a symptom cluster not described in the criteria for any DSM-5 obsessive-compulsive and related disorder, such as obsessional jealousy or olfactory reference disorder. "Unspecified" disorders can refer to symptom clusters that resemble presentations found in a particular DSM-5 chapter but that do not meet criteria for any specific disorder; the unspecified diagnosis is often used when the clinician has insufficient clinical information to make a diagnosis, such as in an emergency evaluation or an initial consultation.

Suggested Readings

Phillips K, Stein DJ (eds): Handbook on Obsessive-Compulsive and Related Disorders. Washington, DC, American Psychiatric Publishing, 2015

Simon N, Hollander E, Rothbaum BO, Stein DJ (eds): The American Psychiatric Association Publishing Textbook of Anxiety, Trauma, and OCD-Related Disorders, 3rd Edition. Washington, DC, American Psychiatric Association Publishing, 2020

CASE 6.1

Depression

Mayumi Okuda, M.D.

Helen Blair Simpson, M.D., Ph.D.

Samuel King, a 52-year-old never-married janitor, presented for treatment of depression. He had been struggling with depressive symptoms for years and had tried fluoxetine, citalopram, and supportive psychotherapy, with minor improvement. He worked full-time but engaged in very few activities outside of work.

When asked how he felt, Mr. King said that his mood was low, he was unable to enjoy things, and he had insomnia, feelings of hopelessness, low energy, and difficulty concentrating and making decisions. He denied current suicidality but added that a few years earlier, he had taken a full bottle of medication with the intent to kill himself. He reported that he had done this during a time that he was abusing alcohol. He denied current alcohol or illicit substance use.

When asked about anxiety, Mr. King said he was worried about contracting diseases such as HIV. Aware of an unusually strong disinfectant smell, the interviewer asked the patient if he had any particular cleaning behaviors related to the HIV concerns. Mr. King paused and clarified that he avoided touching practically anything outside of his home. When further encouraged, Mr. King said that if he even came close to things that he considered potentially contaminated, he had to wash his hands incessantly with household bleach. He described that he felt like "something was still there" in his hands and he had to wash his hands until it felt that he had finally done it "right."

On average, Mr. King washed his hands up to 30 times a day, spending hours on this routine. Physical contact was particularly difficult. Shopping for groceries and taking public transportation were a big problem, and he had almost given up trying to socialize or engage in romantic relationships. These behaviors had only intensified during the COVID-19 pandemic, though a co-worker liked to joke that Mr. King had been cleaning and social distancing for years before it became fashionable.

When asked if he had other worries, Mr. King replied that he had intrusive images of hitting someone, fears that he would say things that might be offensive or inaccurate, and concerns about disturbing his neighbors. To counteract the anxiety produced by these images and thoughts, he constantly replayed prior conversations in his mind, kept diaries to record what he said, and often apologized for fear he might have sounded offensive. When he showered, he made sure that the water in the tub only reached a certain level for fear that if he were not attentive, he would flood his neighbors.

Mr. King used gloves at work and performed well. He had no medical problems. He spent most of his free time at home. Although he enjoyed the company of others, the fear of having to touch something if he was invited to a meal or to another person's home was too much for him to handle.

The examination revealed a casually dressed man who smelled strongly of bleach. He was worried and constricted but cooperative, coherent, and goal directed. He denied hallucinations and other strongly held ideas. He denied a current intention to hurt himself or others. He was cognitively intact. He recognized that his fears and urges were "kinda crazy," but he felt they were out of his control.

Discussion

Mr. King has prominent depressive symptoms as well as obsessions and compulsions. He reports dysphoria, anhedonia, insomnia, hopelessness, anergia, and difficulty concentrating. Although he denies current suicidal thoughts, he has a history of a suicide attempt. These symptoms have persisted much longer than the required 2 weeks, have affected the quality of his life, and do not appear to have been precipitated by substance use or a medical problem. He clearly warrants a major depressive disorder diagnosis.

Evaluation for obsessive-compulsive disorder (OCD) can be less straightforward. Mr. King discussed both his obsessions and his compulsions in a first session, but many patients are less spontaneously revealing. For that reason, an assessment for possible OCD requires specific, tactful questions that can allow people with varying levels of insight to discuss thoughts, feelings, and behaviors that can be embarrassing and private.

DSM-5 defined obsessions as having two related qualities: First, they are recurrent, persistent thoughts, urges, or images that are intrusive and unwanted and generally induce anxiety or distress. Second, the individual tries to ignore, suppress, or neutralize these symptoms through some other thought or action (i.e., by enacting a compulsion).

Mr. King reports multiple obsessions. These include obsessions related to contamination (fear of contracting HIV), aggression (intrusive images of hitting someone), scrupulosity (fear of sounding offensive or inaccurate), and symmetry (exactness in the level of water). He also experienced sensory phenomena, preceding the compulsion to wash his hands; he described a physical sensation of feeling that his hands were contaminated and described a just-right sensation.

Attempts to ignore or suppress the thoughts, urges, or images can take the form of avoidance and lead to significant disability. This is certainly true for Mr. King, who spends hours on his OCD routines and avoids leaving his apartment, engaging in social relationships, and performing the most basic of errands.

DSM-5 made several minor changes to the description of obsessions. For example, the term *urge* is used instead of *impulse* to avoid confusion with impulse-control disorders. DSM-5 also used the term *unwanted* instead of *inappropriate* to reflect the reality that people with OCD view their symptoms with varying degrees of ego-dystonicity. Finally, although obsessions are noted to *generally* cause anxiety or distress, research indicates that not all obsessions result in significant anxiety or distress.

Mr. King also has a number of compulsions. Compulsions are defined as repetitive behaviors (e.g., hand washing) or mental acts (e.g., counting) that the individual feels driven to perform in response to an obsession, or according to rules that must be rigidly applied. These behaviors or mental acts must be aimed at reducing distress or preventing some dreaded event, but they should also be either excessive or realistically unconnected to the anticipated event. He reports multiple compulsions: excessive hand washing, checking (keeping diaries), repeating (clarifying what he said repeatedly), and mental compulsions (replaying prior conversations in his mind).

As is seen for disorders throughout DSM-5, the OCD diagnosis requires that symptoms cause distress or impairment. Typically, OCD is time-consuming (1 hour per day is a guideline) and causes distress and impairment in multiple spheres of the patient's life. Even though Mr. King is able to work, his choice of occupation might have been influenced by his OCD symptoms (few other jobs allow the constant wearing of gloves and frequent use of bleach). Not only are his symptoms time-consuming, but he appears to be a lonely, isolated man, whose life has been significantly ravaged by his OCD.

It is important to explore whether OCD symptoms can be attributable to a substance, a medication, a medical condition, or a comorbid psychiatric condition. From the history, it appears that Mr. King takes no medications, abuses no substances, has no medical illness, and lacks actual physical complaints. None of these seem to be likely contributors.

Recurrent thoughts and repetitive behavior can be found in a variety of other psychiatric diagnoses. To exclude these other diagnoses, the clinician should ask the patient a series of very specific questions. For example, recurrent thoughts, avoidant behaviors, and repetitive requests for reassurance can also occur in anxiety disorders (e.g., generalized anxiety disorder, social anxiety disorder). The obsessions of OCD must also be distinguished from the rumination of major depressive disorder, in which thoughts are usually mood congruent and not necessarily experienced as intrusive or distressing. When OCD is identified, it is useful to specifically explore the possibility of OCD-related disorders (e.g., body dysmorphic disorder, hoarding disorder), which can present similarly to OCD and can also be co-occurring.

In an effort to subcategorize OCD symptoms, the DSM-5 diagnostic criteria listed two specifiers. The first identifies those OCD patients who also have a past or current history of a tic disorder; data suggest that OCD patients with a history of tic disorders may have a different clinical course and response to treatments than OCD patients without a history of tics.

A second DSM-5 specifier relates to insight, which varies significantly among different people with OCD. The three insight specifiers are good or fair; poor; and absent. Mr. King appears to understand that his obsessional beliefs are untrue and so would fall into the most insightful category. Individuals who are completely convinced of the validity of their OCD beliefs would previously have been viewed as delusional, but DSM-5 integrated this cluster of people into the OCD diagnosis with the specifier "with absent insight/delusional beliefs."

Diagnoses

- Obsessive-compulsive disorder, with good or fair insight
- Major depressive disorder

Suggested Readings

Hollander E, Zohar J, Sirovatka, Regier DA (eds): Obsessive-Compulsive Spectrum Disorders: Refining the Research Agenda for DSM-V. Arlington, VA, American Psychiatric Association, 2011

Leckman JF, Denys D, Simpson HB, et al: Obsessive-compulsive disorder: a review of the diagnostic criteria and possible subtype and dimensional specifiers for DSM-5. Depress Anxiety 27(6):507–527, 2010

Shephard E, Stern ER, van den Heuvel OA, et al: Toward a neurocircuit-based taxonomy to guide treatment of obsessive-compulsive disorder. Mol Psychiatry 26(9):4583–4604, 2021

Zandberg LJ, Zang Y, McLean CP, et al: Change in obsessive-compulsive symptoms mediates subsequent change in depressive symptoms during exposure and response prevention. Behav Res Ther 68:76–81, 2015

CASE 6.2

Germs

Dan J. Stein, M.D., Ph.D.
Helen Blair Simpson, M.D., Ph.D.
Katharine A. Phillips, M.D.

Trevor Lewis, a 32-year-old single man living with his parents, was brought to his psychiatric consultation by his mother. She noted that since adolescence, her son had been concerned with germs, which led to long-standing hand-washing and showering rituals. During the prior 6 months, his symptoms had markedly worsened. He had become preoccupied with being infected by COVID-19 and spent the day cleaning not only his body but all of his clothing and linen. He had begun to insist that the family also wash their clothing and linen regularly, and that they keep the windows shut all the time. He allowed no visitors to their home. When the parents were occasionally exposed to other people by going outside, he insisted that they wear their masks in his presence for the ensuing 48 hours. The resulting conflicts had led to the current consultation.

Mr. Lewis had in the past received a selective serotonin reuptake inhibitor and cognitive-behavioral therapy for his symptoms. These had had some positive effects, and he had been able to complete high school successfully. Nevertheless, his symptoms had prevented him from completing college or working outside the home; he had long felt that his home was relatively germ-free in comparison to the outside world. However, over the past 6 months, he had increasingly indicated that home, too, was contaminated, including with COVID-19.

At the time of presentation, Mr. Lewis had no other obsessive-compulsive and related disorder symptoms such as sexual, religious, or other obsessions; appearance or acquisition preoccupations; or body-focused repetitive behaviors. However, in the past he had also experienced obsessions relating to fears of harming himself or others, together with associated checking compulsions (e.g., checking that the stove was switched off). He had a childhood history of motor tics. During high school, he found that marijuana reduced his anxiety. He denied having had access to marijuana and other psychoactive substances since leaving school.

Mr. Lewis was interviewed over video using a telehealth system. He appeared disheveled and unkempt. He was completely convinced that COVID-19 had contaminated his home and that his washing and cleaning were necessary to stay uninfected. When challenged with information about COVID-19's mode of spread, he answered that COVID-19 might come into the home through an open window or the sweat of visitors, and his masked parents could certainly get infected by going to the grocery store. He added that his parents had tried to convince him that he was excessively worried, but he did not believe them. In fact, his worries kept returning even when he tried to think of something else.

There was no evidence of hallucinations or of a formal thought disorder. He denied an intention to harm or kill himself or others. He was cognitively intact.

Discussion

Mr. Lewis is completely convinced that his home is contaminated by COVID-19. He is unable to suppress these preoccupying, intrusive thoughts. He feels obliged to perform unreasonable behaviors in response to his excessive worries. These behaviors consume his day and are socially and occupationally debilitating. He meets the symptomatic criteria for DSM-5 obsessive-compulsive disorder (OCD). Contamination and cleanliness concerns, with subsequent washing and cleaning rituals, are a common symptom dimension in OCD.

DSM-5 listed two specifiers for OCD. The tic-related OCD specifier is based on a growing literature indicating that individuals with OCD and current or past tics have particular distinguishing features, and that the presence or absence of tics helps guide assessment and intervention. Mr. Lewis had a history of motor tics in childhood. DSM-5 also recommends an assessment of insight, particularly specifying whether the individual with OCD has good or fair insight, poor insight, or absent insight/delusional beliefs. The "with absent insight/delusional beliefs" specifier is provided not only for OCD but also for body dysmorphic disorder and hoarding disorder, and appears to be a valid, clinically useful distinguishing feature.

Obsessive thoughts and compulsive behaviors are found in other psychiatric disorders. Patients with illness anxiety disorder (IAD) are preoccupied with having or acquiring a serious illness, and may perform excessive related behaviors, such as seeking reassurance. Mr. Lewis is worried about getting COVID-19, which might prompt the consideration that he has IAD. His cleaning compulsions and checking are more characteristic of OCD, however, and he lacks the somatic symptoms, other health-related concerns, and checking of the body for signs of illness that are commonly found in IAD. Similarly, although patients with generalized anxiety disorder can have worries about their own or others' health, they also have other kinds of worries, and they do not have compulsions.

Patients with delusional disorder do not have the obsessions, compulsions, preoccupations, or other characteristic symptoms of OCD. Conversely, patients with OCD with absent insight/delusional beliefs may appear delusional but do not have other features of psychotic disorders, such as hallucinations or formal thought disorder. Mr. Lewis does not have a substance use or medical history that is associated with psychotic symptoms.

It would be useful to have a more detailed picture of the nature and severity of Mr. Lewis's OCD symptoms, including avoidance and functional impairment. Mr. Lewis was noted to be disheveled and unkempt, for example, which might seem odd for someone with prominent cleanliness concerns. His appearance might be explained, however, if his contamination rituals are so time-consuming that he avoids starting them.

Although Mr. Lewis's diagnosis appears clear, it can be helpful to make use of one of the symptom severity scales designed for OCD, such as the Yale-Brown Obsessive Compulsive Scale, or a scale to measure insight/delusionality, such as the Brown Assessment of Beliefs Scale.

Diagnosis

- Obsessive-compulsive disorder, tic related, with absent insight/delusional beliefs

Suggested Readings

du Toit PL, van Kradenburg J, Niehaus D, Stein DJ: Comparison of obsessive-compulsive disorder patients with and without comorbid putative obsessive-compulsive spectrum disorders using a structured clinical interview. Compr Psychiatry 42(4):291–300, 2001

Eisen JL, Phillips KA, Baer L, et al: The Brown Assessment of Beliefs Scale: reliability and validity. Am J Psychiatry 155(1):102–108, 1998

Goodman WK, Price LH, Rasmussen SA, et al: The Yale-Brown Obsessive Compulsive Scale, I: development, use, and reliability. Arch Gen Psychiatry 46(11):1006–1011 1989

Leckman JF, Denys D, Simpson HB, et al: Obsessive-compulsive disorder: a review of the diagnostic criteria and possible subtypes and dimensional specifiers for DSM-V. Depress Anxiety 27(6):507–527, 2010

Stein DJ, Costa DLC, Lochner C, et al: Obsessive-compulsive disorder. Nat Rev Dis Primers 5(1):52, 2019

CASE 6.3

Appearance Preoccupations

Katharine A. Phillips, M.D.

Vincent Mancini, a 26-year-old single white man, was brought for an outpatient evaluation by his parents because they were distressed by his symptoms. Since age 13, he had been excessively preoccupied with his "scarred" skin, "thinning" hair, "asymmetrical" ears, and "wimpy" and "inadequately muscular" body build. Although he looked normal, Mr. Mancini was completely convinced that he looked "ugly and hideous," and he believed that other people talked about him and made fun of him because of his appearance.

Mr. Mancini spent 5–6 hours a day compulsively checking his disliked body areas in mirrors and other reflecting surfaces such as windows, excessively styling his hair "to create an illusion of fullness," pulling on his ears to try to "even them up," and comparing his appearance with that of others. He compulsively picked his skin, sometimes using razor blades, to try to "clear it up." He lifted weights daily and regularly wore several layers of T-shirts to look bigger. He almost always wore a cap to hide his hair. He had received dermatological treatment for his skin concerns but felt it had not helped.

Mr. Mancini missed several months of high school because he was too preoccupied to do schoolwork, felt compelled to leave class to check mirrors, and was too self-conscious to be seen by others; for these reasons, he was unable to attend college. He became socially withdrawn and did not date "because no girl would want to go out with someone as ugly as me." He often considered suicide because he felt that life was not worth living "if I look like a freak" and because he felt isolated and ostracized because of his "ugliness." His parents expressed concern over his "violent outbursts," which occurred when he was feeling especially angry and distressed over how he looked or when they tried to pull him away from the mirror.

Mr. Mancini reported depressed mood, anhedonia, worthlessness, poor concentration, and suicidal ideation, all of which he attributed to his appearance concerns. To self-medicate his distress over his appearance, he drank alcohol and smoked marijuana. He used protein powder to "build up muscle" but denied use of anabolic steroids or other performance-enhancing drugs or drugs of abuse. He had distressing and problematic anxiety in social situations during his late teens that he attributed to feeling "stupid," but he denied recent social anxiety that was unrelated to his appearance concerns.

Mr. Mancini had no significant medical history and was taking no medication. His mother had obsessive-compulsive disorder (OCD).

Mr. Mancini was neatly dressed and groomed and wore a baseball cap. He had no obvious physical defects. His eye contact was poor. He was oriented and grossly cognitively intact. His affect was irritable; his mood was depressed, with passive suicidal ideation. He had no psychomotor abnormalities; his speech was normal. He was completely convinced that he was ugly and was certain that other people talked about him and laughed at him because of his physical appearance; he had no other psychotic symptoms. He believed his appearance "defects" were real and not attributable to a psychiatric disorder.

Discussion

Mr. Mancini is preoccupied with perceived defects or flaws in his appearance that are not observable or appear only slight to others. In response to his appearance concerns, he performs repetitive behaviors, including compulsively checking his disliked body areas in mirrors and other reflecting surfaces, excessively styling his hair, pulling on his ears, and picking his skin; he also performs repetitive mental acts (i.e., comparing his appearance with that of other people). The preoccupation causes clinically significant distress and functional impairment. According to DSM-5, Mr. Mancini has body dysmorphic disorder (BDD).

BDD is common and affects slightly more females than males. About two-thirds of cases have onset in childhood or adolescence. BDD can involve any body area (often the face or head) and usually involves multiple areas. Preoccupations occur, on average, for 3–8 hours a day. Over the disorder's course, all individuals perform repetitive behaviors or repetitive mental acts (e.g., comparing) intended to fix, check, hide, or obtain reassurance about their perceived defects. Skin picking, intended to improve perceived skin defects, is a common BDD symptom. In such cases, BDD is diagnosed rather than excoriation (skin-picking) disorder.

The appearance preoccupations usually cause functional impairment, which is often marked. Approximately 80% of BDD patients have lifetime suicidal ideation, which often is attributed to BDD, and a quarter or more attempt suicide. Suicidality appears to be more common in BDD than in many other severe psychiatric disorders. Available data, although limited, suggest a markedly elevated suicide rate. Aggressive or violent behavior can occur as a symptom of BDD.

BDD's diagnostic criteria include specifiers indicating degree of insight regarding BDD beliefs: with good or fair insight, with poor insight, and with absent insight/delusional beliefs. Mr. Mancini has absent insight/delusional beliefs because he is completely convinced that he looks ugly. Poor insight is the most common level of insight, and about one-third of individuals diagnosed with BDD have delusional beliefs. Those with delusional BDD beliefs should be diagnosed with BDD rather than a psychotic disorder. Mr. Mancini has BDD-specific delusions of reference; ideas or delusions of reference are present in the majority of individuals with BDD. Other psychotic symptoms typically do not occur as symptoms of BDD.

The diagnostic criteria for BDD also include a specifier for muscle dysmorphia, consisting of preoccupation with the idea that one's body build is too small or insufficiently muscular. This specifier is used even if the person is preoccupied with other body areas. Thus, Mr. Mancini's diagnosis includes this specifier. Muscle dysmorphia is considered a form of BDD rather than an eating disorder, because it meets diagnostic criteria for BDD and not all individuals with muscle dysmorphia have abnormal eating behavior.

BDD shares preoccupations, obsessions, and repetitive behaviors with OCD, but BDD specifically involves perceived appearance flaws. Symmetry preoccupation, which may be an OCD symptom, should be considered a BDD symptom when it involves physical appearance, as in Mr. Mancini's case. BDD and OCD are related disorders—and Mr. Mancini's mother is noted to have OCD—but they have important differences. Differences include poorer insight, more frequent ideas and delusions of reference, and greater suicidality in BDD; greater comorbidity of BDD with major depressive disorder and possibly substance-related disorders; and differences in some of the approaches used in cognitive-behavioral therapy for the two conditions.

Major depressive disorder is the most common co-occurring disorder, often developing secondary to the distress and impairment caused by BDD. Both BDD and major depressive disorder should be diagnosed if criteria are met for both disorders.

When social anxiety and avoidance are attributable to preoccupation with perceived appearance defects, BDD should be diagnosed rather than social anxiety disorder. Social anxiety and avoidance are nearly universal in BDD and are due to these individuals' beliefs or fear that they will be considered ugly, ridiculed, or rejected because of their physical features. However, co-occurring social anxiety disorder is present in more than one-third of individuals with BDD. Mr. Mancini was previously diagnosed with social anxiety disorder because he had social anxiety in high school that was not attributable to his appearance concerns.

Substance use disorders occur in a substantial proportion of individuals with BDD, often as the result of the distress caused by BDD. Mr. Mancini admitted to use of both marijuana and alcohol, although it is not clear whether their use reaches criteria for substance use disorder. From about 20% to more than 40% of people with the muscle dysmorphia form of BDD abuse anabolic-androgenic steroids, which may have dangerous physical and psychological effects. Mr. Mancini denied use of these drugs, but his "violent outbursts" could reflect steroid use that he declined to mention during his initial evaluation.

Diagnosis

- Body dysmorphic disorder, with absent insight/delusional beliefs, with muscle dysmorphia

Suggested Readings

Phillips KA (ed): Body Dysmorphic Disorder: Advances in Research and Clinical Practice. New York, Oxford University Press, 2017

Phillips KA, Stein DJ, Rauch SL, et al: Should an obsessive-compulsive spectrum grouping of disorders be included in DSM-V? Depress Anxiety 27(6):528–555, 2010

Phillips KA, Wilhelm S, Koran LM, et al: Body dysmorphic disorder: some key issues for DSM-V. Depress Anxiety 27(6):573–591, 2010

CASE 6.4

Depression and Anxiety

David Mataix-Cols, Ph.D.
Lorena Fernández de la Cruz, Ph.D.

Wendy Nichols was a 47-year-old single white woman referred to a community mental health care team for the management of a mixed presentation of low mood and generalized anxiety. She had never taken any psychiatric medication but had completed a course of cognitive-behavioral therapy for a previous depressive episode 5 years earlier.

Ms. Nichols's medical history was unremarkable. She lived alone in a two-bedroom apartment and had no family or friends nearby. She had a university degree and worked as a part-time sales assistant in a charity thrift shop. She said she had dated in college but had "somehow been too busy" in recent years.

On initial examination, she was an articulate, well-dressed woman who was coherent and cooperative. She was clearly in a low mood. She complained about poor concentration and difficulties getting organized. She denied any substance misuse.

The clinician noted that Ms. Nichols's purse was filled with bills and other papers. When asked, the patient initially shrugged it off, indicating that she "carried around my office." When the interviewer inquired further, it emerged that Ms. Nichols had had difficulty discarding important business papers, newspapers, and magazines for as long as she could remember. She felt that it all started when her mother got rid of her old toys when she was age 12. Now, many years later, Ms. Nichols's apartment had become filled with books, stationery, crafts, plastic packages, cardboard boxes, and all sorts of other things. She said she knew it was a little crazy, but these items could be handy one day. She said, "Waste not, want not." She also reported that many of her possessions were beautiful, unique, and irreplaceable, or had strong sentimental value. The thought of discarding any of these possessions caused her great distress.

Over a series of interviews, the clinician developed a clearer understanding of the extent of the problem. Rooms in Ms. Nichols's apartment had begun to fill when she was in her early 30s, and by the time of the interview, she had little room to live. Her kitchen was almost entirely full, so she used a mini fridge and a toaster oven that she had wedged into piles of paper in the hallway. She ate her meals in the only available chair. At night, she moved a pile of papers from the bed onto that chair so she could sleep. Ms. Nichols continued to buy from the charity thrift store where she worked and also picked up daily free newspapers that she planned to read in the future.

Embarrassed by the condition of her apartment, she had told no one about her behavior and had invited no one into her apartment for at least 15 years. She also avoided social functions and dating, because—despite being naturally sociable and very lonely—she knew she would be unable to reciprocate with invitations to her home. She was surprised to have told the clinician, because she had not told even her own mother, but she would like help. She declined the clinician's offer of a home visit or a telehealth visit but did offer some photographs of her living room from her telephone's camera. The photographs showed furniture, papers, boxes, and clothes piled from floor to ceiling.

Ms. Nichols described long-standing feelings of sadness and loneliness, as well as anxiety whenever she tried to clean up or whenever someone tried to befriend her. She denied other psychiatric symptoms, including delusions, hallucinations, obsessions, and compulsive behavior.

Discussion

Ms. Nichols has hoarding disorder, a diagnosis first introduced in DSM-5. She has had difficulty discarding possessions for as long as she can remember. Concerned about perceived future use for the items and sentimental attachment, she experiences severe distress at the thought of discarding any of her possessions. These difficulties have resulted in a living space that is barely functional. Apart from the loss of functionality of her home, she is distressed about her social isolation. The case report does not provide evidence that either a medical disorder or another psychiatric condition is responsible for the hoarding behavior.

It is useful to recognize that valuable items are often intermingled with useless or valueless items, so that jewelry and legal documents can be sandwiched between yellowed newspapers. Knowing such details helps the clinician ask the right questions, which is especially useful in trying to elicit history from a patient who is likely to be embarrassed about the behavior. It can be useful to document clutter through the use of photographs, videos, or a home visit. Home visits are recommended for a full evaluation of any potential risks associated with the disorder, such as fire risks or other health hazards.

DSM-5 lists two specifiers for hoarding disorder. The "excessive acquisition" specifier refers to the excessive obtaining of items, whether they be free, bought, or stolen, when clearly these items are not needed or there is no space for them. Because many people with hoarding disorder lack insight into their difficulties, the diagnosis of hoarding disorder includes a specifier for level of insight. Ms. Nichols indicates that her acquisitions and hoarding are reasonable (the items might be useful or have monetary or sentimental value). She has never told her family, much less gone for previous treatment. Ms. Nichols understands that she has a problem and says she wants help, however, so she would be said to have good or fair insight.

It is important to explore whether the accumulation of objects is judged to be a direct consequence of another DSM-5 disorder. If so, hoarding disorder is not diagnosed. For example, excessive accumulation of possessions has been described in obsessive-compulsive disorder and a number of neurodevelopmental (e.g., autism spectrum disorder), neurocognitive (e.g., frontotemporal dementia), and psychotic (e.g., schizophrenia) disorders. None of these other diagnoses seems to fit Ms. Nichols.

The decreased energy in major depressive disorder can lead to messy accumulation, and Ms. Nichols does appear to have a depression. Not only does the case report not go into enough detail to clarify the depression diagnosis (hence, the DSM-5 diagnosis of unspecified depressive disorder), the nearly lifelong hoarding difficulties appear to have preceded her mood symptoms. Thus, hoarding disorder should be diagnosed along with Ms. Nichols's unspecified depressive disorder.

Diagnoses

- Hoarding disorder, with excessive acquisition, with good or fair insight
- Unspecified depressive disorder

Suggested Readings

Frost RO, Steketee G, Tolin DF: Diagnosis and assessment of hoarding disorder. Annu Rev Clin Psychol 8:219–242, 2012

Mataix-Cols D: Clinical practice. Hoarding disorder. N Engl J Med 370(21):2023–2030, 2014

Mataix-Cols D, Fernández de la Cruz L: Hoarding disorder has finally arrived, but many challenges lie ahead. World Psychiatry 17(2):224–225, 2018

Nordsletten AE, Fernández de la Cruz L, Aluco E, et al: A transcultural study of hoarding disorder: insights from the United Kingdom, Spain, Japan, and Brazil. Transcult Psychiatry 55(2):261–285, 2018

Pertusa A, Frost RO, Fullana MA, et al: Refining the diagnostic boundaries of compulsive hoarding: a critical review. Clin Psychol Rev 30(4):371–386, 2010

CASE 6.5

Hair Pulling

Dan J. Stein, M.D., Ph.D.

Zoe Oliver was a 22-year-old single woman who presented to her general practitioner after reading a magazine article about trichotillomania (hair-pulling disorder). She had never previously told anyone other than her mother about her hair pulling, but the magazine had indicated that it was fairly common and treatable. She was pessimistic that anything would work, but she and her mother agreed that she should seek help.

Ms. Oliver's hair pulling most often took place as a ritual when she returned home from her job as a paralegal. She would search for hairs of a particular texture from the crown of her head (though she also pulled from her eyebrows, eyelashes, and pubic region). She felt intense relief if the hair came out with its root. She would then typically bite off the root of the hair and swallow the rest of the hair. She had never experienced any gastrointestinal symptoms after hair swallowing. She said the hair pulling had begun at age 12, and she had never known anyone with similar behaviors.

Ms. Oliver fought hard to stop the behavior and, at times, had been able to stop for several months at a time. When the hair pulling returned, she would again feel ashamed and angry at herself. Scarves and hats covered the bald patch, but she would usually withdraw from friends and boyfriends to avoid being caught.

Even when demoralized about the behavior, Ms. Oliver did not have vegetative symptoms of depression. Aside from fears of being found out, she lacked prominent anxiety. She denied obsessions, compulsions, hoarding, tics, and preoccupations with either bodily defects or having an illness. She also had no history of a range of other body-focused repetitive behaviors, such as lip biting or cheek chewing, in either herself or her close family members.

When asked what she would do if she could not find the "right" kind of hair to pull, she admitted that she would often pick at her skin or at a scab. The scab's coming off in just the right way led to a feeling of relief that was similar to that which she experienced when hair pulling. She would also sometimes chew and swallow her scabs. Ms. Oliver often picked at scabs on her back so that the lesions would not be easily visible to others. Nevertheless, the resultant scarring did lead her to avoid situations like beach parties and dates and other situations where her behavior might be exposed.

Discussion

Ms. Oliver likely meets the diagnostic criteria for both DSM-5 trichotillomania (hair-pulling disorder) and excoriation (skin-picking) disorder. The two disorders are frequently comorbid and have very similar diagnostic criteria. Ms. Oliver pulls out her hair and picks at her skin and scabs, she has made unsuccessful efforts to stop, and both the hair pulling and the skin picking cause significant psychosocial dysfunction. The case report does not indicate that a comorbid condition could be exacerbating either behavior. The diagnoses of trichotillomania and excoriation disorder are frequently missed, both because patients are embarrassed to report symptoms and because clinicians fail to follow up on possible clues, but once the symptoms are clarified, the diagnoses are generally clear-cut.

Although both conditions appear to be having a major impact on her life, Ms. Oliver seems to view her trichotillomania as a more pervasive issue. DSM-5 includes the term *hair-pulling disorder* as an alternative name for *trichotillomania*, in much the same way that *skin-picking disorder* is a synonym for *excoriation disorder*. *Excoriation* does describe the behavior, however, whereas the term *trichotillomania* implies that the hair pulling is a type of mania, which is misleading; thus, many people prefer the term *hair-pulling disorder*.

Ms. Oliver appears to experience tension prior to the hair pulling and skin picking, as well as relief or gratification following the act. Not all individuals with trichotillomania experience such a symptom pattern. In contrast to prior classification systems, including DSM-IV, that categorized trichotillomania as an impulse-control disorder and emphasized that the condition is characterized by prior tension and subsequent relief or gratification, DSM-5 focuses instead on a history of attempts to decrease the hair pulling.

When hair pulling leads to noticeable hair loss, individuals often disguise their bald patches via the use of makeup, scarves, hats, or wigs; therefore, DSM-5 does not require the hair loss to be noticeable. Distress or impairment is emphasized throughout DSM-5, and Ms. Oliver does experience shame and diminished functioning. Ms. Oliver also reports swallowing her hair (trichophagy), which can lead to a trichobezoar and gastrointestinal sequelae, but she does not appear to have experienced any physical complications.

Ms. Oliver seeks out a particular type of hair to pull (and scab to pick), and is fully aware when the hair (or scab) is found, pulled, and eaten. Other individuals pull out hair and pick at skin in a more automatic way. Many individuals with trichotillomania and excoriation disorder have a personal or family history of obsessive-compulsive and related disorders. Others, like Ms. Oliver, do not have such a history. Although trichotillomania and excoriation disorder do seem to lie in the obsessive-compulsive spectrum, there are many clinical differences between these two disorders and obsessive-compulsive disorder.

Multiple psychiatric and nonpsychiatric medical conditions can lead to hair pulling and skin picking. If they are found, then they become the primary diagnosis rather than either trichotillomania or skin picking disorder. For example, if the hair- and skin-focused behaviors are related to an appearance preoccupation, the patient is more likely to have body dysmorphic disorder. Hair loss is found in medical conditions ranging from lupus to alopecia areata; if a patient has evident hair loss and denies hair pulling, a medical workup may detect a systemic illness. Delusional parasitosis and tactile hallucinations can lead to skin picking, as can both cocaine intoxication and scabies infestation, but these do not fit the situation with Ms. Oliver. Finally, Ms. Oliver's behavior does not appear to reflect nonsuicidal self-injurious behavior, which can also lead to skin lesions.

It would be useful to have a more detailed understanding of Ms. Oliver's hair-pulling and skin-picking symptoms. Structured interviews can help ensure that possible comorbidities are recognized, and severity measures may help in the evaluation of these disorders. These instruments can help inform the clinician in regard to both prognosis and treatment. It would also be useful to go beyond the initial report—that Ms. Oliver engages in these behaviors after work to feel better—and better understand pertinent cues and stressors, as well as develop a deeper understanding of the benefits and disadvantages of these behaviors.

Diagnoses

- Trichotillomania (hair-pulling disorder)
- Excoriation (skin-picking) disorder

Suggested Readings

Grant JE, Chamberlain SR: Trichotillomania. Am J Psychiatry 173(9):868–874, 2016
Lochner C, Keuthen NJ, Curley EE, et al: Comorbidity in trichotillomania (hair-pulling disorder): a cluster analytical approach. Brain Behav 9(12):e01456, 2019
Machado MO, Köhler CA, Stubbs B, et al: Skin picking disorder: prevalence, correlates, and associations with quality of life in a large sample. CNS Spectr 23(5):311–320, 2018

CHAPTER 7

Trauma- and Stressor-Related Disorders

INTRODUCTION

John W. Barnhill, M.D.

The chapter on trauma- and stressor-related disorders consists of a cluster of disorders that require identification of a triggering external event. This was a new chapter in DSM-5. Previously, all of the disorders had been listed in other chapters. This chapter also features the only diagnosis that is new to the main DSM-5-TR text: prolonged grief disorder, which in DSM-5 had been listed in the "Conditions for Further Study" chapter in Section III, where it was called persistent complex bereavement disorder.

Posttraumatic stress disorder (PTSD) and acute stress disorder (ASD) were moved from the chapter on anxiety disorders. Both PTSD and ASD are characterized by heterogeneous symptoms, not only anxiety, and one consequence of this classification change was to emphasize the importance of assessing the breadth of reactions to an external trauma or stressor. At the same time, both disorders often present with prominent anxiety, and an alternative conceptualization of both PTSD and ASD would characterize them on an anxiety spectrum of disorders, alongside, for example, obsessive-compulsive disorder, which was also moved from the anxiety disorders into its own chapter in DSM-5.

A PTSD diagnosis requires the presence of symptoms from each of four symptom clusters: intrusion symptoms (previously known as reexperiencing), avoidance symptoms, negative alterations in cognition and mood, and arousal symptoms. DSM-5 more explicitly recognized the heterogeneity of acute post-trauma response by eliminating the requirement that individuals with ASD have symptoms from multiple symptom clusters. Instead, it is necessary to have at least nine of 14 symptoms. In practice, this could mean that one individual with ASD could have all four intrusion symptoms, whereas another might have none.

PTSD and ASD are most clearly delineated by duration, with PTSD persisting at least 1 month after the external event and ASD lasting no more than 1 month. For both PTSD and ASD, the initial stressor criterion now specifies whether the trauma was experienced, witnessed, or experienced indirectly. Unlike DSM-IV, DSM-5 did not require an assessment of the patient's initial subjective response for either disorder. Finally, diagnostic thresholds for PTSD were lowered for children and adolescents, and a preschool subtype was added.

Two of the chapter's disorders—reactive attachment disorder (RAD) and disinhibited social engagement disorder (DSED)—are initially found in childhood, although both may have lifelong consequences. Children with RAD have responded to the absence of expectable caregiving by a cluster of withdrawn and inhibited symptoms, whereas those with DSED have symptoms described as indiscriminately social and disinhibited.

Adjustment disorder had previously served as a residual category for people who were distressed but did not meet criteria for a more discrete disorder. The adjustment disorders were reconceptualized in DSM-5 as an array of stress-response syndromes that occur after exposure to a distressing event. As in DSM-IV, the adjustment disorders should include a specifier that identifies the predominant disturbance (e.g., depressed mood, anxiety, disturbance of conduct, or a combination).

It has long been recognized that it is normal for people to grieve the death of a loved one. Clinicians and researchers have increasingly identified a subgroup of people whose emotional reaction appears to be excessive in intensity for over a year. The diagnosis of prolonged grief disorder has been introduced within the main body of DSM-5-TR to meet this clinical concern.

DSM-5-TR explores the growing evidence that culture affects clinical expression. For example, non-Western groups appear to respond to PTSD with less avoidance and more somatic symptoms such as dizziness and shortness of breath. Although DSM-5-TR emphasizes categories of disorders, it also includes discussion of how developmental issues can affect symptomatology. For example, children younger than 6 years can be traumatized by life-threatening events such as the threat of abandonment, and a primary presenting complaint might be nightmares, with or without traumatic content.

The trauma- and stressor-related disorders can usefully bring together seemingly unrelated symptoms. For example, an adult might present with complaints related to anxiety, depression, paranoia, social isolation, and substance use. Without a careful history that looks for trauma, the clinician might conceptualize the patient as having half a dozen diagnoses rather than a single trauma- and stressor-related diagnosis that synthesizes a disparate set of problems. At the same time, comorbidities are common among the disorders discussed in this chapter, and, if found, should generally be identified along with the disorder directly related to the trauma or stress.

Suggested Readings

Doric A, Stevanovic D, Stupar D, et al: UCLA PTSD reaction index for DSM-5 (PTSD-RI-5): a psychometric study of adolescents sampled from communities in eleven countries. Eur J Psychotraumatol 10(1):1605282, 2019

Lewis-Fernández R, Kirmayer LJ: Cultural concepts of distress and psychiatric disorders: understanding symptom experience and expression in context. Transcult Psychiatry 56(4):786–803, 2019

Shaw JA, Espinel Z, Shultz JM: Care of Children Exposed to the Traumatic Effects of Disaster. Washington, DC, American Psychiatric Publishing, 2012

Simon N, Hollander E, Rothbaum BO, Stein DJ (eds): The American Psychiatric Association Publishing Textbook of Anxiety, Trauma, and OCD-Related Disorders, 3rd Edition. Washington, DC, American Psychiatric Association Publishing, 2020

CASE 7.1

Dangerous Behaviors

Daniel S. Schechter, M.D.

Adriana was a 4-year-old girl referred to an early childhood mental health care clinic for evaluation of "dangerous behaviors." The parents were particularly concerned that Adriana maintained poor boundaries, was impulsive, and was too quick to trust strangers.

Adriana had been adopted from an Eastern European orphanage at age 29 months. At the time of the adoption, Adriana's medical records were reviewed by a local pediatrician, who found no problems aside from growth parameters that were all below the 5th percentile. When the adoptive parents met her at the orphanage, Adriana approached without shyness and visited easily with them. The parents had been pleasantly reassured by the child's happy demeanor and her spontaneous, warm hugs.

Not long after her adoption, Adriana began to clearly seek out her mother for comfort when distressed or hurt. At most other times, however, Adriana did not distinguish between strangers and her family. In the grocery store, she would warmly hug whoever was waiting next to them in line. In group and family settings, she would frequently try to sit in the laps of people she had barely met. Once, at a shopping mall, she tried to leave with another family. Her parents were concerned that this behavior might put her at risk of abduction or abuse.

Compared with other children her age, Adriana had trouble taking turns and sitting for circle time at school. She interrupted, intruded into classmates' play space, and occasionally hit others. Small triggers upset her for prolonged periods. She had trouble soothing herself but would generally calm down if held by her teacher or a parent.

Trauma- and Stressor-Related Disorders   **151**

Adriana lived with her adoptive mother and father and her 12-year-old brother, who was the biological child of her parents. Her mother stayed home for Adriana's first year in the United States, but Adriana had been attending a half-day child care program for the past year. Her mother noted progress in the child's development, although she remained language delayed, with comprehension better than productive language. She was slower than classmates in developing school readiness skills, but her gross and fine motor skills were considered average. Her sleep and appetite were fine. She had gained weight, but her head circumference remained just below the 5th percentile.

On examination, she was a pleasant, well-groomed girl who appeared younger than her age. She spoke little but did appear to pay attention to the interviewer. Within a few minutes, she tried to crawl onto the interviewer's lap.

Discussion

Adriana is a preschool-age child who was referred for "dangerous behaviors" that relate primarily to excess physical familiarity with strangers. The parents worry that these behaviors place Adriana at risk for predation.

The case report also indicates that Adriana has trouble regulating her proximity to other people, both in terms of going too far away from her mother and getting too close to strangers. Even with peers, she "intruded into classmates' play space." The parents apparently felt reassured after first meeting Adriana when she lacked shyness and happily gave them spontaneous, warm hugs. Typically developing children tend to express selective attachment by age 6 or 7 months, however, and show frank reticence in the presence of strangers by age 8 or 9 months. Adriana's seemingly desirable behavior at age 29 months suggests that, in fact, attachment-related psychopathology was already present.

Adriana most likely has a DSM-5 diagnosis of disinhibited social engagement disorder (DSED). In particular, her disinhibited social behaviors cannot be attributed to general impulsivity, and she has all four of the core symptomatic criteria (only two are required): reduced or absent reticence in approaching and interacting with unfamiliar adults; overly familiar behavior; diminished or absent checking back with an adult caregiver after venturing away; and willingness to go off with an unfamiliar adult with minimal or no hesitation.

DSED reflects a change in the diagnostic nomenclature. In DSM-IV, the diagnosis of reactive attachment disorder (RAD) of infancy or early childhood was characterized by a pattern of markedly disturbed and developmentally inappropriate attachment behaviors evident before age 5 years. RAD in DSM-IV was divided into two subtypes: inhibited and indiscriminate. The indiscriminate subtype of RAD was reconceptualized in DSM-5 as disinhibited social engagement disorder, whereas the inhibited form continues to be called reactive attachment disorder. DSM-5 clarified that DSED can be found even among children without disordered attachment—for example, among those who approach their caregiver when stressed or hurt, as Adriana does with her adoptive mother.

Adriana's adoption occurred beyond the age when children typically develop selective attachment. This suggests that she was subject to pathogenic care during a sensitive, if not critical, period of social brain development. For example, a high child-to-caregiver ratio at the orphanage might have limited her opportunities to form selective attachments. One can assume that this early adverse environment, which was likely characterized by neglect, interacted with biological vulnerability. Adriana's inhibitory dyscontrol within social contexts, for example, may indicate abnormalities in the development of the prefrontal and cingulate cortices and related circuits of the brain. Such abnormalities may be associated with risk factors such as prenatal malnutrition or toxicity and/or prematurity, as well as other genetic risk factors.

Adriana also tends to become easily distressed and to have difficulty calming down. Such difficulty with emotion regulation can also be linked to disordered early attachment and pathogenic care. But her ability to self-soothe may also have been affected by her delayed expressive language development, itself an associated feature in support of the diagnosis of DSED according to DSM-5.

Also linked to early—even prenatal—pathogenic care is the description of Adriana's early growth parameters as being below the 5th percentile, with persistence of a small head circumference and the possibility of mild cognitive delays affecting school readiness. Although adequate records are unlikely in Adriana's case, it would be useful to explore the possible role of such factors as malnutrition, maternal substance abuse, and fetal alcohol syndrome. It would also be useful to investigate possible comorbidities, which are frequent in this disorder. For example, some children with DSED also have attention-deficit/hyperactivity disorder (ADHD). It is useful, however, to recall that although both DSED and ADHD may feature impulsivity, DSED is a specific relationship disorder.

Does DSED pathologize outgoing friendliness? The short answer is no. Whereas most young children might smile at or talk to familiar adults, or even unfamiliar adults acknowledged as "safe" by their caregivers (i.e., requiring social referencing), it is developmentally atypical for 4½-year-old children to approach strangers affectionately, to touch, talk, or walk off with them, especially without referencing their caregivers. It is also maladaptive and potentially dangerous! Recognition of DSED is an important step in providing the sort of clinical care that can help this vulnerable cluster of patients whose lives have already been marked by inattention and neglect.

Diagnosis

- Disinhibited social engagement disorder

Suggested Readings

Bowlby J: Attachment and Loss, 2nd Edition, Vol 1: Attachment. New York, Basic Books, 1999

Schechter DS, Suardi F, Manini A, et al: How do maternal PTSD and alexithymia interact to impact maternal behavior? Child Psychiatry Hum Dev 46(3):406–417, 2015

Seim AR, Jozefiak T, Wichstrøm L, et al: Reactive attachment disorder and disinhibited social engagement disorder in adolescence: co-occurring psychopathology and psychosocial problems. Eur Child Adolesc Psychiatry 31(1):85–98, 2022

Zeanah CH, Chesher T, Boris NW; American Academy of Child and Adolescent Psychiatry (AACAP) Committee on Quality Issues (CQI): Practice parameter for the assessment and treatment of children and adolescents with reactive attachment disorder and disinhibited social engagement disorder. J Am Acad Child Adolesc Psychiatry 55(11):990–1003, 2016

CASE 7.2

Two Reactions to Trauma

Matthew J. Friedman, M.D., Ph.D.

Traumatic Event: Bethany Pinsky, age 23, had gone to a theater to see the local premiere of a big-budget movie. As she settled into her seat, waiting for the show to begin, a young man in a ski mask suddenly appeared in front of the screen. Brandishing an assault rifle, he fired directly into the audience. She saw many people get shot, including the woman sitting next to her. People all around began screaming, and there was a confused stampede for the exit door. Terrified, she somehow fought her way to the exit and escaped, uninjured, to the parking lot, where police cars were just arriving.

Charles Quigley, age 25, went to the same movie theater at the same time. He too feared for his life. Hiding behind a row of seats, he was able to crawl to the aisle and sprint to the exit. Although covered in blood, he escaped without physical injury.

Bethany and Charles, 2 Days Later: Two days later, both Ms. Pinsky and Mr. Quigley considered themselves "nervous wrecks." Grateful that they were alive and uninjured, they nevertheless found themselves extremely anxious and on edge. They jumped at the slightest noise. They kept watching television for the latest information about the shooting, but every time there was actual videotaped footage of the event, they experienced panic attacks, broke out into a sweat, were unable to calm down, and could not stop thinking about the traumatic event. They could not sleep at night because of nightmares, and during the day they felt assaulted by intrusive and unwelcome memories of gunshots, screams, and their own personal terror during the event.

Bethany, 2 Weeks Later: Ms. Pinsky had reclaimed most of her pretraumatic thoughts, feelings, and behaviors within 2 weeks. Although traumatic reminders of the shooting sometimes led to a brief panic or physiological reaction, these did not dominate her waking hours. She no longer experienced nightmares. She knew that she would never forget what happened in that movie theater, but for the most part, her life was returning to normal and had returned to the trajectory it had been following before the shootings occurred.

Charles, 2 Weeks Later: Mr. Quigley had not recovered 2 weeks later. He felt emotionally constricted and unable to experience pleasant or positive feelings. He jumped at the slightest sound, he was unable to focus on his work, and his sleep was fitful and marked by traumatic nightmares. He tried to avoid any reminders of the shootings but nevertheless relentlessly recalled the sound of gunfire, the screams, and the sticky feel of the blood pouring out of his neighbor's chest and onto him as he hid behind the seats. He felt episodically disconnected from his surroundings and from himself. He viewed his life as having been changed by this traumatic experience.

Discussion

During the acute aftermath of a traumatic event, almost everyone is upset. The appropriate professional stance at this very early stage is that these are transient reactions that will typically resolve within 2–3 days and from which normal recovery should be expected. Ms. Pinsky's reaction after the shooting falls within the broad range of reactions called *normative stress reactions* in DSM-5. It is a normal response to traumatic stress and not a psychiatric disorder.

Many different symptom presentations may occur in normative stress reactions, but they generally include a combination of the following:

a. *Emotional reactions*, such as shock, fear, grief, anger, resentment, guilt, shame, helplessness, hopelessness, and numbing
b. *Cognitive reactions*, such as confusion, disorientation, dissociation, indecisiveness, difficulty concentrating, memory loss, self-blame, and unwanted memories
c. *Physical reactions*, such as tension, fatigue, insomnia, startle reactions, racing pulse, nausea, and loss of appetite
d. *Interpersonal reactions*, such as distrust, irritability, withdrawal/isolation, feeling rejected/abandoned, and being distant

A significant minority of individuals develop acute stress disorder (ASD), which involves more intense symptoms, during the month after the traumatic event. To meet DSM-5 criteria for ASD following a trauma, an individual must exhibit a minimum of nine of 14 possible symptoms, spread across five categories:

a. *Intrusion symptoms*, such as intrusive distressing memories, recurrent traumatic dreams, dissociative reliving (e.g., flashbacks) of the traumatic event, and intense psychological distress or physiological reactivity to traumatic reminders
b. *Negative mood*, such as an inability to experience positive emotions
c. *Dissociative symptoms*, such as amnesia, and derealization or depersonalization
d. *Avoidance symptoms*, such as avoidance of internal reminders such as trauma-related thoughts or feelings and avoidance of external reminders such as people, places, or situations
e. *Arousal symptoms*, such as insomnia, irritability, hypervigilance, problems of concentration, or exaggerated startle reactions

Depending on which symptom categories are most prominent, patients with ASD can seem quite different from one another. For example, one person with ASD might have all of the intrusion symptoms, whereas another may have none of them.

ASD is distinguished from other psychiatric diagnoses on the basis of a careful history. For example, ASD is diagnosed within the first month after a trauma, whereas posttraumatic stress disorder (PTSD) can only be diagnosed after that first month. Adjustment disorders are also diagnosed in the first month following a trauma, but unlike ASD patients, patients with adjustment disorder do not have 9 of the 14 possible ASD symptoms.

When symptoms are evaluated individually, the variety of ASD symptoms can mislead the clinician. Panic, anxiety, depression, dissociation, and intrusive, obsessional thoughts are all common in ASD, for example, and can lead to consideration of a wide spectrum of disorders. Traumatic brain injury often accompanies and complicates the diagnosis of both ASD and PTSD, especially when the brain injury is relatively subtle and unrecognized. Evaluation of any of these symptoms can be confusing, especially when the trauma is not as obvious as a movie theater shooting. Bringing together seemingly unrelated symptoms into one or two diagnoses can reduce patient confusion, focus treatment, and reduce unnecessary pharmacological treatment.

Diagnoses

- Ms. Pinsky: No diagnosis; normative stress reaction
- Mr. Quigley: Acute stress disorder

Suggested Readings

Bryant RA: Acute stress disorder. Curr Opin Psychol 14:127–131, 2017
Friedman MJ, Bovin MJ, Weathers FW: DSM-5 criteria for PTSD, in Handbook of PTSD: Science and Practice, 3rd Edition. Edited by Friedman MJ, Keane TM, Schnurr PP. New York, Guilford, 2021, pp 19–37
Silov D, Klein L: Cultural, trauma and traumatic stress among refugees, asylum seekers and postconflict populations, in Handbook of PTSD: Science and Practice, 3rd Edition. Edited by Friedman MJ, Keane TM, Schnurr PP. New York, Guilford, 2021, pp 483–500

CASE 7.3

A Car Wreck

Robert S. Pynoos, M.D., M.P.H.
Alan M. Steinberg, Ph.D.
Christopher M. Layne, Ph.D.

Dylan, a 15-year-old high school student, was referred to a psychiatrist for help in dealing with stress from being involved in a serious automobile accident 2 weeks earlier. On the day of the accident, Dylan was riding in the front passenger seat when, as the car was pulling out of a driveway, it was struck by an oncoming SUV that was speeding through a yellow light. The car he was in was hit squarely on the driver's side, which caused the car to roll over once and come to rest right side up. The collision of metal on metal made an extremely loud noise. The driver of the car, a high school classmate, was knocked unconscious for a short period and was bleeding from a gash in his forehead. Upon seeing his injured friend, Dylan became afraid that his friend might be dead. His friend in the back seat of the car was frantically trying to unlatch her seat belt. Dylan's door was jammed, and Dylan feared that their car might catch fire while he was stuck in it. After a few minutes, the driver, Dylan, and the other passenger were able to exit through the passenger doors and move away from the car. They realized that the driver of the SUV was unharmed and had already called the police. An ambulance was on its way. All three were transported to a local emergency room, where they were attended to and released to their parents' care after a few hours.

Dylan had not had a good night's sleep since the accident. He often awoke in the middle of the night with his heart racing, visualizing oncoming headlights. He was having trouble concentrating and was unable to effectively complete his homework. His parents, who had begun to drive him to and from school, noticed that he was anxious every time they pulled out of a driveway or crossed an intersection. Although he had recently received his driving permit, he refused to practice driving with his father. He was also unusually short-tempered with his parents, his younger sisters, and his friends. He had recently gone to see a movie but had walked out of the theater before the movie started; he complained that the sound system was too loud. His concerned parents tried to talk to him about his stress, but he would irritably cut them off. After doing poorly on an important exam, however, he accepted the encouragement of a favorite teacher to go to a psychiatrist.

When seen, Dylan described additional difficulties. He hated that he was "jumpy" around loud noises, and he could not shake the image of his injured and unresponsive friend. He had waves of anger toward the driver of the SUV. He reported feeling embarrassed and disappointed in himself for being reluctant to practice driving. He stated that about 5 years earlier, he had witnessed the near-drowning of one of his younger sisters. Also, he mentioned that this past month was the first anniversary of his grandfather's death.

Discussion

Dylan meets the DSM-5 diagnostic formulation of acute stress disorder (ASD), which requires any 9 of 14 acute stress symptoms. ASD can be diagnosed 3 days after exposure to a traumatic situation; it may be a transient stress response that remits within 1 month or may progress after 1 month to PTSD.

Dylan presents with symptoms of ASD 2 weeks after being involved in a serious automobile accident. His symptoms are associated with clinically significant distress, impairment in social and school functioning, and disengagement from current developmental tasks (e.g., learning to drive). In adolescence, such acute disruption can have immediate and long-term consequences—providing the rationale for prompt diagnosis and intervention.

Dylan's stress-related symptoms include recurrent intrusive distressing memories of the accident; psychological and physiological reactions to reminders; efforts to avoid thinking or having feelings about what happened; avoidance of external reminders that restricts his daily life; a recurrent distressing dream and an accompanying sleep disturbance that leaves him unrested and tired during the day; irritable behavior that disrupts his relationships with parents and friends; problems with concentration that jeopardize school performance during this important high school year; and an exaggerated startle response, which makes him feel childish and different from his friends. Although the driver lost consciousness, Dylan remained fully conscious and showed no signs of a mild traumatic brain injury. There was no persistent disorientation or confusion. Dylan also has no history of a prior anxiety disorder that would explain his symptoms, all of which began after the traumatic event.

Like many adolescents, Dylan is reluctant to discuss his experience or symptoms, in part because doing so makes him feel that something is wrong with him—a concern that adds to his adolescent anxiety over being different from peers. Acute intervention strategies can help adolescents to understand their acute stress reactions, gain skills to manage reminders, and develop plans with their teachers to gradually recover their prior level of academic functioning. Prior traumatic experiences and losses—such as his sister's near-drowning and his grandfather's death—can exacerbate an individual's reactions to a current trauma and can increase a clinician's understanding of the symptom profile.

Diagnosis

• Acute stress disorder

Suggested Readings

Bryant RA, Friedman MJ, Spiegel D, et al: A review of acute stress disorder in DSM-5. Depress Anxiety 28(9):802–817, 2011

Dai W, Liu A, Kaminga AC, et al: Prevalence of acute stress disorder among road traffic accident survivors: a meta-analysis. BMC Psychiatry 18(1):188, 2018

CASE 7.4

Easily Triggered

Lori L. Davis, M.D.

Eric Reynolds, a 75-year-old retired electrician, sought help at the Veterans Affairs outpatient mental health care clinic because of his "very short fuse" and tendency to be "easily triggered." Mr. Reynolds indicated that he had had these symptoms for decades, but that he had finally agreed to get treated because his wife seemed desperate that he get in better control.

Mr. Reynolds indicated that he always felt on guard, especially while in public. When unexpectedly startled by sudden noises, he tended to fly into a rage. That was apparently one reason he had chosen to be a self-employed electrician: he could work by himself. Similarly, he enjoyed hunting and gardening, activities that he could enjoy in quiet solitude.

Reluctantly, he described intrusive memories of watching his fellow soldiers die in the field, which caused him enormous shame, guilt, and sadness, Several times a week, he awakes in a panicky sweat after a combat nightmare, although, as he said, "It's ridiculous. Those guys have been dead for 50 years."

Although these symptoms are very distressing, Mr. Reynolds is most worried about his "hair-trigger" temper. Without cause, he finds himself antagonizing other drivers who cut him off, confronting strangers who stand too close to him in checkout lines, and shifting into "attack mode" when approached from behind by others. He springs into this aggressive mode automatically, without a thought or consideration of the circumstances. Although he keeps a handgun in the console of his car for self-protection, Mr. Reynolds has no intention of harming others. He is always remorseful after a threatening incident and worries that he might inadvertently hurt someone. Most recently, while drifting off to sleep on his physician's examination table, a nurse touched his foot, and he leapt up and began cursing in a threatening manner. He felt as if he were back on guard duty, when he was accidentally dozing, and an incoming mortar round stunned him into action. His reaction scared both the nurse and himself.

Mr. Reynolds's symptoms apparently began soon after he left Vietnam, where he served as a field radio operator. He never sought help for his symptoms, apparently because of his independent and self-reliant nature. After retirement as a self-employed electrician, he spent almost all of his time at home. During these past few years, his wife and adult children became more aware of his various symptoms, including how they were putting a severe strain on his family relationships and overall happiness.

Mr. Reynolds was raised in a loving family that struggled financially as Midwestern farmers. At age 20, Mr. Reynolds was drafted into the U.S. Army and deployed to Vietnam. He described himself as having been upbeat and happy prior to his army induction. He said he enjoyed basic training and his first few weeks in Vietnam, until one of his comrades got killed. At that point, all he cared about was getting home alive, even if it meant killing others. His personality changed from that of a happy-go-lucky farm boy to a terrified, overprotective soldier. Upon returning to civilian life, he managed to get a graduate business degree, but he became a self-employed electrician because of his need to stay isolated in his work. In his retirement, he hoped to volunteer, garden, and get some "peace and quiet." It turned out, however, that his retirement was much like the rest of his adult life: although he could occasionally settle into one of his hobbies, most of his days were filled with tension, guilt, and arguments.

Despite having used alcohol and marijuana during his early adulthood, he had not consumed excessive alcohol for several decades or used marijuana since the age of 30. He had no legal history.

On examination, Mr. Reynolds was a well-groomed man who appeared anxious and somewhat guarded. He was coherent and articulate. His speech was at a normal rate, but the pace accelerated when he discussed disturbing content. He denied depression but was anxious. His affect was somewhat constricted but appropriate to content. His thought process was coherent and linear. He denied all suicidal and homicidal ideation. He had no psychotic symptoms, delusions, or hallucinations. He had very good insight. He was well oriented and seemed to have above-average intelligence.

Discussion

Mr. Reynolds manifests symptoms from all four PTSD symptom categories: intrusive symptoms, persistent avoidance, negative alterations in cognitions and mood associated with the traumatic event, and marked alterations in arousal and reactivity. Mr. Reynolds's primary concerns relate to fear-mediated symptoms, particularly his exaggerated fight-or-flight responses to unexpected stimulation. As is often seen in PTSD, the reaction is out of proportion to the circumstances and can be unpredictable; in other words, the reaction is not premeditated or part of general impulsivity. In addition to hyperreactivity, Mr. Reynolds demonstrates hypervigilance, excessive concern for safety, and anxiety or fear. He has classic reexperiencing symptoms of intrusive memories, nightmares, flashbacks, and physiological reactivity to triggers that resemble or remind him of the traumatic events. Although not present in this patient, suicidality and psychotic symptoms are not uncommon in PTSD and should be evaluated on a regular basis.

As is often the case with PTSD, Mr. Reynolds exhibits a powerful, involuntary reaction to particular kinds of external stimuli. These symptoms of being "easily triggered" are very disturbing for the individual as well as for family members, friends, and caregivers.

Mr. Reynolds's efforts to avoid conflict have progressively narrowed his opportunities in all spheres, including social, family, and hobbies. For example, his decision to work as an electrician rather than to take advantage of his business degree seems based largely on his effort to control his personal space. It would be useful to know more about how Mr. Reynolds's PTSD might be affecting his relationship with his wife. His retirement appears to have worsened his symptoms and propelled him into finally seeking treatment. One possibility is that his wife is now spending more time with him and able to see his reactions more frequently and serves as a force behind his decision to seek treatment. Another possibility is that his retirement was precipitated by the negative consequences of untreated PTSD symptoms on his job-related duties and relationships.

Because people with PTSD have high rates of psychiatric comorbidity, the practitioner should carefully consider other diagnoses. Mr. Reynolds has apparently not consumed excessive alcohol or marijuana in many years, so neither appears related to the exacerbation of his symptoms; however, because substance use is very common in patients with PTSD, special attention should be paid to the possibility of underreporting.

Mr. Reynolds's edgy hyperarousal overlaps somewhat with the dysphoric irritability that can be seen in bipolar II disorder, but his most intense symptoms are reactive and sudden; this contrasts with the multiday periods of manic symptoms such as mood changes, racing thoughts, elevated energy or drive, or a reduced need for sleep. He denies feeling depressed, and his reduced pleasure appears more related to his avoidance of social activities that he previously found enjoyable. He has maintained interest in woodworking and reading, which are consistent with his tendency to self-isolate in a safe and quiet environment.

DSM-5-TR™ Clinical Cases

Like many survivors of trauma, Mr. Reynolds prides himself on his resiliency and independence; such qualities likely served him well in Vietnam and while running his business. That same independence seems to have contributed to his avoidance of mental health treatment despite 50 years of uncomfortable symptoms. It would be useful to further explore his thoughts about stigma, psychotherapy, and PTSD, given that the development of a trusting alliance will be crucial to his treatment.

Diagnosis

- Posttraumatic stress disorder

Suggested Readings

Bryant RA: Post-traumatic stress disorder: a state-of-the-art review of evidence and challenges. World Psychiatry 18(3):259–269, 2019

Moore BA, Pujol L, Waltman S, Shearer DS: Management of post-traumatic stress disorder in veterans and military service members: a review of pharmacologic and psychotherapeutic interventions since 2016. Curr Psychiatry Rep 23(2):9, 2021

Schein J, Houle C, Urganus A, et al: Prevalence of post-traumatic stress disorder in the United States: a systematic literature review. Curr Med Res Opin 37(12):2151–2161, 2021

CASE 7.5

Stressed Out[*]

Cheryl C. Munday, Ph.D.

Jamie Miller Abelson, M.S.W.

Franklin Sims was a 21-year-old single African American man who sought treatment at a university-affiliated community mental health care clinic because he felt "stressed out," withdrawn from friends, and "worried about money." He said he had been feeling depressed for 3 months, and he attributed the "nosedive" to the end

---

[*]This case is dedicated to the memory of James S. Jackson, Ph.D., in recognition of his leadership of research on the mental health of Black Americans.

of a 3-year romantic relationship shortly after he and his girlfriend had seriously discussed marriage.

Mr. Sims, the son of working-class parents, had supported himself financially since high school and was accustomed to feeling nervous about making ends meet. He was angered by his girlfriend's decision to end the relationship, particularly her failure to understand his concerns about establishing financial stability. He increasingly ruminated about money, his grades, and his future.

Mr. Sims was a full-time undergraduate employed as a full-time midnight-shift warehouse worker. He was accustomed to this schedule, but he had increasingly found it difficult to concentrate in class after staying awake all night at the warehouse. When he had a day off, his sleep and energy were fine, and he still enjoyed hanging out with his friends. His appetite was unchanged, and his physical health was good. His grades had recently declined, however, and he had become increasingly discouraged about money and about being his family's first college student. His parents did not understand why he had decided to attend an out-of-state university, and he was increasingly dissatisfied with life on the predominantly white college campus after some recent experiences of racial discrimination. He had not previously sought any type of mental health care services, but a supportive cousin suggested that he see a therapist after he had told her that he sometimes just felt like giving up.

Mr. Sims was an only child—a self-described "good student and popular kid." High school was complicated by his parents' periodic unemployment, financial strains, and related marital difficulties.

He started drinking alcohol and smoking marijuana in ninth grade, but neither had ever caused him difficulty. At the time of the evaluation, he said he occasionally had a beer or marijuana cigarette at parties, but that he didn't have the time, money, or inclination to get intoxicated.

On examination, Mr. Sims was punctual, cooperative, pleasant, attentive, appropriately dressed, and well groomed. He spoke coherently. He appeared generally worried and constricted, but he smiled appropriately several times during the interview. He said he felt bad about his declining grades, but he denied feeling guilty or worthless. He had a quiet, dry sense of humor. He denied current suicidality, homicidality, and psychosis. He was cognitively intact, and his insight and judgment were considered good.

Discussion

The case report indicates that Mr. Sims has felt depressed, angry, withdrawn, and episodically hopeless over the past few months. These problems appear to have developed in response to the breakup with his girlfriend. It would be useful to further explore his recent history, including whether the hopelessness shaded into suicidality, but it appears that his appetite, sleep, and energy are normal. He has had difficulty concentrating and feeling rested, but his schedule would make it difficult not to be sleep deprived, and he appears to rebound quickly when he does get the occasional day off. Although he would not meet DSM-5 criteria for major depressive disorder, he does appear to be suffering and having difficulty functioning. Substance use and medical issues do not appear to be implicated. He appears, therefore, to meet criteria for adjustment disorder with depressed mood.

In addition to learning more about the breakup, it would be important to further explore Mr. Sims's adjustment to a predominantly white university, including the stress of racial discrimination and the likelihood that his parents may not appreciate the difficulties of his situation. It would also be useful to clarify his sleep issues, his depressive and anxiety symptoms, and stress related to family conflict and financial insecurity.

In the course of the evaluation, it would also be helpful to underline his many strengths. For example, until recently he has been able to successfully negotiate a full-time job, a serious relationship, and a full-time academic schedule at a university far from home. Clarifying his resilience is useful both for developing a treatment plan and for reminding Mr. Sims that the evaluator sees him as a young person of promise as well as someone who could use help with his mental health.

It bodes well for his long-term adjustment that Mr. Sims appears motivated for treatment. Young Black men are generally expected to be strong and independent, and norms of masculinity make it difficult for them to seek help or talk about their feelings. For Mr. Sims, coming to the counseling center would not have been an easy step to take. The success of Mr. Sims's eventual treatment is likely based at least partly on his alliance with a therapist who is comfortable with issues specific to Mr. Sims's gender, race, and ethnicity. For example, Mr. Sims is an academic striver with considerable desire for personal growth, but it would not be surprising if he maintained an ambivalent perspective on his achievement orientation. As a first-generation college student, his parents' emotional support may be compromised by their limited familiarity with higher educational demands. In his culture, studying hard can be seen as a "white" endeavor, and complaining of psychological distress can be seen as a sign of masculine weakness.

As a young man striving to maintain financial independence and to consolidate masculine social roles, increased recognition of everyday racial discrimination may exacerbate the stressful impact of his girlfriend's rejection. Diagnostically, an adjustment disorder reflects an immediate stress response and may portend a more long-term, more severe psychological outcome. Therapeutically, it would be important to address the personal meaning of his loss and the potential chronicity of everyday racial discrimination as he attempts to consolidate a gender role that is consistent with peer culture, racial group identity, and racial and cultural norms. Seeking therapy could therefore be perceived by him both as a further blow to his sense of emotional resilience and as an important source of support in adjusting to the loss of his girlfriend. Therapeutic support of his long-term future goals could prove to be a protective factor against the long-term impact of persistent racial discrimination and of future psychological distress.

Diagnosis

- Adjustment disorder with depressed mood, acute stressor

Suggested Readings

Assari S, Moazen-Zadeh E, Caldwell CH, Zimmerman MA: Racial discrimination during adolescence predicts mental health deterioration in adulthood: gender differences among Blacks. Front Public Health 5:104, 2017

Goodwill JR, Taylor RJ, Watkins DC: Everyday discrimination, depressive symptoms, and suicide ideation among African American men. Arch Suicide Res 25(1):74–93, 2021

Hoggard LS, Powell W, Upton R, et al: Racial discrimination, personal growth initiative, and African American men's depressive symptomatology: a moderated mediation model. Cultur Divers Ethnic Minor Psychol 25(4):472–482, 2019

Strain JJ: The psychobiology of stress, depression, adjustment disorders and resilience. World J Biol Psychiatry 19(suppl 1):S14–S20, 2018

Watkins DC, Neighbors HW: An initial exploration of what "mental health" means to young black men. The Journal of Men's Health & Gender 4(3):271–282, 2007

CASE 7.6

Lung Cancer

Anna Dickerman, M.D.
John W. Barnhill, M.D.

The psychiatric consultation-liaison service at a large hospital was asked to "rule out depression" in Gabriela Trentino, a 65-year-old woman with recurrent lung cancer, after she was noted to display sad affect and tearfulness on morning rounds.

Ms. Trentino was a widowed Italian American homemaker with two grown sons. She had just been admitted to the medical service for shortness of breath. She was subsequently found to have a unilateral pleural effusion. Ms. Trentino had already been through several rounds of chemotherapy over the prior few months. At the time of the consultation, she was awaiting the results of thoracentesis to assess for pulmonary metastases.

Interviewed separately, Ms. Trentino and her two sons agreed that until this hospitalization, she had never previously been especially depressed or anxious but had instead been the family's "rock." She had never seen a therapist, taken psychiatric medication, or used alcohol, opiates, or illicit drugs. Her family history was notable for a father who drank to excess, which she described as the reason she had never tasted alcohol.

On examination, the patient was a well-groomed woman sitting in bed with an oxygen nasal cannula in place, wringing her hands and dabbing at her eyes with a wet tissue. She was cooperative and coherent. She was visibly dysphoric, with a constricted, worried affect. She reported being extremely worried about the pending thoracentesis study. She knew that metastases could mean "a death sentence" and said, "I want to be alive for my son's marriage this year." She added tearfully, "I've been through so much with the illness already.... When is it going to stop?"

Ms. Trentino endorsed poor sleep and impaired concentration since her admission to the hospital 5 days earlier. She had been eating less than usual. She said she was "too sad and worried" to do her usual daily crossword. She denied confusion and psychotic symptoms. She appeared cognitively intact, and her Montreal Cognitive Assessment score was 29 out of 30, with 1 lost point for incorrect recall of an object after 5 minutes. She adamantly denied suicidal ideation, again speaking of her love for her two children.

Ms. Trentino's vital signs were notable for an oxygen saturation of 94% on room air (corrected to 99% on nasal cannula), and her chest X ray showed a large left-sided pleural effusion. Neurological examination was unremarkable. Her basic lab results were otherwise within normal limits. Collateral information from nursing staff indicated that she rang her call bell frequently throughout the day to ask about medication and test details.

Discussion with the patient's family members revealed appropriate concern about their mother's health, as well as frustration over her psychological state. As one of the sons told the psychiatric consultant, "We understand this is a stressful time for Mom, but all she does in the hospital is cry all day and keep on asking us the same questions over and over again. She's usually the pillar of the family, and now she's needy and pessimistic. Can you do something?"

Discussion

Ms. Trentino presents with depressive and anxious symptoms in clear temporal relation to a major stressor (rehospitalization for malignancy with the possibility of progression of disease). The patient, her family, and the hospital staff indicate that her presentation is clinically significant, affecting both her and her care. The most likely DSM-5 diagnosis is adjustment disorder with mixed anxiety and depressed mood.

In addition to adjustment disorder, several other diagnoses are also possible. Her medical team is concerned that she has a depression. Ms. Trentino does endorse four major depressive signs and symptoms (depressed mood most of the day, decreased appetite, insomnia, and poor concentration), and these are affecting her quality of life. To meet DSM-5 criteria for major depressive disorder, however, one must have five depressive symptoms for 2 weeks, and Ms. Trentino has had only four symptoms for less than 1 week. If Ms. Trentino's symptoms intensify slightly and persist, she would likely qualify for a major depressive disorder diagnosis.

Ms. Trentino also displays significant anxiety. She describes difficulty concentrating, feelings of being on edge, and poor sleep. By report, Ms. Trentino never had significant anxiety until she was faced with the recent potentially life-threatening illness. The acuity makes an underlying anxiety disorder unlikely.

Brain metastases and paraneoplastic syndrome are not unusual in lung cancer and could cause anxiety and depression. Neither of these devastating complications tends to occur, however, without other neurological abnormalities and delirium. In consultation with neurology and oncology, a brain scan and/or paraneoplastic panel might be warranted.

Ms. Trentino's hypoxemia—presumably secondary to her pleural effusion—may have contributed to her anxiety. The anxiety has persisted after correction of her oxygen saturation, but dysregulated oxygenation can often cause anxiety.

Medications can also cause anxiety and depression. Although the team should look throughout the medications list, the search should focus particularly on the use of and withdrawal from steroids, opiates, and benzodiazepines.

Adjustment disorder was reclassified in DSM-5 into the chapter on trauma- and stressor-related disorders. Life-threatening illness is an example of such a stressor. For Ms. Trentino to warrant a diagnosis of acute stress disorder, her symptoms would need to intensify. A posttraumatic stress disorder diagnosis would require both an intensification of symptoms and a duration of greater than 1 month.

If Ms. Trentino's worries interfere with her treatment, she might qualify for an additional DSM-5 diagnosis: psychological factors affecting other medical conditions. At the moment, however, she has been compliant with treatments and interventions.

Diagnosis

- Adjustment disorder with mixed anxiety and depressed mood

Suggested Readings

Bachem R, Casey P: Adjustment disorder: a diagnosis whose time has come. J Affect Disord 227:243–253, 2018

O'Donnell ML, Agathos JA, Metcalf O, et al: Adjustment disorder: current developments and future directions. Int J Environ Res Public Health 16(14):2537, 2019

CASE 7.7

Overdose

Megan Mroczkowski, M.D.

Cynthia R. Pfeffer, M.D.

Hannah, a 16-year-old white girl with no past psychiatric history, was brought to the hospital emergency department following an overdose of unknown amounts of sedating medications. Upon arrival, Hannah had a Glasgow Coma Scale score of 8, indicating severe compromise. She was intubated and admitted to the pediatric intensive care unit. After stabilization over several days, she was admitted to an inpatient psychiatric unit. Current regulatory practice mandates suicide screening for all patients; in this case, Hannah screened positive for suicidal ideation, plan, and attempt on the Columbia Suicide Severity Rating Scale (C-SSRS).

While Hannah was intubated, her parents and her best friend agreed that she appeared to have been in her usual good mood until the evening of the overdose. The best friend reported that a different friend had texted Hannah that she had seen Hannah's boyfriend kissing another girl. Within a couple of hours of reading that text, Hannah was found by her parents, confused and barely arousable. On her desk was a note: "I just want to sleep forever." The parents immediately called an ambulance.

Psychiatric history was notable for an absence of depression, suicidal ideation, self-injurious behaviors, mania, or psychosis. She had no previous psychiatric contacts, hospitalizations, or psychotherapy. According to her parents and her best friend, Hannah never used cigarettes, alcohol, marijuana, or other illicit drugs. She had no legal history

Hannah lived with her parents and two younger sisters. Her academic performance as an eleventh grader at a local public school was stellar. She reported that she hoped to be a physician or attorney. Her best friend said she had been cheerful earlier in the day. Family psychiatric history was notable for her mother having an anxiety disorder for which she was prescribed clonazepam and alprazolam. As a late adolescent, the mother had also made two suicide attempts by medication overdose. Her father had chronic back pain from a sports injury, for which he took oxycodone. Extended family history was notable for a paternal uncle with an alcohol use disorder. No one in the extended family had committed suicide.

After she was extubated, Hannah said she felt fine, and that the suicidal feelings were completely gone. She also said that she had been doing well until the minute she read about her boyfriend kissing another girl. Hannah denied having any disturbances of mood, anxiety, sleep, appetite, energy, or concentration, either at the time of the evaluation or in the weeks leading up to the overdose. She denied somatic complaints, psychotic features, and any history of self-injury, such as cutting. She denied any history of trauma or substance use. She recalled that the thought to die came "out of the blue," and that she immediately wrote the suicide note and gathered medications from her parents' medicine cabinet. In retrospect, she was horrified by the overdose and grateful that she was alive.

Hannah continued to deny depression and suicidality throughout her hospitalization. She was discharged to outpatient care within the hospital clinic. No psychotropic medication was prescribed. She was seen weekly for cognitive-behavioral therapy that focused on coping skills when angry or disappointed. After 6 months, Hannah was noted to be doing well and to have been consistently free of suicidal ideation, intent, or behavior. At that point, Hannah, her parents, and the psychologist agreed to end the treatment, with the understanding that she would restart treatment should she experience any trouble coping.

Discussion

Until the evening of the overdose, Hannah appears to have been a happy, highly functional teenager. After she received the text about her boyfriend, she became immediately suicidal, wrote the note, and took a serious overdose of sedating medications that she had taken from her parents' medicine cabinet.

By all accounts, Hannah's overdose had been completely unanticipated. She had no known history of depression, anxiety, or trauma. She had no history of substance use, self-injurious behavior, or suicidal ideation. She did not seem to have personality traits that might predispose her to a suicide attempt. Hannah's mother had an anxiety disorder and a history of two suicide attempts by overdose as an adolescent, but Hannah herself had apparently been a "cheerful" friend and "stellar" student.

In regard to making a diagnosis, it appears that Hannah has developed marked, out-of-proportion, and impairing distress in response to a stressor. There is no evidence of another psychiatric disorder. Therefore, Hannah's symptoms seem to best fit the criteria for a DSM-5 diagnosis of adjustment disorder with depressed mood.

As is true for almost all DSM diagnoses, the diagnostic criteria for adjustment disorder do not mention suicidal ideation or behavior. Even in diagnoses in which suicidality is listed as one of multiple potential symptoms in the criteria (e.g., major depressive disorder, borderline personality disorder), it is not a required part of the diagnosis. Instead, DSM discusses suicidality and self-destructive behavior in the descriptive text accompanying the diagnostic criteria for disorders that are associated with high rates of suicidal behavior.

DSM-5 included proposed criteria for suicidal behavior disorder and nonsuicidal self-injury in the Section III chapter "Conditions for Further Study." Although nonsuicidal self-injury was expanded to "nonsuicidal self-injury *disorder*" in DSM-5-TR, the criteria sets themselves have not changed. As was true in DSM-5, criteria for both conditions essentially require only the presence of a particular behavior (together with the absence of several exclusionary criteria). In other words, although it may be important for the clinician to specifically evaluate whether and to what degree the individual has contemplated suicide or considered self-harm, the diagnosis of suicidal behavior disorder requires only a suicide attempt, and the diagnosis of nonsuicidal self-injury disorder requires only some sort of self-inflicted physical harm.

In an important change from DSM-5, DSM-5-TR also added suicidal behavior and nonsuicidal self-injury to the Section II chapter "Other Conditions That May Be a Focus of Clinical Attention," which provides ICD-10-CM codes for conditions, behaviors, circumstances, or problems that are not mental disorders per se but can affect the course, prognosis, or care of a disorder (examples include family problems, economic hardship, and nonadherence to medical treatment). The addition of these behaviors to the Section II chapter as codable conditions has important ramifications for medical recordkeeping. For example, coding for suicidal behavior in the medical chart allows the clinician to document and monitor suicidal behavior that may or may not be associated with a specific psychiatric diagnosis. Such codes can also help future clinicians to more rapidly evaluate potentially ambiguous situations. For example, if Hannah returns to the hospital in an altered state of consciousness but without a readily available collateral historian, clinicians will be reminded by the codes in her chart to look for an overdose.

In the Section III "Conditions for Further Study" chapter, the text accompanying the proposed criteria for suicidal behavior disorder lists specifiers that can be helpful not just in documentation but also in assessment. These specifiers characterize the violence, lethality, and degree of planning associated with an attempt. For example, Hannah's overdose would be categorized as "nonviolent," in contrast to behavior such as a self-inflicted gunshot wound. While the degree to which she intended to actually kill herself may not be clear, her overdose would be considered of high lethality because it required intubation and an admission to the intensive care unit. Finally, her overdose would be considered impulsive, rather than well-planned-out.

Time frame is an additional specifier. Hannah will be considered to have a "current" suicidal behavior disorder for 12 months after the overdose. Because the risk of an additional suicide attempt remains high for 2 years after an attempt, the disorder would be categorized as "in early remission" between 13 and 24 months after this event. If all goes well, Hannah's suicidal behavior disorder will be considered to be in remission by the time that she is a freshman in college.

Diagnoses

- Adjustment disorder with depressed mood
- Suicidal behavior disorder

Suggested Readings

Miller AB, Prinstein MJ: Adolescent suicide as a failure of acute stress-response systems. Annu Rev Clin Psychol 15:425–450, 2019

Nestadt PS, Triplett P, Mojtabai R, Berman AL: Universal screening may not prevent suicide. Gen Hosp Psychiatry 63:14–15, 2020

Rodway C, Tham SG, Turnbull P, et al: Suicide in children and young people: can it happen without warning? Journal of Affective Disorders 275:307–310, 2020

CASE 7.8

Burnout

John W. Barnhill, M.D.

Isaac Ulysse, a 29-year-old surgery resident at a large urban hospital, was referred to his employee assistance program because of "burnout." Dr. Ulysse's supervisors had become concerned about his appearing increasingly distracted and sad. After performing very well at their medical school and during the first 2 years of surgery training, Dr. Ulysse was now manifesting some problems, with his most recent performance review being notable for uncharacteristic sloppiness and lateness. Dr. Ulysse had shrugged off two referrals, but after being told that he was being released from work until he got clearance from psychiatry, he agreed to an evaluation.

Dr. Ulysse stated that he was fine, "just a little burned out." He'd always prided himself on having more energy than everyone else, but he'd started getting worn down during the COVID-19 pandemic. He said he was sleeping poorly, was always tired, and was having trouble concentrating. After about 20 minutes, he asked if he could leave, that he felt better already. The psychiatrist explained that she would need to meet with him at least a few times before she could allow him to go back to work.

Reminded that he wasn't yet ready to go back to work, Dr. Ulysse appeared to slump in his seat. When the psychiatrist asked him to say more, he replied that he hated being this way, hated being weak.

He said he knew he had burnout. He'd read up on it, and he felt exhausted, cynical about his being a "cog in the medical-industrial complex," and less able to finish his daily work. He thought he might also have a depressive disorder, given that he was sad just about every day and also felt tired, worthless, and unable to sleep and concentrate normally. He said this had been going on for 12 or 18 months, but he'd been "good at hiding things until recently." Dr. Ulysse asked whether the psychiatrist could diagnose him with burnout, since he'd prefer not to get a label that is a "career killer, at least for a surgeon." He said he would be completely adherent with an antidepressant medication if the psychiatrist would let him go back to work. When asked if he felt suicidal, he responded that he had always thought that was a ridiculous question: "If you're really serious about suicide, why tell somebody who has 911 on speed dial? But no, I'm not going to kill myself."

At this point, the psychiatrist asked for more background information. Dr. Ulysse was the only child born to a pharmacist and a French professor, who had left Haiti when he was born. He had grown up in a suburban area where he was often the only Black child in his grade. When asked if that was difficult for him, he looked skeptical. "Yeah," he said, "I know all about microaggressions and structural racism, all that stuff, but my strategy was to always be smarter, funnier, nicer, and more athletic than everybody else. I always had a confident smile on my face, and now nothing makes me happy. My nickname at my fancy high school was Superman. I literally dated the homecoming queen, and nobody seemed to mind about the Black/white thing." At that point, he laughed and added, "well, except for my Gran, my dad's mother, who lived with us when I was growing up. She thought I was asking for trouble."

After a few moments of silence, Dr. Ulysse began to quietly cry. When asked to say more, he explained that his parents worked "all the time" when he was young, so his grandmother lived with them and took care of him throughout his school years. She had died of COVID-19 about 18 months earlier. Since then, he described thinking about her "all the time".and having become increasingly preoccupied by his failure to convince her to get the COVID vaccine.

He said he knew it was ridiculous, but he had partially believed her when she had insisted that she was able to protect everyone in the family from the virus. "Did I mention my Gran was a Catholic witch, and a very good one?" Dr. Ulysse added that although he knew she was dead, part of him continued to expect her to walk through the door, and he looked up multiple times every day, expecting her to be there. He spent long hours reviewing his inability to convince her to get the vaccine as well as his decision not to visit her for months for fear of infecting her. He awoke with nightmares most nights. He didn't remember the content of the dreams very well, but they tended to be about his grandmother disappearing and him being unable to help. He noted that he had become increasingly angry and bitter at colleagues, his parents, and his ex-girlfriend. Since she had moved out of their apartment 6 months earlier, he hadn't spoken to her or seen any of his friends. His parents called frequently and have tried to "kidnap" him for a weekend with family, but they appear to have gotten frustrated that he was being so stubborn. He said that he was okay watching TV—where he focused on "pestilence and wars"—but he just felt too numb to talk to people. He also stated that he barely knew who he was anymore, and that his job as a surgery trainee had come to seem irrelevant if it meant that he couldn't even help his family. Although he was definitely not going to kill himself, and he knew the whole idea was "stupid," he did daydream almost every day about being dead so that he could see his grandmother again.

Discussion

Under threat of suspension from his duties as a surgery resident, Dr. Ulysse accepted a psychiatric evaluation for what he called burnout. *Burnout* is a widely used term that is included in the *International Classification of Diseases*, Eleventh Revision (ICD-11), as an occupational phenomenon rather than a medical/psychiatric disorder. DSM-5-TR has no "burnout" diagnosis. Burnout is defined in ICD-11 as a syndrome that grows out of workplace stress and features three overlapping criteria: exhaustion, distance or cynicism toward one's job, and reduced efficacy at work. Dr. Ulysse appears to meet these basic criteria for burnout, although the psychiatrist continues the evaluation to better understand his situation.

In addition to fulfilling criteria for burnout, Dr. Ulysse describes a cluster of depressive symptoms. He has felt depressed and anhedonic most of the day, nearly every day, for more than a year. Although not all of the criteria for major depressive disorder (MDD) are evaluated in the case report, Dr. Ulysse does mention insomnia, fatigue, inappropriate guilt, concentration difficulties, and recurrent thoughts of death. Because his symptoms have lasted less than 2 years, he would not meet criteria for persistent depressive disorder, but he does appear to meet criteria for MDD.

Dr. Ulysse relates his symptoms specifically to the death of his grandmother, however, and he describes intense symptoms since she died 18 months earlier. He might, therefore, meet criteria for prolonged grief disorder, which is the only diagnosis that was added to DSM-5-TR's official section on diagnostic criteria and codes. Previously, the same diagnosis had been described in DSM-5's "Conditions for Further Study" chapter in Section III as "persistent complex bereavement disorder."

Prolonged grief disorder is a maladaptive grief response that can be identified 12 months after the death of a loved one. The grief response involves a cluster of symptoms that occur most days, including almost every day during the preceding month—intense longing for the deceased, as well as at least three of eight symptoms that are directly related to the death (in other words, if Dr. Ulysse indicated that some of his symptoms were lifelong and not recently intensified, they would not be counted toward the diagnosis of prolonged grief disorder). These eight symptoms are as follows:

- Identity disruption (feeling as though part of oneself has died)
- A marked sense of disbelief about the death
- Avoidance of reminders that the person is dead
- Intense emotional pain (anger, bitterness, guilt)
- Difficulty reintegrating into one's personal relationships and activities
- Emotional numbness
- A sense that life is meaningless
- Intense loneliness

As is true throughout DSM-5-TR, the symptoms must also cause clinically significant distress or impairment in social, occupational, or other areas of functioning.

The normal grief experience varies significantly, and DSM-5-TR emphasizes that the nature, duration, and severity of the bereavement reaction must clearly exceed the reaction that would be expected given the social and cultural context.

In regard to Dr. Ulysse, he appears to have experienced symptoms almost every day for over a year, and his response has led both to serious distress and to a global impairment in functioning. In addition, many of his symptoms appear to fit core criteria for prolonged grief disorder and be directly related to his grandmother's death: he feels as though part of himself has died (identity disruption); he has a sense that she is not actually dead; he feels intense emotional pain; he has had uncharacteristic difficulty with his relationships and activities; he feels that his job is meaningless; and he feels intense loneliness. He appears, therefore, to meet criteria for prolonged grief disorder.

It would be useful to obtain a better understanding of Dr. Ulysse cultural background. Haitian by birth, he casually mentions that his grandmother is a "Catholic witch." We do not have much relevant information, but it would not have been unusual for Dr. Ulysse's Haitian grandmother to have integrated beliefs from the Catholic Church and Haitian *vodou* (voodoo). Although he grew up in an affluent suburb and was trained as a physician in the United States, Dr. Ulysse would likely have absorbed some of the beliefs of his primary childhood caretaker, his grandmother. For example, she may have heavily valued dreams, which might intensify his reactions to the frequent nightmares in which he fails to save her from COVID-19. Although it would be helpful to have a clearer picture of the patient's cultural issues, his reaction does appear to be maladaptive within his culture; for example, his parents have gotten worried enough about him that they have been actively trying to pull him out of his isolation.

Dr. Ulysse might provisionally be given two diagnoses: MDD and prolonged grief disorder. Further evaluation might allow the clinician to meaningfully distinguish between the two disorders. Although there is much symptomatic overlap between the two disorders, the distress in prolonged grief disorder is focused on feelings of loss and separation from a loved one rather than reflecting a generalized low mood. Given the above clinical information, it seems most reasonable to provisionally diagnose him with both disorders.

Regardless of his specific diagnosis, Dr. Ulysse symptoms appear to be intensified by the stigma he associates with mental illness. A surgeon with a nickname of "Superman," he appears to be ashamed of his current situation, which likely intensifies his sense of isolation and hopelessness. Prolonged grief disorder is associated with elevated rates of suicidal ideation, and, while he denies that he would ever kill himself, he does describe daydreams of dying so he can be reunited with his grandmother. Without a therapeutic intervention, he is certainly at risk for self-injury as well as prolonged distress and dysfunction. The evaluating psychiatrist should resist Dr. Ulysse's request to be diagnosed with burnout. It may be tempting to accede to the request of a colleague, and "burnout" may feel less stigmatizing to Dr. Ulysse than MDD or prolonged grief, but downplaying Dr. Ulysse's symptoms would be both fraudulent and potentially dangerous, given that an inaccurate diagnosis could lead to a substandard treatment plan and poor outcome.

Finally, Dr. Ulysse is also at risk for a substance use disorder. The case report does not mention anything about substances, but it would not be unusual if he had tried to self-medicate his insomnia, sadness, and fatigue so that he could function at his customary level. Sedating drugs (e.g., alcohol, marijuana, benzodiazepines) might have been used to promote sleep or relaxation, for example, whereas stimulants (e.g., amphetamines, cocaine) might have been used to help restore energy, concentration, and a more upbeat mood. If any of these drugs have been used, his symptoms might have fallen into an intensely dysfunctional cycle. Furthermore, Dr. Ulysse is unlikely to spontaneously report the use of drugs and excessive amounts of alcohol; even if legal, excess use is not just stigmatized within medicine but also potential grounds for dismissal from the training program. The nature of this psychiatric evaluation is not entirely clear, but if it is a mandatory evaluation prior to his being allowed back to work, it is likely that he will be required to submit to a toxicology screen (if, indeed, such a screen has not already been done).

Dr. Ulysse may find the evaluation stressful, but successful identification of his psychiatric disorder(s) is likely to be an important first step in developing an effective treatment plan.

Diagnoses

- Major depressive disorder
- Prolonged grief disorder

Suggested Readings

Bryant RA, Kenny L, Joscelyne A, et al: Treating prolonged grief disorder: a randomized clinical trial. JAMA Psychiatry 71(12):1332–1339, 2016

Casey PR, Strain JJ: Trauma- and Stressor-Related Disorders: A Handbook for Clinicians. Arlington, VA, American Psychiatric Association Publishing, 2016

Maciejewski PK, Maercker A, Boelen PA, Prigerson HG: "Prolonged grief disorder" and "persistent complex bereavement disorder", but not "complicated grief", are one and the same diagnostic entity: an analysis of data from the Yale Bereavement Study. World Psychiatry 15(3):266–275, 2016

Molina N, Viola M, Rogers M, et al: Suicidal ideation in bereavement: a systematic review. Behav Sci (Basel) 9(5):53, 2019

Prigerson HG, Shear MK, Reynolds CF III: Prolonged grief disorder diagnostic criteria—helping those with maladaptive grief responses. JAMA Psychiatry 79(4):277–278, 2022

World Health Organization: International Statistical Classification of Diseases and Related Health Problems, 11th Edition (ICD-11). Geneva, World Health Organization, 2019/2021

CHAPTER 8

Dissociative Disorders

INTRODUCTION

John W. Barnhill, M.D.

Commonly encountered in people with a variety of psychiatric diagnoses (and in many people without a diagnosis), dissociative symptoms can affect consciousness, memory, identity, emotion, perception, body representation, and behavior. Dissociative experiences are common, affecting perhaps half the population at some point. Although they are common, symptoms can be vaguely experienced and poorly recalled, so they are often overlooked by clinicians. Many or most dissociative episodes are fleeting or do not cause significant distress or dysfunction, and therefore do not warrant a specific DSM-5 diagnosis. Nevertheless, identification of dissociative experiences can help make sense of sometimes-confusing symptoms.

DSM-5 describes three specific dissociative disorders—dissociative identity disorder, dissociative amnesia, and depersonalization/derealization disorder—as well as two more general categories of dissociative disorder—other specified and unspecified. All are frequently associated with physical, emotional, and/or sexual trauma and abuse, and it is not at random that the DSM-5 chapter on dissociative disorders is located immediately after the chapter that focuses on trauma- and stressor-related disorders.

Dissociative identity disorder (DID) refers to the presence of two or more distinct personality states. Formerly known as "multiple personality disorder," DID involves a discontinuity in the sense of self and the sense of agency, perception, cognition, and/or sensory-motor functioning. DID also involves memory gaps that transcend ordinary forgetting. Some cultural groups may view DID as "possession" by spiritual beings external to the person, but the disturbance should not be diagnosed as pathological if it conforms to broadly accepted cultural or religious practices. Furthermore, DID is generally not applicable to children who have imaginary playmates or who are otherwise engaging in normal imaginative play. As is often the case with all dissociative disorders, people with DID tend to present with other psychiatric issues, including depression, anxiety, substance abuse, self-injury, posttraumatic stress disorder, and non-epileptic seizures. Patients may conceal or not be aware of memory gaps and other discontinuities, which further complicates the psychiatric evaluation.

In contrast to DID, which involves organization of different personalities via dissociative processes, other dissociative diagnoses are perhaps more common and less controversial. Dissociative amnesia involves an inability to recall important autobiographical information that is generally related to a specific stressor or trauma. It can be associated with nonepileptic seizures or other functional neurological symptoms (e.g., DSM-5-TR functional neurological symptom disorder [conversion disorder]). DSM-5 removed dissociative fugue as a separate disorder and included it as a specifier for dissociative amnesia. Fugue states are notable for the inability to recall important autobiographical memories (e.g., personal identity) and can include wandering away from home while maintaining an ability to function adequately.

A detached and unreal sense of oneself (depersonalization) or the outside world (derealization) is relatively common, with a reported lifetime population prevalence of 50%. To meet criteria for depersonalization/derealization disorder, however, the symptoms must be persistent (generally lasting at least 1 month) and/or recurrent. Reality testing should be spared. As with other DSM-5 diagnoses, impairment and/or distress is also required, so occasional "spacing out" is not necessarily a disorder.

DSM-5 provides a diagnostic option—"other specified dissociative disorder"—for presentations that do not meet full criteria for DID, dissociative amnesia, or depersonalization/derealization disorder. For example, the diagnosis "other specified dissociative disorder (identity disturbance due to prolonged and intense coercive persuasion)" can be given when an individual has dissociative effects following an intense experience such as brainwashing, long-term political imprisonment, or indoctrination into a cult. Acute dissociative reactions to stressful events can have a variety of dissociative manifestations when viewed cross-sectionally but are notable for their brevity; they can clear within days. If they persist for more than 1 month, the individual likely warrants a different diagnosis (e.g., depersonalization/derealization disorder).

Suggested Readings

Laddis A, Dell PF, Korzekwa M: Comparing the symptoms and mechanisms of "dissociation" in dissociative identity disorder and borderline personality disorder. J Trauma Dissociation 18(2):139–173, 2017 27245196

Lewis-Fernández R, Martínez-Taboas A, Sar V, et al: The cross-cultural assessment of dissociation, in Cross-Cultural Assessment of Psychological Trauma and PTSD (International and Cultural Psychology Series). Edited by Wilson JP, Tang CS. Boston, Springer, 2007, pp 279–317

Lippard ETC, Nemeroff CB: The devastating clinical consequences of child abuse and neglect: increased disease vulnerability and poor treatment response in mood disorders. Am J Psychiatry 177(1):20–36, 2020

Lyssenko L, Schmahl C, Bockhacker L, et al: Dissociation in psychiatric disorders: a meta-analysis of studies using the Dissociative Experiences Scale. Am J Psychiatry 175(1):37–46, 2018

CASE 8.1

Sad and Alone

Richard J. Loewenstein, M.D.

Judith Vaughan was a 29-year-old special education teacher who sought a psychiatric consultation because "I'm tired of always being sad and alone."

The patient reported chronic, severe depression that had not responded to multiple trials of antidepressants and mood stabilizer augmentation. She reported greater benefit from psychotherapies based on cognitive-behavioral therapy and dialectical behavior therapy. Electroconvulsive therapy had been suggested, but she had refused. She had been hospitalized twice for suicidal ideation and severe self-cutting that required stitches.

Ms. Vaughan reported that previous therapists had focused on the likelihood of trauma, but she casually dismissed the possibility that she had ever been abused. It had been her younger sister who had reported "weird sexual touching" by their father when Ms. Vaughan was 13. There had never been a police investigation, but her father had apologized to the patient and her sister as part of a resultant church intervention and an inpatient treatment for alcoholism and "sex addiction." She denied any feelings about these events and said, "He took care of the problem. I have no reason to be mad at him."

Ms. Vaughan reported little memory for her life between the ages of about 7 and 13 years. Her siblings would joke about her inability to recall family holidays, school events, and vacation trips. She explained her amnesia by saying, "I don't remember anything because nothing happened."

She reported a "good" relationship with both parents. Her father remained "controlling" toward her mother and still had "anger issues," but had been abstinent from alcohol for 16 years. On closer questioning, Ms. Vaughan reported that her self-injurious and suicidal behavior primarily occurred after visits to see her family or when her parents surprised her by visiting.

Ms. Vaughan described being "socially withdrawn" until high school, at which point she became academically successful and a member of numerous teams and clubs. She did well in college. She excelled at her job and was regarded as a gifted teacher of autistic children. She described several friendships of many years. She reported difficulty with intimacy with men, experiencing intense fear and disgust at any attempted sexual advances. Whenever she did get at all involved with a man, she felt intense shame and a sense of her own "badness," although she felt worthless at other times as well. She tended to sleep poorly and often felt tired.

She denied use of alcohol or drugs. She added that even the smell of alcohol made her feel like throwing up.

On mental status examination, the patient was well groomed and cooperative. Her responses were coherent and goal directed, but often devoid of emotional content. She appeared sad and constricted. She described herself as "numb." She denied hallucinations, confusion, and a current intention to kill herself. However, thoughts of suicide were "always around."

More specific questions led Ms. Vaughan to deny that she had ongoing amnesia for daily life, particularly denying ever being told of behavior she could not recall, unexplained possessions, subjective time loss, fugue episodes, or inexplicable fluctuations in skills, habits, and/or knowledge. She denied a sense of subjective self-division, hallucinations, inner voices, or passive influence symptoms. She denied flashbacks or intrusive memories, but she did report recurrent nightmares of being chased by "a dangerous man" from whom she could not escape. She reported difficulty concentrating, although she was "hyperfocused" at work. She reported an intense startle reaction. She said that she often found herself silently counting and singing rather than let herself daydream. She added that she was very careful, checking multiple times every night to ensure that her doors were locked. When she got anxious, she found that rearranging her furniture helped her feel safer.

Discussion

Ms. Vaughan reports persistently depressed mood, insomnia, fatigue, feelings of worthlessness, and suicidality. It is not surprising that she has received serial treatments for major depressive disorder, nor is it surprising that these treatments have not been particularly successful.

In addition to her depressive symptoms, the patient describes symptoms and historical events that hint at additional issues. Although Ms. Vaughan's younger sister was the one who reported their father for "weird sexual touching," he had apologized to her as well as to her sister. Ms. Vaughan has a history of severe self-cutting that occurs when she sees her family. Sexual intimacy leads to feelings of disgust and shame, and as a result—despite having sought treatment because she feels sad and alone— Ms. Vaughan avoids men. She has recurrent nightmares of being chased by "a dangerous man." She denies having been abused, but she describes a 6-year autobiographical memory gap that seems to have ended at the exact time that her father was sent away for inpatient treatment of alcoholism and "sex addiction." Even the smell of alcohol makes her want to throw up.

Given this information, it is not surprising that previous therapists have "focused on the likelihood of trauma." In particular, the apparent child sexual abuse in conjunction with a 6-year memory deficit conforms well to a DSM-5 diagnosis of dissociative amnesia (DA).

In contrast to the memory failures associated with intoxications and neurocognitive disorders, DA involves problems with autobiographical memory: what I did, where I went, what I thought or felt, and so forth. The most common presentation of DA is *localized* dissociative amnesia, an inability to remember a specific period of time or event, such as all of second grade. In *selective* dissociative amnesia, memory is preserved for some of the events during a circumscribed period of time, such as some retained memories from second grade, but with amnesia for all or part of the actual trauma.

DA is associated with physical and sexual abuse, and its extent seems to increase with increased severity, frequency, and violence of the abuse.

DA can be difficult to distinguish from other trauma-related diagnoses because disorders such as posttraumatic stress disorder (PTSD) also feature memory loss in the context of trauma. If the memory loss is the core symptom and involves a period that extends well beyond the actual trauma, then DA should be coded separately from a PTSD diagnosis. Ms. Vaughan's memory loss extended over 6 years, which conforms to the period of presumed sexual abuse. In addition, she describes intrusive thoughts (nightmares), avoidance (of dating and sex), negative alterations in cognitions and moods (belief in her own "badness"), and hyperarousal/hyperreactivity (startle reaction). In other words, she also meets criteria for PTSD and so warrants a comorbid diagnosis.

A subgroup of DA patients will also have significant obsessive-compulsive disorder symptoms, and Ms. Vaughan describes recurrently counting, singing, checking, and arranging, all in an effort to avert danger.

Another subgroup of patients will have far broader amnesia, called generalized dissociative amnesia (GDA). This loss of memory can expand to encompass an entire life, including personal identity, fund of knowledge, and memory for skills. Longitudinal observation of people with GDA shows that many will meet diagnostic criteria for DSM-5 dissociative identity disorder (DID).

DID is notable for a disruption of identity characterized by two or more distinct personality states. These states involve a marked discontinuity in the sense of self as well as clinically relevant memory gaps. Although Ms. Vaughan does not recall much of elementary school, she denies experiencing typical DID symptoms such as suddenly finding herself somewhere without recalling having gotten there (dissociative fugue); unexplained appearance or disappearance of possessions; being told of unrecalled behavior; and inexplicable fluctuations in skills, capacities, and knowledge (e.g., being able to play music at one time but being unable to access this skill at another). In addition, individuals with DID tend to experience symptoms such as hearing inner voices, depersonalization/derealization, a subjective sense of self-division, behaviors related to switching or shifting of identity states, and symptoms related to overlap or interference between identity states. Although these symptoms warrant longitudinal investigation, Ms. Vaughan specifically denied them and is unlikely to have DID.

The diagnostic interview with people with DA is unusual. They rarely volunteer information about memory problems. They commonly minimize the amnesia and its connection to traumatic events. Perhaps most important, discussion of even the possibility of trauma can induce intense anxiety, flashbacks, nightmares, and somatic memories of the abuse. Tact, pacing, and timing are critical, and an overzealous pursuit of "truth" can inflict psychological harm on a person who is still suffering from abuse endured many years earlier.

Diagnoses

- Dissociative amnesia
- Major depressive disorder, chronic, with suicidal ideation
- Posttraumatic stress disorder

Suggested Readings

Brand BL, Loewenstein RJ, Spiegel D: Dispelling myths about dissociative identity disorder treatment: an empirically based approach. Psychiatry 77(2):169–189, 2014

Lanius RA, Vermetten E, Pain C (eds): The Impact of Early Life Trauma on Health and Disease: The Hidden Epidemic. Cambridge, UK, Cambridge University Press, 2010

Loewenstein RJ: Dissociation debates: everything you know is wrong. Dialogues Clin Neurosci 20(3):229–242, 2018

CASE 8.2

Feeling Unreal

Daphne Simeon, M.D.

Ken Waldron, a 20-year-old college sophomore, was referred by his resident advisor (RA) to the school's mental health care clinic after he appeared depressed in the weeks following a breakup with his girlfriend. Mr. Waldron did not attend the evaluation session, telling his RA that "everybody gets bummed after a breakup—I'll be fine." When Mr. Waldron seemed "strange and out of it," his RA made another appointment and then accompanied Ken to the meeting.

In that initial session, Mr. Waldron was hesitant but revealed that he had been crushed by the breakup. While he had previously been an excellent student, he'd quit doing homework and just looked out the window during class. He noticed that his grades had declined markedly, but "I don't seem to care." Although he said he felt lonely, he also admitted to steadily deleting incoming texts, so that he rarely communicated with his friends and family.

When asked to describe other symptoms of depression, Mr. Waldron replied that he didn't have anything to say. He said that his mind felt blank, "as usual." He added that he also felt increasingly detached from his physical body, going about his daily activities "like a robot." He said he felt so disconnected that he often wondered if he were dead or living in a dream, or just had "no self."

Mr. Waldron said that he'd been depressed for a few weeks after the breakup. He said he'd never been in love before and was shocked when Jill told him she needed "time apart." For weeks afterward, he felt sad and a little desperate, but he'd continued to see friends and go to class; however, at some point, things began to change. He said he started feeling numb, unreal, and disconnected, but it was all a little fuzzy.

Mr. Waldron described a time-limited bout of extreme anxiety in tenth grade. At that time, panic attacks had begun and then escalated in severity and frequency over 2 months. During those attacks, he had felt very detached, as if everything around him was unreal. The symptoms sometimes lasted for several hours and were reminiscent of his current complaints. The onset appeared to coincide with his mother's entry into a psychiatric hospital. When she was discharged, all of his symptoms cleared rapidly. He did not seek treatment at that time.

Mr. Waldron also described experiencing transient feelings of unreality in elementary school, just after his parents divorced and his father left young Jason and his mother, who had a diagnosis of paranoid schizophrenia. His childhood was significant for pervasive loneliness and the sense that he was the only adult in the family. His mother was only marginally functional, with a few actively psychotic episodes. His father rarely visited but did provide enough money for them to continue to live in reasonable comfort. Jason often stayed with his grandparents on weekends, but in general, he and his mother lived a very isolated life. He did well in school and had a few close friends, but he largely kept to himself and rarely brought friends home. Jill would have been the first girlfriend to meet his mother.

Mr. Waldron denied using any drugs, in particular cannabis, hallucinogens, or ketamine, and his urine toxicology was negative. Although his home life featured emotional neglect by both parents and emotional abuse when his mother was actively psychotic, he denied physical or sexual abuse. He denied any psychiatric history of mania, psychosis, or other past psychiatric symptoms, except as described above. He also specifically denied amnesia, blackouts, multiple identities, hallucinations, paranoia, and other unusual thoughts or experiences.

Results of routine laboratory tests, a blood toxicology screen, and a physical examination were normal, as were a brain magnetic resonance imaging scan and an electroencephalogram. Consultations with an otorhinolaryngologist and a neurologist were noncontributory.

Discussion

Mr. Waldron is experiencing persistent detachment from his physical body, mind, and emotions and has a pervasive sense of "no self." During these experiences, his reality testing remains intact. The history indicates that there are no medical causes for these symptoms, and psychiatric comorbidity does not account for them. The symptoms are persistent, and his functioning is significantly impaired. Mr. Waldron meets criteria for DSM-5 depersonalization/derealization disorder.

Mr. Waldron has had similar symptoms twice before, but neither episode appears to have met criteria for depersonalization/derealization disorder. Mr. Waldron's first episode, in elementary school, was triggered by his father's abandonment; his symptoms reportedly lasted only a few days. Although the DSM-5 criteria do not specify a minimum duration for depersonalization/derealization disorder, they indicate that symptoms must be "persistent or recurrent."

The second episode occurred in the context of 2 months of escalating panic attacks precipitated by his mother's psychiatric hospitalization. Although these symptoms met the duration criteria for depersonalization/derealization disorder, they occurred exclusively in the context of another psychiatric condition (panic disorder), and they resolved with the resolution of the other psychiatric disorder.

Mr. Waldron's most recent episode, however, shows the classic features of depersonalization/derealization disorder: the experiences have persisted for several months after resolution of the short-lived depressive episode; the experiences are not associated with another psychiatric, substance use, or medical disorder; and reality testing remains intact during the experiences. Notably, the second episode of symptoms was more heavily weighted toward derealization, whereas the third and clinically diagnostic episode was more heavily weighted toward depersonalization. Incorporating evidence from recent research in the field, DSM-5 combined depersonalization and derealization symptoms into a single disorder that can consist of either one set—or, more commonly, both sets—of symptoms.

Before the diagnosis can be made, other potential psychiatric and medical causes need to be explored and excluded. Given his mother's schizophrenia, one alternative explanation would appear to be a psychotic disorder or a schizophrenia prodrome. Mr. Waldron seems to have maintained his social and academic functioning until the depersonalization worsened, and he also maintained reality testing despite the symptoms; therefore, he lacks criteria for a current psychotic diagnosis.

Additionally, in any patient with a dissociative presentation, all possible types of dissociative symptoms must be assessed. Depersonalization/derealization symptoms are very common in dissociative identity disorder and can occur in dissociative amnesia as well. Notably, Mr. Waldron denied symptoms of amnesia or identity alteration.

Like many patients with depersonalization/derealization disorder, Mr. Waldron does not consider his suffering delusional, but instead is convinced of its "physical" nature. Such a conviction can often lead to extensive medical workups that may be more reassuring to patients than helpful in identifying a medical etiology. Young people with typical presentations and without risk factors or abnormal findings on physical and neurological examinations are highly unlikely to be harboring some underlying medical or neurological illness. The workup may help these patients proceed with psychiatric treatment, but it can sometimes be useful for the psychiatrist to temper the enthusiasm of other physicians who may suggest prolonged or invasive testing.

It is also useful to recognize that Mr. Waldron is a college student who originally presented with depressive symptoms following a breakup. Without the friendly persistence of his resident advisor and the tactful inquiry by the clinician at the mental health clinic, recognition of Mr. Waldron's dissociative symptoms would have been significantly delayed, as would the development of an effective treatment plan. Effective treatment is always important, of course, but a delayed or inaccurate diagnosis in an adolescent can lead to difficulties in school, work, and relationships, as well as in the young person's internal sense of self. These difficulties not only can be temporarily challenging and painful but also can have a powerfully negative effect on the young person's life trajectory.

Dissociative disorders tend to be associated with childhood maltreatment. In comparison with people with other dissociative disorders, patients with depersonalization/derealization disorder tend to report trauma that is less extreme and often of an emotional nature rather than physical or sexual. Mr. Waldron's history is typical in that he clearly experienced emotional neglect and periodic emotional abuse, but he denied physical or sexual trauma. An initial working hypothesis might be that Mr. Waldron's recent episode stemmed from these childhood experiences in combination with his vulnerability to panic and depression and the impact of losing his first real girlfriend.

Diagnosis

• Depersonalization/derealization disorder

Suggested Readings

Choi KR, Seng JS, Briggs EC, et al: The dissociative subtype of posttraumatic stress disorder (PTSD) among adolescents: co-occurring PTSD, depersonalization/derealization, and other dissociation symptoms. J Am Acad Child Adolesc Psychiatry 56(12):1062–1072, 2017

Simeon D, Abugel J: Feeling Unreal: Depersonalization Disorder and the Loss of Self. New York, Oxford University Press, 2008

Thomson P, Jaque SV: Depersonalization, adversity, emotionality, and coping with stressful situations. J Trauma Dissociation 19(2):143–161, 2018

CASE 8.3

Dissociations

Roberto Lewis-Fernández, M.D.

Lourdes Zayas, a 33-year-old Puerto Rican woman born in the United States, was brought to the emergency room (ER) after she became distraught and tried to swallow bleach.

The patient, who had no previous psychiatric history, had apparently been doing fine until the day before, when her fiancé was murdered in a drug-related incident in Puerto Rico. Her family reported that Ms. Zayas reacted initially with inordinate calm. Concerned, relatives discreetly followed her around in their small apartment for several hours. She did not speak but instead engaged in repetitive, unnecessary tasks such as folding and unfolding clothes.

That afternoon, standing at the washing machine, she had cried out, grabbed a bottle of bleach, and tried to drink from it. Her brother knocked it away. She fell to the ground, shaking, screaming, and crying. This episode lasted a few seconds, after which she "lay as if dead" for a few minutes. The family recalled no tonic-clonic movements, tongue biting, or loss of sphincter control. When the ambulance arrived, Ms. Zayas was crying softly, repeating the name of her fiancé, and was generally unresponsive to questions. After medical staff treated mild burns to her lips, she was triaged to the psychiatry department.

Over the next few hours, Ms. Zayas became more responsive. During a clinical interview done in Spanish, she reported being struck "numb" (*insensible*) by the news of her fiancé's death and described a sense of being disconnected from her body, her emotions, and her surroundings. These symptoms were still present in the ER but diminished over several hours. She also described amnesia for what occurred from the moment when she cried out and her vision went "dark" (*oscura*), to when she "awoke" in the ER.

While being kept under observation for 24 hours, Ms. Zayas had two more episodes of sudden agitation, crying, and screaming, during which she attempted to scratch her face and to leave the room. Because she responded quickly to verbal intervention and reassuring physical contact, she was not given medications or placed in restraints, but was kept on one-to-one observation. Her laboratory test results were unremarkable, as were an electroencephalogram and a lumbar puncture.

On examination, she was crying softly, her mood was sad, and she said she did not remember making a suicide attempt. She was oriented to time, person, and place; had no psychotic symptoms; and denied current suicidal ideation.

Ms. Zayas was transferred to an inpatient psychiatric unit for evaluation. She initially had difficulty falling asleep and had sad, scary dreams about her fiancé. She denied recalling anything from the hours after she tried to swallow bleach. She made efforts to avoid thinking about her fiancé and was disturbed by intrusive recollections of their time together, but she never met DSM-5 criteria for acute stress disorder or major depressive disorder. Her symptoms had improved significantly after 1 week. She took no medications at the hospital and was discharged after 10 days with follow-up to outpatient care. She attended a single appointment 1 month later, at which point she and her family agreed that she was episodically sad about the death of her fiancé but essentially back to her normal self. At that point, she was lost to follow-up.

Discussion

Different clinicians might try to conceptualize Ms. Zayas's symptoms in different ways. Because her fiancé's murder was undoubtedly traumatic, a clinician might try to fit her symptoms into one of the diagnoses listed among the DSM-5 trauma- and stressor-related disorders. Another clinician might recognize psychotic symptoms and try to find a diagnosis among the schizophrenia spectrum and other psychotic disorders. Another might try to find a depressive or anxiety-related disorder that fits the symptomatology. Still another might look for a personality disorder or a preexisting personality vulnerability that could have led to these symptoms.

By staying close to the provided information, however, one can develop a more parsimonious explanation. In response to news of the murder, Ms. Zayas went "numb" and walked around the apartment for hours repetitively folding and unfolding clothes. She described being disconnected from her body, emotions, and surroundings. She was thwarted when she tried to drink bleach and then fell to the ground, shaking and crying. She had amnesia for the event, saying she awoke hours later in the ER. She then went on to have several days of intrusive, unwelcome memories and nightmares, as well as recurrent depersonalization and derealization experiences, but she was essentially back to her normal self within a week or two.

Ms. Zayas had an acute dissociative reaction. Listed as an example of other specified dissociative disorder, this DSM-5 diagnosis describes a cluster of people who respond to a stress with acute, transient dissociative symptoms that might include some combination of the following: constriction of consciousness; depersonalization; derealization; perceptual disturbances (e.g., time slowing, macropsia); micro-amnesias; transient stupor; and alterations in sensory-motor functioning (e.g., analgesia, paralysis). Ms. Zayas reported constriction of consciousness (brooding with repetitive behaviors), depersonalization, derealization, transient stupor, and micro-amnesia.

In some individuals, an acute episode becomes recurrent, especially when repeated stressors precipitate new acute reactions. In other individuals, the acute condition resolves with minimal sequelae.

Acute dissociative episodes may be comorbid with other psychiatric diagnoses, or they may be an isolated reaction in an otherwise normally functioning person. They have also been described as part of a heterogeneous cluster of syndromes from around the world. A similar dissociative episode might be labeled a "falling out" in the southern United States or an "indisposition" in Haiti. Throughout Latin America, similar episodes are called *ataque de nervios* (attack of nerves), which is the term that Ms. Zayas and her family used throughout her hospitalization. The revised "Culture and Psychiatric Diagnosis" chapter in DSM-5-TR Section III has an entry on *ataque de nervios*, including the diagnoses potentially associated with this condition.

Fear of this type of reaction presumably led the family to monitor Ms. Zayas closely after she received the news of her fiancé's murder, and helped prevent greater harm from the bleach. *Ataques* are very common, with a lifetime prevalence of about 10% in Puerto Ricans living in the United States. They are considered to be expected, even normal, reactions when precipitated by discrete and overwhelming stressors, such as in Ms. Zayas's case. A lifetime history of *ataque* is, however, associated with higher rates of mental health–related disability, suicidal ideation, and outpatient mental health care. Ms. Zayas's *ataque,* therefore, suggests potential vulnerability to psychiatric sequelae. In this particular case, Ms. Zayas and her family should be counseled that she may be at risk for another attack in the context of another stressor and would also be at risk for a delayed onset of posttraumatic stress disorder.

The DSM-5-TR Core Cultural Formulation Interview, a standardized protocol for conducting an individual cultural assessment, can help clinicians understand Ms. Zayas's and her family's perspectives about the situation and facilitate development of a negotiated treatment plan.

Diagnosis

• Other specified dissociative disorder (acute dissociative reactions to stressful events)

Suggested Readings

Guarnaccia PJ, Lewis-Fernández R, Martínez Pincay I, et al: Ataque de nervios as a marker of social and psychiatric vulnerability: results from the NLAAS. Int J Soc Psychiatry 56(3):298–309, 2010

Lewis-Fernández R, Kirmayer LJ: Cultural concepts of distress and psychiatric disorders: understanding symptom experience and expression in context. Transcult Psychiatry 56(4):786–803, 2019

Lewis-Fernández RL, Aggarwal NK, Hinton L, Hinton DE, Kirmayer LJ (eds): DSM-5 Handbook on the Cultural Formulation Interview. Arlington, VA, American Psychiatric Publishing, 2016

Lim RF (ed): Clinical Manual of Cultural Psychiatry, 2nd Edition. Arlington, VA, American Psychiatric Publishing, 2015

CHAPTER 9

Somatic Symptom and Related Disorders

INTRODUCTION

Anna Dickerman, M.D.
John W. Barnhill, M.D.

Somatic symptom disorder (SSD) is a DSM-5 diagnosis that describes a cluster of patients who have distressing somatic symptoms along with excessive thoughts, feelings, or behaviors related to these symptoms. SSD is an umbrella term intended to describe most of the patients who had previously held the diagnoses of somatization disorder, pain disorder, and hypochondriasis, which appeared in the DSM-IV chapter on somatoform disorders. A key difference is that diagnosing SSD requires a search for positive symptoms, such as distress and dysfunction, rather than a search for a negative (ruling out medically unexplained symptoms). Patients with SSD can—and often do—have physiologically based medical diagnoses, but the new diagnosis allows the clinician to focus on the distress and dysfunctional thoughts, feelings, and behaviors rather than the validity of patients' medical complaints.

The DSM-5 chapter on somatic symptom and related disorders also includes illness anxiety disorder, functional neurological symptom disorder (conversion disorder), psychological factors affecting other medical conditions (PFAOMC), and factitious disorder, as well as the "other specified" and "unspecified" somatic symptom and related disorder categories.

For each of these disorders, the clinician should try to understand the patient's own perspective on the somatic experience, which is almost inevitably filtered through multiple lenses, including culture, health literacy, and previous health care experiences. When possible, DSM-5-TR text attempts to reduce the stigma and perceived criticism that can become part of a psychiatric diagnosis.

For example, the term *hypochondriasis* was eliminated in DSM-5 because it was deemed pejorative and counterproductive to the development of a therapeutic alliance. It is also a term with a long, complex history that led to a broad spectrum of ideas about its meaning and etiology. DSM-5 divided hypochondriasis into two diagnostic clusters. Most people with DSM-IV hypochondriasis have significant health anxiety in the presence of significant somatic symptoms; in DSM-5, these people are described as having SSD. Perhaps 25% of individuals with elevated health anxiety lack significant somatic complaints; they are diagnosed with illness anxiety disorder (IAD), which was new in DSM-5.

DSM-5 takes a similar approach to individuals who appear to have abnormal thoughts, feelings, and behaviors in the context of pain. Individuals who would have been diagnosed with a DSM-IV pain disorder generally fall under the DSM-5 SSD umbrella, with the specifier "with predominant pain." Some people with abnormal thoughts, feelings, and behaviors related to pain may be best conceptualized as having DSM-5 PFAOMC, a diagnosis that was previously included in the DSM-IV chapter "Other Conditions That May Be a Focus of Clinical Attention." PFAOMC refers to a condition in which psychological or behavioral factors adversely influence a medical condition. An example would be denial of the significance of chest pain, leading to delayed medical intervention for a myocardial infarction.

The exploration of medically unexplained symptoms was deemphasized in DSM-5, and most of the disorders in this chapter do not require that the clinician rule out physiologically based medical conditions. DSM-5-TR functional neurological symptom disorder (previously known as conversion disorder) is somewhat different. Its symptomatic criteria include altered voluntary motor or sensory function along with evidence that there is incompatibility between the symptom and recognized neurological or medical conditions. Specifiers for functional neurological symptom disorder can be used to describe symptoms (e.g., weakness or seizures), duration (e.g., acute or persistent), and the presence or absence of a relevant psychological stressor.

Factitious disorder is the conscious production of false signs or symptoms. As with functional neurological symptom disorder, exploration of possible factitious disorder requires that the clinician consider the possibility that the patient's symptoms are not based on physiologically mediated illness. Such an approach need not be inevitably adversarial, and it is useful to balance the necessary skepticism with professional curiosity when the patient's presentation does not seem to be making sense.

As seen throughout DSM-5, the chapter on somatic symptom and related disorders includes an "unspecified" category that is best used when symptoms are suggestive but information is limited. The "other specified" category is used when clinicians make a decision that an individual has characteristic features of a specific somatic symptom and related disorder and has significant distress and/or dysfunction but does not quite meet the stated criteria for that particular disorder. For example, a patient might meet all the criteria for SSD or IAD but have had symptoms for less than the required 6 months; the patient would then be noted to have brief SSD or brief IAD. The other two diagnoses within this other specified category are IAD without excessive health-related behaviors and pseudocyesis (i.e., false pregnancy).

Anxiety and depressive disorders are each identified in about half of the somatic symptom and related disorders. Posttraumatic stress disorder and obsessive-compulsive disorder are also commonly identified in people with SSD. Identification of comorbidities can be crucial to the development of a strong alliance and a workable treatment plan.

All of these disorders involve a prominent focus on physical concerns, and so it is not surprising that they are most commonly found in medical rather than mental health care settings. These disorders are often accompanied by an unusual degree of clinical uncertainty, which can lead to a zealous search for the "real" cause of the problem. In general, DSM-5 encourages clinicians to focus on the patient rather than on the detection of falsehood. Although it may be useful to check a pregnancy test to detect pseudocyesis or an electroencephalogram during what appears to be a psychogenic nonepileptic seizure (previously called *pseudoseizure*), a skeptical search for "the truth" is often futile and can lead to mistrust, a fractured alliance, and termination of the treatment. Instead, DSM-5 encourages clinicians to apprehend the individual's relationship to the symptoms from cognitive, behavioral, and affective perspectives. In so doing, the clinician not only can develop an accurate and nonjudgmental understanding of the patient but also can begin the process of treatment.

Suggested Readings

Bagayogo IP, Interian A, Escobar JI: Transcultural aspects of somatic symptoms in the context of depressive disorders. Adv Psychosom Med 33:64–74, 2013

Bailer J, Kerstner T, Witthöft M, et al: Health anxiety and hypochondriasis in the light of DSM-5. Anxiety Stress Coping 29(2):219–239, 2016

Löwe B, Gerloff C: Functional somatic symptoms across cultures: perceptual and health care issues. Psychosom Med 80(5):412–415, 2018

MacKinnon RA, Michels R, Buckley PJ: The psychosomatic patient, in The Psychiatric Interview in Clinical Practice, 3rd Edition. Arlington, VA, American Psychiatric Publishing, 2015, pp 499–512

Newby JM, Hobbs MJ, Mahoney AEJ, et al: DSM-5 illness anxiety disorder and somatic symptom disorder: comorbidity, correlates, and overlap with DSM-IV hypochondriasis. J Psychosom Res 101:31–37, 2017

CASE 9.1

Pain and Depression

James A. Bourgeois, O.D., M.D.

Michelle Adams, a 51-year-old former hairdresser, came to a psychiatric clinic at the urging of her primary care doctor. A note sent ahead revealed that she had been tearful and frustrated at her last medical appointment, and her doctor, who had been struggling to control the patient's persistent back pain, felt that an evaluation by a psychiatrist might be helpful.

Greeting Ms. Adams in the waiting room, the psychiatrist was struck by both her appearance and her manner: here was a woman with shaggy silver hair and dark sunglasses, seated in a wheelchair, who offered a limp handshake and a plaintive sigh before asking the psychiatrist if he would mind pushing her wheelchair into his office. She was tired from a long commute, and, she explained, "Nobody on the street offered to help me out. Can you believe that?"

Once settled, Ms. Adams stated that she had been suffering from unbearable back pain for the previous 13 months. On the night "that changed everything," she had locked herself out of her apartment and, while trying to climb in through a fire escape, had fallen and fractured her pelvis, coccyx, right elbow, and three ribs. Although she did not require surgery, she was bed-bound for 6 weeks and then underwent several months of physical therapy. Daily opioid medication had been only moderately helpful. She had seen "a dozen" doctors of various specialties and tried multiple treatments, including anesthetic injections and transcutaneous electrical nerve stimulation therapy, but her pain was unrelenting. Throughout this ordeal and for years previously, Ms. Adams smoked cannabis daily, explaining that a joint enjoyed in hourly puffs "softened" her pain and helped her to relax. She did not drink alcohol or use other illicit drugs.

Prior to the accident, Ms. Adams had worked at a neighborhood salon for more than 20 years. She was proud to have had a large number of devoted clients, and she relished the camaraderie with her colleagues, whom she referred to as "my real family." She had been unable to return to work since her accident on account of the pain. "These doctors keep telling me I'm good to go back to work," she said with visible anger, "but they don't know what I'm going through." Her voice broke. "They don't believe me. They think I'm lying."

She added that although friends had initially reached out after the accident, lately they had seemed less sympathetic. She let incoming telephone calls go to voice mail most of the time because she just did not feel up to socializing on account of the pain. In the previous month, she had stopped bathing daily and gotten slack about cleaning her apartment. Without the structure of work, she often found herself up until 5:00 A.M., and pain woke her several times before she finally got out of bed in the afternoon. As for her mood, she said, "I'm so depressed it's ridiculous." She often felt hopeless of any possibility of living without pain but denied ever thinking of suicide. She explained that her Catholic faith prevented her from considering taking her own life.

Ms. Adams had never seen a psychiatrist before and did not recall ever having felt depressed prior to her accident, although she described a "hot temper" as a family trait. She spoke of only one meaningful romantic relationship, many years previously, with a woman who was emotionally abusive. When asked about any legal difficulties, she revealed several arrests for theft in her 20s. She was "in the wrong place at the wrong time," she said, and was never convicted of a crime.

Discussion

Ms. Adams presents with a history of pain since her fall the year before. She has received care, rehabilitation, and various invasive outpatient procedures, yet her pain, and its associated socially limiting dysfunction, persist and have escalated. She has become, in a crescendo of psychiatric comorbidity, increasingly depressed, to the point where she now manifests mood, motivation, self-care, and sleep symptoms. It would be necessary to elicit more information in order to confirm a diagnosis of major depressive disorder, but she does appear likely to meet diagnostic criteria.

In addition, Ms. Adams uses cannabis daily. She appears to have become behaviorally dependent on it for its mildly analgesic and anxiolytic properties. She does not seem to see it as a problem. Nevertheless, she is chronically depressed, unmotivated, and poorly functional, and is using, daily, an illicit substance known to induce exactly those effects. She likely qualifies, therefore, for a cannabis use disorder diagnosis in accordance with DSM-5. It would also be useful to explore the possibility of a cannabis-induced major depressive disorder, connecting these illnesses.

In addition to the depressive disorder and the cannabis use disorder, Ms. Adams appears to experience disproportionate thoughts, feelings, or behaviors related to her pain and physical debility. They have persisted for more than a year and are quite debilitating. Ms. Adams qualifies, therefore, for DSM-5 somatic symptom disorder (SSD), with a specifier of "predominant pain." In her case, the pain has taken on a life of its own, far after the initial medical recovery period. It is important to recall that pain disorder is no longer considered a separate illness in DSM-5 but instead is viewed as one of the SSDs.

As illustrated in this case, it is common for patients with SSDs to develop secondary depressive and substance use disorders. In terms of phenomenology, it is often useful to approach such cases by sequentially ascertaining the "tri-morbidity" of somatic symptom (pain in this case), depressive disorder, and substance use disorder. As presented in this unfortunately quite common narrative, the patient was functioning well without apparent disabling psychiatric illness or substance use until the emergence of overwhelming and persistent pain. Therefore, the "primary" psychiatric illness is the SSD, with depressive and substance use disorder "derivative" from the initial somatic symptom presentation.

The diagnostic phase is often marked by multiple potential pitfalls. Patients with SSDs will usually be seen in primary care or nonpsychiatric specialty medical clinics and may balk at a psychiatric referral. Although only tangentially suggested in Ms.

Adams's history, excess use of opioid analgesia often becomes the initial psychiatric focus, as well as the initial potential conflict. Psychiatrists may find themselves in a power struggle over the use of prescription opioids within minutes of first meeting the patient. Thus, patients like Ms. Adams are at risk of not receiving thorough clinical evaluations for readily treatable disorders, such as depressive and substance use disorders, and therefore of not beginning the process of reconceptualizing their pain from a debilitating catastrophe to a chronic, but manageable, symptom.

Diagnoses

- Somatic symptom disorder, with predominant pain, persistent, moderate to severe
- Cannabis use disorder
- Major depressive disorder, single episode, chronic

Suggested Readings

Bourgeois JA, Kahn D, Philbrick KL, Bostwick JM, et al: Casebook of Psychosomatic Medicine. Washington, DC, American Psychiatric Publishing, 2009

Jaracz J, Gattner K, Jaracz K, Górna K: Unexplained painful physical symptoms in patients with major depressive disorder: prevalence, pathophysiology and management. CNS Drugs 30(4):293–304, 2016

CASE 9.2

Somatic Complaints

James L. Levenson, M.D.

Norma Balaban, a 37-year-old married woman who worked as an administrative assistant to a university dean, was referred by her primary care physician for evaluation of depression and multiple somatic symptoms. She had been generally healthy, other than binge eating and obesity, until a year earlier and had undergone gastric bypass surgery 6 years earlier.

As she entered the consulting room, Ms. Balaban handed the psychiatrist a three-page summary of her physical concerns. Nocturnal leg spasms and daytime leg aches had been her initial concerns. She then developed sleep difficulties that led to "brain fog" and head heaviness. She had intermittent cold sensations in her extremities, face, ears, eyes, and nasal passages. Pulsating sensations in her eyes were, she thought, more pronounced after a poor night's sleep. In recent months, she had developed difficulty urinating, menstrual irregularity, and multiple muscle complaints, including right gluteal pain with a burning sensation into her right thigh. She also had neck stiffness with accompanying thoracic back spasms.

Ms. Balaban's primary care physician had evaluated the initial symptoms and then referred her to a rheumatologist and a neurologist. The rheumatologist diagnosed mechanical back pain without evidence of inflammatory arthritis. She had also diagnosed possible migraines with peripheral neuropathic and ocular symptoms. The neurologist noted that Ms. Balaban was also being evaluated by a neurologist and a neuro-ophthalmologist at a nearby medical center. The other neurologist concluded her evaluation with a provisional diagnosis of "atypical migraine variant," noting that "the patient seemed to also have a significant degree of depression, which might be aggravating the symptoms or even be an underlying precipitating factor." A review of tests done at the two medical centers indicated that Ms. Balaban had received the following essentially normal tests: two electroencephalograms, an electromyogram, three brain and three spinal magnetic resonance images, two lumbar puncture studies, and serial laboratory exams. Psychiatric consultation had been recommended, but the patient declined until repeatedly urged by her primary care physician.

Ms. Balaban initially spoke to the psychiatrist primarily about her physical complaints. She was very frustrated that despite having seen several specialists, she had received no clear diagnosis, and she was still very concerned about her symptoms. She had started taking fluoxetine and gabapentin, prescribed by her primary care physician, and experienced partial improvement in her mood and some of her pains. She found it difficult to concentrate and complete her work and was spending a lot of time on the internet researching her symptoms. For the past several months, she had kept a spreadsheet that tried to link her symptoms to her blood pressure and pulse.

She also felt bad about not spending enough time with her children or husband, but just did not have the energy. She acknowledged bouts of depressed mood over the prior year with some anhedonia and occasional thoughts of suicide (she had considered crashing her car), but no anorexia or guilt. She described having experienced premenstrual depressive symptoms for about a year.

Ms. Balaban had been treated for postpartum depression 6 years earlier after the birth of her second child. Family history was significant for cancer, depression, and hypertension.

Ms. Balaban lived with her husband and their daughters, ages 10 and 6 years. Her husband was being treated for depression. The patient had graduated from college and was the longtime administrative assistant to a dean at the local university. She grew up in a small town in a rural area. She reported a happy childhood and denied any experiences of physical or sexual abuse. There was no history of a substance use disorder.

On mental status examination, the patient was alert, casually but neatly dressed, cooperative, and not at all defensive. Her mood and affect were depressed, and she demonstrated psychomotor retardation. There were no abnormalities of thought process or content, no abnormalities of perception, and no evident cognitive dysfunction.

Discussion

Ms. Balaban devotes an inordinate amount of time and energy to thinking about, documenting, and seeking care for her physical symptoms. Those symptoms are distressing to her and interfere with her ability to function. She has been symptomatic at least 6 months. She meets criteria for DSM-5 somatic symptom disorder (SSD).

SSD was a new diagnosis in DSM-5 and reflects significant change from earlier classification systems. SSD symptoms can begin at any age, although the excess concern about somatic symptoms should generally persist at least 6 months. DSM-5 also emphasizes the importance of abnormal thoughts, feelings, and behaviors in response to the somatic symptoms, rather than whether there is a medical cause for the physical symptoms.

Ms. Balaban's large number of seemingly unrelated physical symptoms do suggest a psychiatric condition. It is possible that she has undiagnosed medical conditions that could account for some of her symptoms (e.g., restless legs syndrome, hypothyroidism), but it is difficult to conceive of a single diagnosis that could account for all of them. However, identifying a medical explanation for her symptoms would not preclude diagnosing SSD. She would still probably be viewed as having disproportionate and persistent thoughts, feelings, or behaviors related to her symptoms and health concerns. In other words, the core issue in SSD is not the specific somatic symptoms or their etiology, but rather the patient's emotional, cognitive, and behavioral response to the symptoms.

One ramification of this shift from the DSM-IV to the DSM-5 diagnosis is that the latter is not grounded in the *absence* of an explanation. The effort to prove that the patient lacks a pertinent medical diagnosis can lead to excessive testing, as seen in Ms. Balaban's situation. In addition, extensive negative testing can lead to an adversarial situation, in which the physician states or implies that there is nothing wrong with the patient. Such testing is counterproductive, as it reinforces the patient's belief that there is an as-yet-undiscovered explanation, leading the patient to press for still more testing and referrals. This tends to lead to further testing and/or "doctor shopping" and additional strain on the doctor-patient relationship. When a psychiatric diagnostic label is eventually attached after the multiple evaluations and testing, the patient is likely to view the diagnosis as pejorative or demeaning and to feel dismissed. If properly explained, a diagnosis of SSD should sidestep this conflict. Patients with SSD generally do have medical problems, but the psychiatric focus becomes the ways their thoughts, feelings, and behaviors have developed in response to their physical complaints.

Ms. Balaban has many of the cognitive features typically found in SSD, including excessive attention to physical symptoms, attribution of normal bodily sensations to a pathological cause, catastrophizing about illness, a self-concept of having a weak body, very low tolerance of pain and other somatic complaints, and fear that normal physical activity will damage her body.

She also has characteristic emotional features of SSD, including health anxiety, negative affectivity, desperation, and demoralization. Her keeping a spreadsheet of her symptoms, blood pressure, and heart rate is a typical behavioral feature of SSD, as are her repeated efforts to seek medical care and reassurance, her excessive internet searches, and her avoidance of normal physical activity.

DSM-5-TR™ Clinical Cases

Patients who present with excessive physical complaints often have additional psychiatric diagnoses from outside the somatic symptom and related disorders category. Although Ms. Balaban does not appear to meet full criteria for the diagnosis of major depressive disorder, she has prominent depressive symptoms, including some suicidal ideation. She also has a history of postpartum depression requiring psychiatric care. This history brings up the possibility of undiagnosed bipolar disorder as well as a possible depressive disorder diagnosis. Ms. Balaban also has a history of binge-eating disorder that should not be neglected. Further evaluation of Ms. Balaban would focus on exploring current and past depression, mania, and hypomania as well as considering possible eating, sleep, and opioid use disorders.

Diagnosis

• Somatic symptom disorder

Suggested Readings

Löwe B, Levenson J, Depping M, et al: Somatic symptom disorder: a scoping review on the empirical evidence of a new diagnosis. Psychol Med 52(4):1–17, 2021
Newby JM, Hobbs MJ, Mahoney AEJ, et al: DSM-5 illness anxiety disorder and somatic symptom disorder: comorbidity, correlates, and overlap with DSM-IV hypochondriasis. J Psychosom Res 101:31–37, 2017
Rief W, Martin A: How to use the new DSM-5 somatic symptom disorder diagnosis in research and practice: a critical evaluation and a proposal for modifications. Annu Rev Clin Psychol 10:339–367, 2014

CASE 9.3

Chronic Lyme Disease

Robert Boland, M.D.

Oscar Capek, a 43-year-old man, was brought by his wife to an emergency room (ER) for what he described as a relapse of his chronic Lyme disease. He explained that he had been fatigued for a month and bedridden for a week. Then, saying he was too tired and confused to give much information, he asked the ER team to call his psychiatrist.

The psychiatrist reported that he had treated Mr. Capek for more than two decades. He first saw Mr. Capek for a panic attack. It resolved with surprisingly small doses of clonazepam. After that, however, Mr. Capek continued to see him for help coping with his chronic illness. Initially a graduate student pursuing a master's degree in accounting, Mr. Capek dropped out of school over worries that the demands of his studies would exacerbate his disease. Since that time, his wife, a registered nurse, had been his primary support. He supplemented their income with small accounting jobs but limited these lest the stress affect his health.

Mr. Capek usually felt physically and emotionally well. He deemed his occasional fatigue, anxiety, and concentration difficulties "controllable" and did not require treatment. Mr. Capek was typically averse to psychotropic medications and took a homeopathic approach to his disease, including exercise and proper nutrition. When his panic symptoms would reemerge, he used small doses (e.g., one-quarter of a 0.5-mg lorazepam pill). His psychiatric sessions were commonly concerned about his underlying disease; he often brought articles on chronic Lyme disease for discussion and was active in a local Lyme disease support group.

Mr. Capek's symptoms would occasionally worsen. However, these worsenings occurred less than yearly, and these "exacerbations" usually related to some apparent stress. The worst episode had been 1 year earlier, when his wife briefly left him following his revelation of an affair. Mr. Capek expressed shame about his behavior toward his wife—both the affair and his inability to support her. He subsequently cut off contact with the other woman and attempted to expand his accounting work. The psychiatrist speculated that similar stress was behind his current symptoms.

The psychiatrist communicated regularly with Mr. Capek's internist. His Lyme disease tests had thus far been negative. When the internist reported this, Mr. Capek became defensive and produced literature on the inaccuracy of Lyme disease testing. Eventually, the internist and the psychiatrist agreed on a conservative treatment approach with a neutral stance regarding the disease's validity.

On examination, Mr. Capek was a healthy, well-developed adult male. He was anxious and spoke quietly with his eyes closed. He frequently lost his train of thought, but with encouragement and patience, he could give a detailed history consistent with the psychiatrist's account. Physical examination findings were unremarkable, and a standard laboratory screen was normal except for a slightly low hemoglobin value. The medical team chose to defer further Lyme testing, given the patient's many past negative tests. However, on hearing about the low hemoglobin, Mr. Capek became alarmed, dismissed reassurances, and insisted that the team investigate this further.

Discussion

Mr. Capek insists that he has a disabling disease despite more plausible explanations. His insistence is undeterred by negative testing and contributes to chronic health anxieties and poor functioning. Previous systems of categorization, including DSM-IV, would have considered Mr. Capek to have "hypochondriasis," but DSM-5 took a different approach.

DSM-5 dropped the diagnosis of hypochondriasis, in part because it had a pejorative connotation that was not conducive to an effective doctor-patient relationship.

Also, the diagnosis tended to encourage an excessive effort to "prove a negative." Patients who, in the past, would have been diagnosed with hypochondriasis are now usually diagnosed with one of two DSM-5 disorders: somatic symptom disorder (SSD) or illness anxiety disorder (IAD). DSM-5 suggests that most patients previously diagnosed with hypochondriasis will now be diagnosed with SSD, with only about one-quarter to one-third of that group being diagnosed with IAD.

The DSM-5 authors intended IAD to describe patients with a conviction that they have a severe illness, coupled with prominent health anxieties and excessive health-related behaviors or maladaptive avoidance. Physical symptoms in IAD are either completely absent or only mild in intensity. In contrast, SSD features an excessive or maladaptive response to somatic symptoms.

Mr. Capek's symptoms appear to fit IAD best. Although he does have occasional symptoms, he usually feels healthy; the chief problem is that Mr. Capek believes he has an underlying disease and has organized his life to avoid triggering it. Moreover, his behavior toward the likely insignificant hemoglobin test demonstrates his hypersensitivity toward any indication of worsening health. This maladaptive approach to his assumed illness, along with his preoccupation with the disease, appears to be his central pathology.

As with any diagnosis—and especially those under the umbrella of somatic symptom and related disorders—there are many essential rule-outs. Most important to eliminate is the possibility of a yet-undiscovered medical illness. Even if Lyme disease is unlikely, there are several recognized albeit ill-defined syndromes—including chronic fatigue, immune dysfunction syndrome, and fibromyalgia—that, although easily overlooked, seem to characterize a subset of patients who do not easily fit into alternative categories. The psychiatrist needs to consider undiagnosed medical illnesses and not move too quickly to an SSD diagnosis, because once a physician attributes the patient's symptoms to a psychiatric diagnosis, the medical workup tends to cease. In this case, the availability of an extended medical and psychiatric history increases diagnostic confidence.

Multiple psychiatric diagnoses are possible. Mr. Capek has a history of recurrent, problematic panic attacks, and so he likely meets criteria for panic disorder. Comorbid psychiatric disorders are common in IAD, and approximately two-thirds of individuals with the disorder will have another mental disorder, most commonly generalized anxiety disorder, panic disorder, obsessive-compulsive disorder (OCD), or a depressive disorder. A single interview would likely be insufficient to identify IAD co-occurring with another acute mental illness, given that many mental disorders can initially present with primarily somatic symptoms. Recognition of co-occurring psychiatric disorders often takes time, tact, and a thorough psychiatric history.

Mr. Capek's illness worry persists despite the lack of supporting evidence, which brings up the possibility that he is psychotic. Admittedly, it can be difficult to judge where somatic preoccupation ends and a delusion begins. However, Mr. Capek's ideas do not attain the rigidity and intensity seen in the somatic delusions that are part of delusional disorder, schizophrenia, and major depressive disorder with psychotic features; furthermore, his illness concern is plausible and lacks the bizarre quality generally found in delusions. In reminding his doctor that a Lyme test is not perfect, Mr. Capek is not irrational but instead is merely overvaluing an unlikely explanation.

It is not inappropriate to consider disorders of falsification, such as factitious disorder or malingering, in the differential. However, experience with this patient suggests that Mr. Capek's illness worry is distressing and disabling for him. Thus, any short-term benefit he has gained from not working seems greatly outweighed by the disabling nature of his symptoms.

Also, DSM-5 reminds us that cultural and social norms can play a role in a person's response to distressing symptoms, as many cultures devalue psychological suffering, seeing only physical suffering as being "worthy" of medical attention. Although Mr. Capek never discussed his Central European heritage in detail, it could also affect how his family reacted to his symptoms.

A key diagnostic issue is whether Mr. Capek is best conceptualized with IAD or OCD. Mr. Capek does appear "obsessional," but his focus is on health concerns. He does not have other symptoms often found in OCD, such as fears of contamination. IAD is therefore a better diagnostic fit than OCD.

Especially useful in confirming the presence of an IAD (and excluding multiple other potential psychiatric diagnoses) is the collateral information obtained from a psychiatrist who has known Mr. Capek for decades.

Historically, a diagnosis within the somatoform or somatic disorders cluster would require some assessment of potential rationales behind the disorder (i.e., the gains that result from the debility). DSM-5 dropped this criterion because of its subjectivity. Nevertheless, in conceptualizing Mr. Capek's situation, it is difficult not to consider the reinforcing role of certain types of secondary gain. Although the patient is suffering from his disorder, it has relieved him from many responsibilities and provides a potential excuse for inappropriate behaviors. Undermining these reinforcing factors must be a part of any meaningful treatment. As DSM-5 reminds us, medical iatrogenesis can also contribute to a disorder, as overzealous providers may reinforce the sick role with excessive referrals and diagnostic testing. The psychiatrist can play a vital role by helping to reduce this reinforcement and by encouraging the patient and the medical team to pursue a conservative, nonjudgmental approach.

Diagnoses

- Illness anxiety disorder, care-seeking type
- Panic disorder

Suggested Readings

Rachman S: Health anxiety disorders: a cognitive construal. Behav Res Ther 50(7–8):502–512, 2012

Scarella TM, Boland RJ, Barsky AJ: Illness anxiety disorder: psychopathology, epidemiology, clinical characteristics, and treatment. Psychosom Med 81(5):398–407, 2019

Sirri L, Grandi S: Illness behavior. Adv Psychosom Med 32:160–181, 2012

CASE 9.4

Seizures

Jason P. Caplan, M.D.
Theodore A. Stern, M.D.

Paulina Delcampo, a 32-year-old single woman with epilepsy that was first diagnosed during adolescence, was admitted to an academic medical center after her family found her convulsing in her bedroom. Before she was taken to the emergency room (ER), emergency medical services administered several doses of lorazepam, with no change in her condition. On arrival at the ER, a loading dose of fosphenytoin was administered to her; it stopped the convulsive activity. Blood tests obtained in the ER revealed therapeutic levels of her usual antiepileptics and no evidence of any infection or metabolic disturbance. Urine toxicology screens were negative for the use of illicit substances. Ms. Delcampo was admitted to the neurology service for further monitoring.

During her admission, a routine electroencephalogram (EEG) was ordered. Shortly after the study began, Ms. Delcampo began convulsing; this prompted administration of intravenous (IV) lorazepam. When the EEG was reviewed, no epileptiform activity was identified. Ms. Delcampo was placed on video-EEG (vEEG) monitoring, and her antiepileptics were tapered and discontinued. In the course of her monitoring, Ms. Delcampo had several episodes of convulsive motor activity; however, none was associated with epileptiform activity on the EEG. Psychiatric consultation was requested.

On interview, Ms. Delcampo denied prior psychiatric evaluations, diagnoses, or treatments. She denied having depressed mood or any disturbance of sleep, energy, concentration, or appetite. She reported no thoughts of harming herself or others. She endorsed no signs or symptoms consistent with mania or psychosis. There was no family history of psychiatric illness or substance abuse. Her examination revealed a well-groomed woman, sitting on her hospital bed with EEG leads in place. She was pleasant and engaged, and she made good eye contact. Cognitive testing revealed no deficits.

Ms. Delcampo noted that she had recently moved to the state to begin graduate school; she was excited about starting her studies and "finally getting my career on track." She denied any recent specific psychosocial stressors other than her move and said, "My life is finally where I want it to be." She was future oriented and concerned about the impact that her seizures might have on her long-term health. She was worried that a protracted hospitalization might cause her to miss the first day of classes (only a week away from the time of the interview). Moreover, she was quite concerned about the costs of her hospitalization because her health insurance coverage did not begin until the school semester commenced and the payment for extended benefits coverage from her previous employer would have a significant impact on her budget.

When the findings of the vEEG study were discussed with Ms. Delcampo, she quickly became quite irritable, asking, "So, everyone thinks I'm just making this up?" She was not calmed by her treaters' attempts to clarify that they did not believe her to be faking her symptoms or by their reassurance that her symptoms might be helped by structured therapy. Ms. Delcampo pulled her EEG leads from her scalp, dressed herself, and left the hospital against medical advice.

Discussion

In DSM-5-TR, the diagnosis of functional neurological symptom disorder (formerly conversion disorder) describes a syndrome of one or more symptoms of altered sensory or motor function that cause significant distress or impairment of function and that cannot be accounted for by a recognized medical or neurological condition. As seen in DSM-5, the historical criterion requiring identification of stressors, conflicts, or other psychological factors believed to precipitate or exacerbate the presenting symptoms is no longer required for the diagnosis. DSM-5-TR allows for further diagnostic clarification by including seven specifiers to characterize the medically unexplained presenting symptoms, along with a specifier for mixed symptoms. DSM-5-TR also includes specifiers for the duration of symptoms: acute (less than 6 months) and persistent (more than 6 months).

The differential diagnosis of patients presenting with medically unexplained symptoms is lengthy. Presentations marked by significant worry or by behaviors prompted by the perception of illness or symptoms may be due to a somatic symptom disorder or illness anxiety disorder. If the patient may be deliberately producing symptoms, the differential diagnosis includes factitious disorder and malingering.

Ms. Delcampo presents with chronic convulsive episodes that are not associated with epileptiform EEG findings. Although it is not uncommon for a patient with nonepileptic seizures (NES) to also be diagnosed with epileptic seizures (most experts agree that the prevalence of comorbid NES in epilepsy is about 10%), most patients found to have NES do not need ongoing treatment with antiepileptic medications. Likely due to the dramatic nature of the presentation and the costs involved in hospital care, the NES variant of functional neurological symptom disorder garners much of the attention in the professional literature, although this condition accounts for only around one-fourth of all functional neurological symptom disorder presentations. Despite the fact that even recent editions of textbooks have made reference to the phenomenon of *la belle indifférence* (i.e., an apparent lack of concern exhibited by the patient regarding his or her symptoms) as being indicative of a functional neurological symptom disorder diagnosis, available evidence does not support the use of this symptom in discriminating between primary neurological and functional illness.

If functional neurological symptom disorder is diagnosed, clinicians should be aware of the common co-occurring findings of depression, chronic pain disorders, fatigue, and a history of abuse.

There is also increasing evidence for a variety of biomarkers in individuals with functional neurological symptom disorder. Although patients may become angry upon learning of a diagnosis of functional neurological symptom disorder, the discussion should focus on the good news: 1) they will not be exposed to unnecessary medications or studies, and 2) treatment, in the form of structured therapy, is available.

Diagnosis

- Functional neurological symptom disorder (conversion disorder) with attacks or seizures, persistent

Suggested Readings

Asadi-Pooya AA: Incidence and prevalence of psychogenic nonepileptic seizures (functional seizures): a systematic review and an analytical study. Int J Neurosci Jun 28, 2021:1–6 [online ahead of print]

Jones LL, Rickards H: History of abuse and psychogenic nonepileptic seizures: a systematic review. Seizure 92:200–204, 2021

Perez DL, Matin N, Williams B, et al: Cortical thickness alterations linked to somatoform and psychological dissociation in functional neurological disorders. Hum Brain Mapp 39(1):428–439, 2018

CASE 9.5

Abdominal Pain

Joseph F. Murray, M.D.

A hospital-based psychiatric consultation-liaison service was called to assess possible depression in Rebecca Ehrlich, a 24-year-old woman who had been hospitalized 2 days earlier for severe abdominal pain. She had been admitted through the emergency room for the latest flare-up of her underlying Crohn's disease. The consultation was called after the nurses became concerned that she was sad and lonely and was having a difficult time adjusting to her medical condition.

Ms. Ehrlich was interviewed by the medical student on the psychiatry service. The patient indicated that the pain was excruciating and that she was neither sad nor lonely but was simply visiting from out of town, so no one knew she was even in the hospital. She told the medical student that her only previous therapy had been in college, when she went to student health services to get help for anxiety about test taking and her career choice. She had successfully completed a short course of cognitive-behavioral therapy, and the anxiety had not reappeared. She denied any other psychiatric history and had never taken psychiatric medication. In college, she studied psychology and worked part-time as a hospital orderly. Ms. Ehrlich had considered a career in medicine or nursing and asked the student how he had decided to go to medical school.

Ms. Ehrlich reported that she had previously worked regularly and had "quite a few friends," but that the recurrent abdominal pain had wrecked her social life and her job prospects. She had lost a job the year before because of absenteeism and had missed several job interviews due to her Crohn's flares. She had dated as a teenager but had been in no relationships since starting college. These things "were not the end of the world, but how would you feel?" As a member of an online bowel disorders support group, Ms. Ehrlich e-mailed other members on a daily basis. She added that the only person in the family who "got" her was an aunt who also had Crohn's disease.

The primary medical team was having difficulty obtaining collateral information from previous physicians, but the medical student was able to contact Ms. Ehrlich's mother. She did not know the exact names or phone numbers of her daughter's medical providers but did recall some of the hospitals and could recall, approximately, some of the physicians' names. She added that her daughter had not wanted her to be involved in her care and had not told her she was out of town, much less that she was in the hospital. She did say that the Crohn's disease had been diagnosed 2 years earlier, during her daughter's last semester of college. The mother estimated that Ms. Ehrlich had been hospitalized at least six times, in contrast with the daughter's report of two earlier hospitalizations. Neither the gastrointestinal (GI) team nor the medical student was able to locate Ms. Ehrlich's primary gastroenterologist, whose name the patient could spell only phonetically.

On examination, Ms. Ehrlich was cooperative and conversant, and appeared comfortable. Her speech was fluent. She appeared calm and unworried about her upcoming procedures. Her thought process was linear. She denied paranoia, hallucinations, or suicidality. Attention and both recent and remote memory were intact. She acknowledged that it had been difficult living with Crohn's disease, but she was optimistic that her symptoms would improve. She denied depressive symptoms. She looked sad at the beginning of the interview, but she appeared more engaged and euthymic the more she talked. She could not explain why the team was unable to locate her doctor and became irritated when the medical student pressed more specifically to elicit further details about her prior care. She was taken to have an endoscopy and a colonoscopy at the end of the interview.

Ms. Ehrlich's endoscopy and colonoscopy results were normal. That evening, the medical student from psychiatry sat in with the GI team as they reviewed the normal results with the patient. She said she was relieved there was no longer anything seriously wrong with her. The GI team told her that she could be discharged the next morning and that she should have her internist call them. She readily agreed.

After the GI team left, Ms. Ehrlich told the student that she was "feeling better already." She quickly removed her own intravenous line and started to get dressed. The student went to get the primary GI team. When they returned, the patient was gone.

The medical student spent much of the next day calling hospitals and physicians that met descriptions provided by the patient and her mother. That afternoon, one of the physicians called back and indicated that he had treated Ms. Ehrlich 6 months earlier at a hospital near her mother's home. That admission was strikingly similar: after a short hospitalization, she quickly fled from the hospital after a normal colonoscopy.

Discussion

The diagnosis of factitious disorder describes a cluster of behaviors in Ms. Ehrlich that might otherwise have remained confusing. Ms. Ehrlich meets all of the DSM-5 criteria for factitious disorder: she presents herself as ill by falsifying symptoms; there are no obvious rewards to the hospitalization; and there is not an obvious alternative diagnosis such as a psychotic disorder. Although Ms. Ehrlich's inability to verify specific past providers might have been a clue to the possibility of deceit, confirmation of the diagnosis came only after Ms. Ehrlich's discharge, when the intrepid medical student was able to clarify a recurrent pattern of dishonesty.

The motivation for the "falsification" and "deceptive behavior" in factitious disorder is not clear. DSM-5 indicates that the symptoms exist without obvious external rewards. In contrast, DSM-IV described the motivation factor for factitious disorder as the assumption of the sick role. Although Ms. Ehrlich may well have been seeking the care of the members of the hospital staff, there is no way of knowing the sorts of subconscious (and conscious) motivators that might be at play. It does appear, however, that Ms. Ehrlich has factitious disorder rather than malingering, a diagnosis that is also notable for conscious symptom production. Malingering differs from factitious disorder in that the former is motivated by concrete factors such as money, housing, and substances of abuse. In practice, there may be multiple and shifting motives in any single case. For example, Ms. Ehrlich might have been subconsciously motivated by taking on the sick role but might also have enjoyed the ready access to intravenous opiates.

Subjective complaints such as psychiatric symptoms and pain are easier to feign. Patients with factitious disorder may claim depression, for example, following the death of a loved one who has not died. They may add blood to a urine sample, ingest insulin or warfarin, inject fecal matter, or claim to have had a seizure. It is very easy to learn how to mimic diseases. Ms. Ehrlich could have learned about Crohn's disease from her aunt, from her work as an orderly, from a support group, or from an internet search. Indeed, some patients with factitious disorders might share their medical stories with others online (or even in person) without necessarily engaging medical providers.

It is not surprising that clinicians frequently have a strong negative countertransference to a patient who falsifies symptoms. Such patients exploit clinicians' desire to care for the sick by pretending to be ill. It is incumbent on all providers to remember that patients with factitious disorder *are* quite ill, but not in the way they pretend.

Medical illness presents in many ways, and it is obviously important to explore a range of possible diagnoses. On the other hand, the possibility of deceit—whatever the patient's underlying motivation—should lead health professionals to pay attention when symptoms are not making sense. Overly extensive and sometimes risky tests and procedures can be an iatrogenic consequence of medical diligence. Given that up to 1% of the hospitalized population is estimated to have factitious disorder, one need not be a cynic to include it in the differential diagnosis.

Diagnosis

• Factitious disorder, recurrent episodes

Suggested Readings

Bass C, Wade DT: Malingering and factitious disorder. Pract Neurol 19(2):96–105, 2019

Pulman A, Taylor J: Munchausen by internet: current research and future directions. J Med Internet Res 14(4):e115, 2012

Yates GP, Feldman MD: Factitious disorder: a systematic review of 455 cases in the professional literature. Gen Hosp Psychiatry 41:20–28, 2016

CASE 9.6

Breathlessness

Janna Gordon Elliott, M.D.

Sofia Fredholm was a 22-year-old woman with cystic fibrosis who was brought to the hospital with symptoms of respiratory distress. On the fourth day of her hospitalization, the intensive care unit called a psychiatric consultation for "noncompliance with treatment." The patient was refusing nebulizer treatments and noninvasive ventilation, and was consistently found to be hypoxic and hypercarbic. The patient told the psychiatrist that she could not tolerate wearing a mask on her face for nebulizer administration or ventilation because it made her "really anxious" and, she said, it caused her to feel more short of breath. She had been sleeping poorly and waking frequently with breathlessness and panic. She described feeling worried that she was getting sicker the longer she stayed in the hospital and she wanted to go home. When she asked her providers for help, she reported, all they would do was ask her to "put her mask back on."

In gathering a history, the consultant learned that Ms. Fredholm had grown up with her parents and two older healthy siblings in a town outside of the large city where this hospital was located. Her mother, originally from Puerto Rico, was a school nurse, and had taken on primary responsibility for Ms. Fredholm's medical care, including administering her daily pulmonary treatments. She referred to this, when Ms. Fredholm was a child, as their "playtime"; she would sing songs and tell her stories. As she grew up, Ms. Fredholm sometimes resisted her mother's help, telling her parents she wanted to be "out like a normal kid," although she would regularly decline invitations to parties and sleepovers at the last minute and stay home, saying she was having trouble breathing. From reviewing the chart, the consultant noted an elevated carbon dioxide level, and doses of a β-agonist for bronchodilation prior to her antibiotics, which were all given by nebulizer.

During the psychiatric interview, Ms. Fredholm was continuously adjusting her oxygen face mask, taking it off for a few minutes, and then stopping to say she was too short of breath to continue talking. She was breathing fast and appeared tremulous and distractible. She repeatedly glanced through the open door of her room and wondered aloud when her mother would be getting back from lunch in the cafeteria. She and her mother, she said, knew how to manage her symptoms better than the doctors did. At home, she was able to use her face mask or mouthpiece for saline nebulizer treatments without any problem. She also found it helpful to breathe over an herbal steam bath her mother would prepare. She was sure she would feel better in a couple of days, adding "they are just making me more anxious by not listening to me."

Later that night, because of rising carbon dioxide levels, Ms. Fredholm was intubated.

Discussion

The case of Ms. Fredholm illustrates how physiological and psychological factors interact in complex ways to influence symptoms, emotions, behaviors, and the delivery and outcome of medical treatment. On a surface level, we see Ms. Fredholm resisting or delaying elements of her treatment, followed by suboptimal management and a negative result (intubation). With further inspection, we can identify more details that clarify why we are in this situation and, perhaps, what to do to improve it. Her behavior seems to be related to mood states (i.e., anxiety) and emotionally laden beliefs (i.e., that others cannot care for her as well as she and her mother can) that each affect how she makes and communicates choices, and how she and her medical team interact. The responses to anxiety—voluntary ones, such as removing constricting ventilatory devices that increase the subjective feeling of dyspnea, and involuntary ones, like increasing rate of ventilation and autonomic activation—may exacerbate the experience of anxiety, while also worsening her physiological status. The physiological changes may similarly contribute to more impulsive decision-making or behaviors. The addition of the pretreatment β-agonist may also increase sympathetic arousal, and the sense of anxiety. At home, she is able to tolerate her treatments, and thus benefit from them, whereas here in the hospital, the cycle described above does not allow her to utilize the offered treatments enough to benefit from them; in fact, she is feeling even worse. This experience—which may be like many she's had before, given the chronicity and severity of her illness—feels counterproductive to her and reinforces the belief that she is better off at home than in the hospital.

The DSM-5 diagnosis of psychological factors affecting other medical conditions (PFAOMC) describes a cluster of patients who have a medical problem that is adversely affected by psychological or behavioral factors. These factors include psychological distress, patterns of interpersonal interaction, coping styles, and maladaptive coping strategies such as denial of symptoms and poor adherence to medications, diagnostic tests, and treatments. The diagnosis is reserved for situations, like that of Ms. Fredholm, in which the psychological and/or behavioral issues have a direct effect on the course or outcome of the medical condition.

The differential diagnosis for PFAOMC is broad, and will depend on the specific situation. Other somatic symptom disorders, anxiety disorders (including separation anxiety disorder), adjustment disorder, a personality disorder, medical- and substance-related anxiety disorders, or mild delirium might all be considered in the case of Ms. Fredholm.

Somatic symptom disorder (SSD), illness anxiety disorder (IAD), and factitious disorder also present with a blurring of psychological and physical signs and symptoms and commonly leave the clinician with the impression that the patient's medical issues are in some way related to underlying emotional issues. In contrast to PFAOMC, SSD and IAD focus on situations in which the perception of—or fear of—physical symptoms or illness influences emotions and behavior, rather than the reverse. People with factitious disorder induce medical complications by their behavior, but theirs is a conscious effort at deception.

Many psychiatric conditions—including substance use disorders, substance-induced disorders, and psychotic, mood, and anxiety disorders—are associated with behaviors that can worsen a co-occurring medical condition. In such cases, the other psychiatric condition should generally be noted rather than PFAOMC. In other situations, the diagnosis of PFAOMC can be useful to include, even for a patient with another relevant psychiatric diagnosis. For example, individuals with rigid, manipulative, or otherwise "difficult" personalities frequently have problematic responses to medical illness, often with deleterious effects on their medical care. These patients are well described by the diagnosis of PFAOMC, often in addition to a diagnosis reflecting their maladaptive character traits, such as a personality disorder. Making use of the PFAOMC diagnosis focuses clinical attention on ways in which personality traits might contribute to the *current* clinical problem and suggests interventions that might help to facilitate more effective treatment.

The diagnoses of anxiety disorder due to another medical condition, depressive disorder due to another medical condition, and substance-induced anxiety or depressive disorder, in which physiological changes directly cause anxiety and mood symptoms, respectively, may also overlap with PFAOMC. Ms. Fredholm's respiratory issues and the β-agonists she' has received are presumably contributing to her anxiety. In a case like this, it might be useful to frame the situation from both perspectives, articulating how the medical and medication factors may be contributing (and therefore important to address), while emphasizing how these fit into the broader picture of the cycle of emotions, beliefs, behaviors, and physical changes that are leading to a worsening of the patient's medical status.

PFAOMC can also be a useful construct in individuals with insecure attachments or maladaptive coping styles that might stem from a variety of developmental factors, often including the experience of growing up with a chronic illness. Such patients might excessively seek, obstruct, or devalue their care or care providers; by recognizing the diagnosis of PFAOMC, clinicians may develop more of a sense of empathy, alliance, and engagement with a patient who may otherwise be seen as simply "difficult."

Denial of medical illness, too, is commonly seen in clinical settings and can be subsumed under the diagnosis of PFAOMC. Denial may include conscious and unconscious elements; may impact medical care and prognosis substantially; and can take a variety of forms, ranging from complete disavowal of one's medical condition to subtle renunciations of the medical reality (e.g., the skin cancer survivor who regularly "forgets" to apply sunscreen).

Cultural factors may similarly impact the course of medical care. In this case, there is the suggestion that Ms. Fredholm and her mother engage in practices approved or endorsed by a culture of origin—herbal steam baths for shortness of breath, or *fatiga*. For individuals of Latin American descent, there also may be greater reliance on the family for medical decision making (part of the broader value of *familismo*, or familism). At times, there can be an assumption on the part of medical providers that such cultural practices or conventions impede standard Western (allopathic) medical treatment. However, it is more common to find that culture-based practices are used in a way that is complementary to (i.e., used in addition to) the allopathic care. In addition, these practices may improve adherence and engagement, by personalizing and giving context to the overall care of the illness. A patient's use of culture-sanctioned practices, even in situations where their use delays or impedes aspects of the medical treatment plan or impacts outcome, should not be used to support a diagnosis of PFAOMC.

PFAOMC is an unusually heterogeneous diagnostic category. Nevertheless, by making explicit a situation in which psychological and behavioral factors are negatively affecting a medical condition, the diagnosis can allow for more effective patient care.

Diagnosis

- Psychological factors affecting other medical conditions

Suggested Readings

Compas BE, Jaser SS, Dunn MJ, Rodriguez EM: Coping with chronic illness in childhood and adolescence. Annu Rev Clin Psychol 8:455–480, 2012

Groves MS, Muskin PR: Psychological responses to illness, in The American Psychiatric Publishing Textbook of Psychosomatic Medicine and Consultation-Liaison Psychiatry, 3rd Edition. Edited by Levenson JL. Washington, DC, American Psychiatric Association Publishing, 2019, pp 53–82

Juckett G: Caring for Latino patients. Am Fam Physician 87(1):48–54, 2013

National Center for Complementary and Integrative Health, National Institute of Health: Complementary, Alternative or Integrative Health: What's in a Name? (Fact Sheet). April 2021. Available at: https://www.nccih.nih.gov/health/complementary-alternative-or-integrative-health-whats-in-a-name. Accessed July 4, 2022.

Stanton AL, Revenson TA, Tennen H: Health psychology: psychological adjustment to chronic disease. Annu Rev Psychol 58:565–592, 2007

CHAPTER 10

Feeding and Eating Disorders

INTRODUCTION

John W. Barnhill, M.D.

Until the publication of DSM-5, half of the people in eating disorder specialty clinics did not meet criteria for either of the two specific eating disorder categories—anorexia nervosa or bulimia nervosa—and instead received the nonspecific diagnosis of eating disorder not otherwise specified (EDNOS). This percentage swelled even further in general psychiatric outpatient settings. A large percentage of patients with impairment and distress related to eating problems were left, therefore, without a diagnosis that specifically described their condition.

DSM-5 made multiple changes to help subdivide the eating disorder population into coherent and evidence-based subgroups. For example, binge-eating disorder (BED) was moved out of DSM-IV Appendix B ("Criteria Sets and Axes Provided for Further Study") and into the main body of the DSM-5 text. The criteria for anorexia nervosa (AN) remained conceptually unchanged but were expanded in two ways. First, the requirement for amenorrhea was eliminated. Second, a previous core AN criterion, the expressed fear of weight gain, is not always present in people who appear to display robust symptoms of AN; in order to remedy this quandary, DSM-5 added an alternative to the "expressed fear" criterion: the individual may manifest persistent behavior that interferes with weight gain. This alternative criterion allows the diagnosis of people whose behavior is indicative of AN but who have impaired insight, suboptimal levels of cooperation or transparency, or alternative rationales for food restriction. Bulimia nervosa (BN) also stayed conceptually the same in DSM-5, but the threshold for diagnosis was lowered by reducing the frequency of binge eating and compensatory behavior from twice to once weekly.

The diagnosis avoidant/restrictive food intake disorder (ARFID) was introduced in DSM-5 to describe people who restrict or avoid food in a way that leads to significant impairment but who do not meet criteria for AN. A broad and inclusive category, ARFID includes individuals who previously met criteria for the DSM-IV diagnosis feeding disorder of infancy or early childhood. ARFID describes a cluster of patients who are generally children and adolescents but who can be any age.

By adding BED to the main text, reducing the threshold for a diagnosis of AN and BN, and creating the ARFID diagnosis, DSM-5 intended to more clearly describe subpopulations of patients who would previously have been recognized as having an eating disorder causing impairment but would have been characterized within the uninformative category of EDNOS. Furthermore, evidence indicates that individuals who meet the more flexible criteria are, in meaningful ways, similar to those who meet the older criteria. Controversy centers on whether this expansion of the criteria for eating disorder diagnoses might "pathologize" people who do not have actual problems with eating. As is the case throughout DSM-5, diagnostic criteria require the presence of significant distress and/or impairment. Individuals within a normal range of eating behaviors should not receive a diagnosis.

Many patients with clinically relevant eating problems do not meet full criteria for a specific eating disorder. For example, an individual may meet all criteria for AN—including significant weight loss—but remain at a normal or above-normal weight. Such a presentation would warrant a diagnosis of specific eating disorder (atypical anorexia nervosa). Other specific eating disorders include bulimia or binge eating of low frequency or duration; purging without binge eating; and night eating syndrome. Finally, the diagnosis "unspecified feeding or eating disorder" is intended to describe individuals who have an apparent eating disorder but do not meet full criteria for a specific disorder, perhaps because of an inadequate amount of confirmatory information (e.g., in an emergency room setting).

Pica refers to the persistent, clinically significant eating of nonnutritive, nonfood substances. Pica is often identified in adults with intellectual development disorder as well as in typically developing children. Worldwide surveys indicate that 30% of pregnant women ingest nonnutritive substances such as ice and clay; food insecurity and vitamin deficiency appear to increase the risk for pica in these pregnant women.

Rumination disorder refers to the recurrent regurgitation of food, which can be seen in infants as well as throughout the life cycle. Pica and rumination disorder can be diagnosed with comorbid psychiatric conditions such as autism spectrum disorder, intellectual developmental disorder, and schizophrenia, as long as the eating disorder reaches a threshold of clinical significance.

Notably, DSM-5 clarifies a hierarchy of diagnoses so that only a single feeding or eating disorder diagnosis can be made for any particular individual (with the exception that pica can be comorbid with any other feeding or eating disorder). The overall eating disorder hierarchy is AN, BN, ARFID, BED, and rumination disorder. In other words, anorexia nervosa takes precedence over the others, and if AN is diagnosed, the individual cannot also have, for example, binge-eating disorder.

DSM-5-TR™ Clinical Cases

Suggested Readings

Fawcett EJ, Fawcett JM, Mazmanian D: A meta-analysis of the worldwide prevalence of pica during pregnancy and the postpartum period. Int J Gynaecol Obstet 133(3):277–283, 2016

Smith AR, Zuromski KL, Dodd DR: Eating disorders and suicidality: what we know, what we don't know, and suggestions for future research. Curr Opin Psychol 22:63–67, 2018

Zipfel S, Giel KE, Bulik CM, et al: Anorexia nervosa: aetiology, assessment, and treatment. Lancet Psychiatry 2(12):1099–1111, 2015

CASE 10.1

Stomachache

Susan Samuels, M.D.

Thomas, an 8-year-old boy with a mild to moderate intellectual developmental disorder, was brought into the emergency room (ER) by his parents after his abdominal pain of the past several weeks had worsened over the prior 24 hours. His parents reported that he had developed constipation, with only one bowel movement in the past week, and that he had vomited earlier in the day. Teachers at his special education classroom for children with intellectual developmental disorders had written a report earlier in the week indicating that Thomas had been having difficulties since soon after transferring from a similar school in a different state about 4 months earlier. The teachers and parents agreed that Thomas often looked distressed, rocking, crying, and clutching his stomach.

One week earlier, a pediatrician had diagnosed an acute exacerbation of chronic constipation. Use of a recommended over-the-counter laxative was not helpful, and Thomas began to complain of nighttime pain. The discomfort led to a diminished interest in his favorite hobbies, which were video games and sports. Instead, he tended to stay in his room, playing with army men figurines that he had inherited from his grandfather's collection. Aside from episodes of irritability and tearfulness, he was generally doing well in school, both in the classroom and on the playground. When not complaining of stomachaches, Thomas ate well and maintained his position at about the 40th percentile for height and weight on the growth curve.

Thomas's past medical history was significant for constipation and stomachaches, as well as for intermittent headaches. All of these symptoms had worsened several months earlier, after the family moved from a house in semirural Florida into an old walk-up apartment in a large urban city in a different state. He shared a room with his younger brother (age 6 years), the product of a normal, unexpected pregnancy, who was enrolled in a regular education class at the local public school. Thomas said his brother was his "best friend." Thomas was adopted at birth, and nothing was known of his biological parents except that they were teenagers unable to care for the child.

On medical examination in the ER, Thomas was a well-groomed boy sitting on his mother's lap. He was crying and irritable and refused to speak to the examiner. Instead, he would repeat to his parents that his stomach hurt. On physical examination, he was afebrile and had stable vital signs. His physical examination was remarkable only for general abdominal tenderness, although he was difficult to assess because he cried uncontrollably through most of the exam.

An abdominal X ray revealed multiple small metallic particles throughout the gastrointestinal tract, initially suspected to be ingested high-lead paint flakes, as well as three 2-centimeter-long metallic objects in his stomach. A blood lead level was 20 μg/dL (whereas normal level for children is <5 μg/dL). More specific questioning revealed that Thomas, being constipated, often spent long stretches on the toilet by himself. His parents added that although the bathroom was in the process of being renovated, its paint was old and peeling. Consultants decided that the larger foreign bodies in the stomach might not safely pass and could be accounting for the constipation. Endoscopy successfully extricated three antique toy soldiers from Thomas's stomach.

Discussion

Thomas is an 8-year-old child with intellectual developmental disorder who was brought to an ER with abdominal pain, chronic constipation, irritability, and changes in mood and functioning. All of these symptoms followed his move to a new city and school 4 months earlier. The differential diagnosis for such complaints is broad and includes psychiatric causes, but the first priority is to do a thorough medical workup to search for sources of pain that the child might not be able to explain (e.g., ear infections, urinary tract infections).

When abdominal pain and constipation are the chief complaints, an abdominal radiograph generally reveals intestines full of stool. Such a result would prompt a more aggressive bowel regimen, as was recommended the week before by his pediatrician. Thomas's X ray, however, was unusual in that it revealed not only the residue of lead-based paint chips but also three small toy soldiers.

The persistent eating of nonnutritive, nonfood substances is the core feature of pica. To meet DSM-5 criteria, the ingestion must be severe enough to warrant clinical attention. Pica is most commonly comorbid with intellectual developmental disorder and autism spectrum disorder, although it can also be found in other disorders, such as schizophrenia and obsessive-compulsive disorder. As seen in Thomas, there is typically no aversion to food in general, and he continued to maintain his position on the growth chart.

Pica does not refer simply to the mouthing and occasional ingestion of nonfood objects that is common in infants, toddlers, and individuals with developmental delay.

Instead, pica refers to chronic and clinically relevant ingestion of objects such as clay, dirt, string, or cigarette butts. Pica can be extremely dangerous. In Thomas's case, for example, he could have experienced a gastrointestinal perforation from the soldiers. In addition, he was eating lead-based paint as well as the soldiers (which, being his grandfather's, could also have been made of lead). The acute lead exposure likely contributed to his abdominal pain, whereas chronic ingestion could be neurologically catastrophic in this boy who already has intellectual developmental disorder.

In addition to having the abdominal pain, Thomas was isolating himself from his classmates and brother and was irritable and tearful. It is possible that these behaviors are reflections of his pain, but they appear to be signs of psychological stress. The pica itself could also be a sign of stress, especially if it began only after the move from Florida. Psychosocial stressors frequently cause multiple physical symptoms in children, especially in those with intellectual developmental disorder. Thomas might also qualify, therefore, for a diagnosis of adjustment disorder with depressed mood. If his mood changes are determined to be secondary to the toxic levels of lead in his bloodstream, then a more accurate diagnosis might be a substance-induced depressive or anxiety disorder. In the ER setting, however, the clinician would likely defer making depressive, anxiety, or adjustment disorder diagnoses until having a chance to evaluate Thomas when he was not in acute abdominal distress.

Diagnoses

- Pica
- Intellectual developmental disorder, mild to moderate

Suggested Readings

Samsel CB, Walter HJ, DeMaso DR: Rumination and pica, in Nelson Textbook of Pediatrics, 21st Edition. Edited by Kliegman RM, St Geme JW III. Philadelphia, Elsevier, 2019, pp 204–205

Sturmey P, Williams DE: Pica in Individuals with Developmental Disabilities (Autism and Child Psychopathology Series, Matson JL, series editor). Switzerland, Springer International Publishing, 2016

Williams DE, McAdam D: Assessment, behavioral treatment, and prevention of pica: clinical guidelines and recommendations for practitioners. Res Dev Disabil 33(6):2050–2057, 2012

CASE 10.2

Drifting Below the Growth Curve

Eve K. Freidl, M.D.

Evelyn Attia, M.D.

Uma, an 11-year-old girl in a gifted and talented school, was referred to an eating disorder specialist by a child psychiatrist who was concerned that Uma had drifted below the 10th percentile for weight. The psychiatrist had been treating Uma for perfectionistic traits that caused her significant anxiety. Their sessions focused on anxiety, not on eating behavior.

Uma's eating difficulties started at age 9, when she began refusing to eat and reporting a fear that she would vomit. At that time, her parents sought treatment from a pediatrician, who continued to evaluate her yearly, explaining that it was normal for children to go through phases. At age 9, Uma was above the 25th percentile for both height and weight (52 inches, 58 pounds), but by age 11, she had essentially stopped growing and had dropped to the 5th percentile on her growth curves (52.5 inches, 55 pounds).

The only child of two professional parents who had divorced 5 years earlier, Uma lived with her mother on weekdays and with her nearby father on weekends. Her medical history was significant for her premature birth at 34 weeks' gestation. She was slow to achieve her initial milestones but by age 2 was developmentally normal. Yearly physical examinations had been unremarkable with the exception of the recent decline of her growth trajectory. Uma had always been petite, but her height and weight had never fallen below the 25th percentile for stature and weight for age on the growth chart. Uma was a talented student who was well liked by her teachers. She had never had more than a few friends, but recently she had stopped socializing entirely and had been coming directly home after school, reporting that her stomach felt calmer when she was in her own home.

For the prior 2 years, Uma had eaten only very small amounts of food over very long durations of time. Her parents had tried to pique her interest by experimenting with foods from different cultures and of different colors and textures. None of this seemed effective in improving her appetite. They also tried to let her pick restaurants to try, but Uma had gradually refused to eat outside of either parent's home. Both parents reported a similar mealtime pattern: Uma would agree to sit at the table but then spent her time rearranging food on her plate, cutting food items into small pieces, and crying if urged to eat another bite.

When asked more about her fear of vomiting, Uma remembered one incident, at age 4, when she ate soup and her stomach became upset and then she subsequently vomited. More recently, Uma had developed fear of eating in public and ate no food during the school day. She denied any concerns about her appearance and said that she had first become aware of her low weight at her most recent visit to the pediatrician. When educated about the dangers of low body weight, Uma became tearful and expressed a clear desire to gain weight.

Discussion

Uma is an 11-year-old girl whose height and weight have both flattened over the preceding 2 years. Yearly medical exams have been noncontributory, and the cause appears to be that Uma eats very small amounts of food, very slowly. The initial trigger for the food refusal appears to have been a fear of vomiting, but for two years, she has eaten minimally despite a stated interest in gaining weight. She has also stopped socializing, and so the eating problem is having a significant impact on her psychosocial functioning.

In contrast to individuals with anorexia nervosa (AN), Uma does not report any fear of gaining weight or becoming fat and does not deny the seriousness of her current low body weight. Her diagnosis, therefore, is avoidant/restrictive food intake disorder (ARFID), a diagnosis that first appeared in DSM-5.

ARFID is a relatively broad category intended to describe a cluster of people who do not meet criteria for AN but whose avoidance or restriction of food leads to health problems, psychosocial dysfunction, and/or significant weight loss. In the case of children like Uma, the diminished food intake might result in a flattening of the growth trajectory rather than weight loss.

The distinction between ARFID and AN may be uncertain when individuals deny a fear of weight gain but instead offer diverse explanations for food restriction, such as somatic complaints (e.g., abdominal discomfort, fullness, lack of appetite), religious motives, desire for control, or desire for familial impact. Longitudinal assessment may be necessary to clarify the diagnosis, and ARFID may precede AN in some people.

A diagnosis of ARFID is likely to present during childhood or adolescence, but people of any age can have this disorder. Three main subtypes have been described: inadequate overall intake in the presence of an emotional disturbance such that the emotional problem interferes with appetite and eating but the avoidance does not stem from a specific motive; restricted range of food intake (sometimes referred to as "picky eating"); and food avoidance due to a specific fear such as fear of swallowing (functional dysphagia), fear of poisoning, or—as in Uma's case—fear of vomiting.

Uma will not eat in public and has gradually isolated herself from her friends and social situations. Such behavior might be consistent with an anxiety disorder. For example, the fear of vomiting could reflect a specific phobia, and the avoidance of friends might reflect social anxiety disorder. Although any anxiety disorder may be concurrent with an eating disorder, a diagnosis of ARFID is likely a more parsimonious explanation in Uma's case. As outlined in DSM-5-TR, ARFID should be diagnosed in the presence of symptoms compatible with another diagnosis when the severity of the eating disturbance exceeds that routinely associated with the other condition and warrants additional clinical attention.

In Uma's case, a variety of other disorders should also be considered during the evaluation. These include medical, structural, and neurological disorders that can impede eating; obsessive-compulsive disorder; and depressive and anxiety disorders that might have emerged in the context of her parents' divorce and her progression toward puberty. Although any of these might be further explored, none of them seem immediately pertinent to Uma's weight loss.

Diagnosis

• Avoidant/restrictive food intake disorder

Suggested Readings

Bryant-Waugh R, Markham L, Kreipe RE, Walsh BT: Feeding and eating disorders in child-hood. Int J Eat Disord 43(2):98–111, 2010

Katzman DK, Norris ML, Zucker N: Avoidant restrictive food intake disorder. Psychiatr Clin North Am 42(1):45–57, 2019

Strand M, von Hausswolff-Juhlin Y, Welch E: A systematic scoping review of diagnostic valid-ity in avoidant/restrictive food intake disorder. Int J Eat Disord 52(4):331–360, 2019

CASE 10.3

Headaches and Fatigue

Jennifer J. Thomas, Ph.D.

Anne E. Becker, M.D., Ph.D.

Valerie Gaspard was a 20-year-old single woman who had recently immigrated to the United States from West Africa with her family to do missionary work. She presented to her primary care physician complaining of frequent headaches and chronic fatigue. Her physical examination was unremarkable except that her weight was only 78 pounds and her height was 5 feet 1 inch, resulting in a body mass index (BMI) of 14.7 kg/m^2. Ms. Gaspard also reported having missed two menstrual periods in the past 6 months. Unable to find a medical explanation for Ms. Gaspard's symptoms and concerned about her extremely low weight, the physician referred Ms. Gaspard to the hospital eating disorders program.

On presentation for psychiatric evaluation, Ms. Gaspard was cooperative and pleasant. She expressed concern about her low weight and denied fear of weight gain or body image disturbance: "I know I need to gain weight. I'm too skinny," she said. Ms. Gaspard reported that she had weighed 98 pounds prior to moving to the United States 1 year earlier and said she felt "embarrassed" when her family members and even strangers told her she had grown too thin. Notably, everyone else in her U.S.-dwelling extended family was either of normal weight or overweight.

Despite her stated motivation to be at a healthy weight, Ms. Gaspard's dietary recall revealed that she was consuming only 600 calories per day. The day before the evaluation, for example, she had eaten only a small bowl of macaroni pasta, a plate of steamed broccoli, and a cup of black beans. Her fluid intake was also quite limited, typically consisting of only two or three glasses of water daily.

Ms. Gaspard provided multiple reasons for her poor intake. The first was lack of appetite: "My brain doesn't even signal that I'm hungry," she said. "I have no desire to eat throughout the whole day." The second was postprandial bloating and nausea: "I just feel so uncomfortable after eating." The third was the limited choice of foods permitted by her religion, which advocates a vegetarian diet. "My body is not really my own. It is a temple of God," she explained. The fourth reason was that her preferred sources of vegetarian protein (e.g., tofu, processed meat substitutes) were not affordable within her limited household budget. Ms. Gaspard had not completed high school and had a minimum-wage position, working part-time at a clerical job at her church.

Ms. Gaspard denied any other symptoms of disordered eating, including binge eating, purging, or other behaviors intended to promote weight loss. However, in regard to exercise, she reported that she walked for approximately 3–4 hours per day. She denied that her activity was motivated by a desire to burn calories. Instead, Ms. Gaspard stated that because she did not have a car and disliked waiting for the bus, she traveled on foot to all work and leisure activities.

Ms. Gaspard reported no other notable psychiatric symptoms apart from the history of inadequate food intake and excessive physical activity. She appeared euthymic and did not report any symptoms of depression. She denied using alcohol or illicit drugs. She noted that her concentration was poor but expressed hope that a herbal supplement she had just begun taking would improve her memory. When queried about past treatment history, she reported that she had briefly seen a dietitian about 6 months earlier when her family began "nagging" her about her low weight, but she had not viewed the meetings as helpful.

Discussion

Ms. Gaspard presents with headache, fatigue, and a 20-pound weight loss since immigrating to the United States 1 year earlier. Her primary care physician identified a low BMI and irregular menses. As an explanation for eating only 600 calories per day, Ms. Gaspard says that she is generally not hungry, and, when she does eat, she feels bloated and nauseous. Furthermore, she explains that her religion advocates a very healthy diet, and she cannot afford much food. In addition, she describes walking 3–4 hours per day because she cannot afford a car and does not like waiting for the bus. Although she seems to have a plausibly normalizing explanation for the activities that have led to the weight loss, it is notable that no one else in her family (with whom she shares communal resources) is below a normal weight. Aside from reduced intake and excessive exercise, no medical cause was identified that would cause her to fall far below a normal BMI. Her weight loss appears to have significant psychosocial ramifications, but her diagnosis is not immediately clear.

A variety of disorders might be considered. For example, major depressive disorder can be associated with appetite loss. Ms. Gaspard is euthymic, however, and actively engaged in her missionary work.

Avoidant/restrictive food intake disorder (ARFID) might present with weight loss, triggered by gastrointestinal discomfort. However, Ms. Gaspard did not mention a specific fear of vomiting or stomach pain as the primary rationale for food restriction; instead, she noted gastrointestinal discomfort as one of many potential contributors to her limited intake. Ms. Gaspard's complaints of bloating and nausea are common among people who chronically undereat, for whatever reason, and are often associated with delayed gastric emptying or whole-gut transit time.

Does Ms. Gaspard meet criteria for anorexia nervosa (AN)? The first criterion for AN is significantly low weight. Ms. Gaspard's BMI of 14.7 places her below the first BMI centile for U.S. females of her age and height. Furthermore, her BMI is well below the World Health Organization's lower limit of 18.5 kg/m^2 for adults. Her weight is so low that her menses have become irregular.

Ms. Gaspard's low food intake (600 calories per day) and high level of physical activity (3–4 hours per day) are at odds with her stated desire to gain weight, regardless of how earnest her pronouncements may sound. Her lack of follow-through with an earlier dietary intervention and her subsequent presentation to primary care for help in managing the symptoms associated with her dehydration and malnutrition (i.e., headaches, fatigue, poor concentration) suggest that she may not grasp the seriousness of her low weight. Furthermore, Ms. Gaspard's characterization of her family's appropriate concern as "nagging" indicates that she may not truly recognize the health consequences of her significantly low weight.

Moreover, her myriad explanations for her restricted dietary intake (ranging from lack of hunger to forgetfulness to lack of resources) slightly undermine the credibility of each individual rationale. Following Ms. Gaspard over time to ascertain that her behaviors are persistent would help confirm the AN diagnosis.

She specifically acknowledges that she knows she needs to gain weight, however, and there is no evidence that she is consciously losing weight in order to look thinner. Given this information, Ms. Gaspard would not have met DSM-IV criteria for AN because of her lack of fat phobia and her continued (albeit irregular) menses. She does, however, meet the updated DSM-5 criteria for AN. It is important to note that amenorrhea (i.e., lack of menses for 3 months or more) was a DSM-IV criterion for AN but was omitted from DSM-5 because of research suggesting that low-weight eating-disorder patients who menstruate regularly exhibit the same level of psychopathology exhibited by their counterparts who have amenorrhea.

A second criterion for AN is either an intense fear of fatness or persistent behavior that interferes with weight gain despite being at a significantly low weight. Ms. Gaspard's reasons for refusing food are inconsistent with the intense fear of weight gain that DSM-IV characterized as the sine qua non of AN. However, many low-weight patients—especially those from non-Western cultural backgrounds—do not explicitly report weight and shape concerns.

An elevated risk of developing eating disorders following immigration from a non-Western to a Western country has been found among some populations and has been attributed to increased exposure to Western beauty ideals as well as stressors associated with acculturation.

Culture-based differences—encompassing prevailing local norms that govern many aspects of life, including dietary and meal patterns, aesthetic ideals for body shape and weight, embodiment of core cultural symbols and standards for social conduct and behavior, self-agency and self-presentation, and somatic idioms of distress—potentially influence the experience, manifestation, and articulation of eating pathology. For example, a narrative that links restrictive eating behaviors to weight management goals can be easily formulated by a patient whose social context associates prestige with thinness, stigmatizes obesity, and assigns high value to achievement and autonomy.

The determinative cultural underpinnings of conventional AN presentations are perhaps best illustrated in Sing Lee's work from Hong Kong documenting "non-fat-phobic anorexia nervosa," a variant of eating disorder that strongly resembles DSM-IV AN except for its absent fear of weight gain. Lee and colleagues argued that fear of fatness had insufficient cultural salience for many of their patients, who rationalized extreme dietary restriction differently but nonetheless reached a dangerously low weight. Evidence that an absence of fat phobia may be associated with a more benign clinical course raises compelling questions not only about cultural mediation but also about cultural moderation of eating pathology. Globalized commerce and communication have opened avenues for broad exposure to what Sing Lee termed a "culture of modernity," and eating disorders are now recognized as having a broad geographical distribution. The revised DSM-5 diagnosis of AN can now be applied to individuals like Ms. Gaspard who exhibit persistent behavior that interferes with weight gain, even if they do not explicitly endorse fat phobia. Such presentations are widespread, encompassing regions in both the Global South and the Global North and including the United States, where Ms. Gaspard presents for care.

Although she does meet criteria for AN, Ms. Gaspard does not manifest behaviors sometimes found in AN. For example, she does not engage in binge eating (i.e., she denies eating large amounts of food while feeling out of control) or purging (i.e., she denies self-induced vomiting or misuse of enemas, laxatives, diuretics, or other medications). Therefore, her presentation is consistent with the restricting subtype of AN.

Diagnosis

- Anorexia nervosa, restricting type

Suggested Readings

Becker AE, Thomas JJ: Eating pathology in Fiji: phenomenologic diversity, visibility, and vulnerability, in Revisioning Psychiatry: Cultural Phenomenology, Critical Neuroscience, and Global Mental Health. Edited by Kirmayer LJ, Lemelson R, Cummings CA. Cambridge, UK, Cambridge University Press, 2015, pp 515–543

Izquierdo A, Plessow F, Becker KR, et al: Implicit attitudes toward dieting and thinness distinguish fat-phobic and non-fat-phobic anorexia nervosa from avoidant/restrictive food intake disorder in adolescents. Int J Eat Disord 52(4):419–427, 2019

Lee S: Reconsidering the status of anorexia nervosa as a Western culture–bound syndrome. Soc Sci Med 42(1):21–34, 1996

Norris ML, Harrison ME, Isserlin L, et al: Gastrointestinal complications associated with anorexia nervosa: a systematic review. Int J Eat Disord 49(3):216–237, 2016

CASE 10.4

Out of Control

James E. Mitchell, M.D.

Wanda Hoffman was a 24-year-old woman who was referred to a psychiatrist by her internist. She said she felt sad, worthless, and lonely. She reported that she needed to improve her diet and exercise but felt out of control. She added that she had gone to her internist several times in recent months for stomachaches, and he finally insisted that she see a psychiatrist.

Ms. Hoffman had been living alone since her college graduation 2 years earlier. She had recently been promoted in her job as an accountant, and said that she enjoyed her work. She mentioned having some friends from high school and being interested in dating, but she felt too tired and sad to do much besides meet up for a quick dinner after work. She was unable to exercise because of low energy, slept poorly, and frequently had stomachaches. These symptoms and the resulting social dysfunction had caused her to feel increasingly isolated, lonely, and sad. She often found herself feeling worthless and wondering how she was going to get through the week, but she denied suicidal intent or plan.

She said she had accepted the psychiatric referral so that she could get an antidepressant medication, but "it had to be one that didn't cause weight gain. Hopefully, I could get one that would cause weight loss, instead." Ms. Hoffman added that she couldn't get back to her ideal weight despite lots of effort. When asked about the effort, Ms. Hoffman grew quiet but did eventually answer: "I wasn't going to talk about this, but I'm a 'failed anorexic.' I can diet for about half a day, but by dinner, I'm starving, so I eat everything I can find, and then I throw up. It's mortifying."

Ms. Hoffman reported that she had started dieting at about age 13; she noted that, in retrospect, she was "being ridiculous," and that her weight had been fine. She said her downfall really began when she started "stress eating" in college. When she realized she had gained 10 or 15 pounds, she began to routinely skip breakfast. She often skipped lunch as well, but then, famished, she would overeat in the late afternoon and evening.

By the end of her sophomore year, Ms. Hoffman had started inducing vomiting, a practice she learned about in a magazine. She had developed her current eating pattern during her junior year and continued it after graduation: no breakfast; a "light" lunch; an "average" dinner, often with friends; and then she'd rush back to her apartment for a second dinner and a pint or two of ice cream, followed by self-induced vomiting.

Discussion

Ms. Hoffman presents with depressed mood, anhedonia, poor sleep, low energy, physical complaints, feelings of worthlessness, and diminished concentration. She denies suicidal intent or plan, but she does have thoughts of death. Therefore, she meets criteria for DSM-5 major depressive disorder.

In addition, Ms. Hoffman reluctantly mentions that she is a "failed anorexic" and that her eating is out of control. She said she started dieting when she entered adolescence, and by college, she had begun starving herself in the morning after eating too much the night before. Because her eating got out of control in the evening, she began to purge. As the cycle intensified after college, she sought psychiatric help because of the social dysfunction and physical and psychological distress.

Ms. Hoffman's history and symptoms are characteristic of bulimia nervosa (BN), which features several core criteria: recurrent binge eating, recurrent inappropriate compensatory mechanisms to prevent weight gain, and a self-evaluation that is unduly influenced by body shape and weight. In addition, these symptoms must have occurred weekly for at least 3 months.

Binge eating is defined as feeling out of control while eating an unusually large amount over a discrete period of time (e.g., an hour or two) rather than snacking throughout the day. If Ms. Hoffman felt significant distress from this eating behavior but did not have compensatory weight loss behaviors (e.g., purging), she would likely meet criteria for binge eating disorder.

As it stands, however, Ms. Hoffman engages in self-induced vomiting, which is common for people with BN. This behavior usually begins out of fear that the binge eating will result in weight gain, with the subsequent vomiting seen as a way of eliminating this risk. Early in the course of the illness, most patients induce vomiting with their fingers, but they often develop the capacity to vomit at will.

It would be useful to ask Ms. Hoffman whether she uses other weight loss methods. For example, some patients with BN use laxatives to induce diarrhea, a strategy that is unlikely to cause weight loss but is quite likely to induce dehydration, stomachaches, and malaise. Other individuals with BN use diuretics, diet pills (e.g., amphetamines), or nonprescribed substances (e.g., cocaine) to limit weight gain.

Most people with BN tend to seek help because of complications of the disorder rather than because of dissatisfaction with their eating behavior. For example, medical complications commonly include dehydration and electrolyte abnormalities such as hypochloremia and metabolic alkalosis, and, more rarely, hypokalemia. These complications can lead to feelings of fatigue, headache, and poor concentration. Rare but serious medical complications include gastric dilatation and esophageal rupture.

As appears to be the case with Ms. Hoffman, BN is commonly comorbid with major depressive disorder. Other common comorbidities include anxiety disorders, substance use problems (often involving alcohol), and personality disorders.

Although Ms. Hoffman sought help from a psychiatrist, she did so through her internist, and it is common for people with BN to present to their primary care physicians with vague medical complaints. Notably, the health care practitioners who are often in the best position to identify patients with BN are dentists, who find evidence of obvious enamel erosion.

Diagnoses

- Bulimia nervosa
- Major depressive disorder

Suggested Readings

Mason TB, Lesser EL, Dolgon-Krutolow AR, et al: An updated transdiagnostic review of social cognition and eating disorder psychopathology. J Psychiatr Res 143:602–627, 2021

Pearson CM, Wonderlich SA, Smith GT: A risk and maintenance model for bulimia nervosa: from impulsive action to compulsive behavior. Psychol Rev 122(3):516–535, 2015

van Eeden AE, van Hoeken D, Hoek HW: Incidence, prevalence and mortality of anorexia nervosa and bulimia nervosa. Curr Opin Psychiatry 34(6):515–524, 2021

CASE 10.5

Weight Gain

Susan L. McElroy, M.D.

Yasmine Isherwood, a 55-year-old married woman, had been in psychiatric treatment for 6 months for an episode of major depressive disorder. She had responded well to a combination of psychotherapy and medications (fluoxetine and bupropion), but she began to complain of weight gain. She was at her "highest weight ever," which was 140 pounds (her height was 5 feet 5 inches, so her BMI was 23.3).

The psychiatrist embarked on a clarification of Ms. Isherwood's eating history, which was marked by recurrent, distressing episodes of uncontrollable eating of large amounts of food. The overeating was not new but seemed to have worsened while she was taking antidepressants. She reported that she often worked late in her job as marketing director for a large software company, and that the eating episodes often occurred on one of 2 days per week that she happened to get home before her husband, a cardiologist at a local hospital. These "eating jags" were notable for a sense that she was out of control. She ate rapidly and alone, until uncomfortably full. She would then feel depressed, tired, and disgusted with herself. She usually binged on healthy food but also had "sugar binges" where she ate primarily sweets, especially ice cream and candy. She denied current or past self-induced vomiting, fasting, or misuse of laxatives, diuretics, or weight-loss agents. She reported exercising for an hour almost every day but denied being "addicted" to it. She did report that in her late 20s, she had become a competitive runner. At that time, she ran an average of about 35 miles per week, despite a lingering foot injury that eventually forced her to shift to swimming, biking, and the elliptical machine.

Ms. Isherwood stated that she had binged on food "for as long as I can remember." She was "chunky" as a child but stayed at a normal weight throughout high school (120–125 pounds) because she was so active. She denied a history of anorexia nervosa. At age 28, when she was competitively running, she reached her lowest adult weight of 113 pounds. At that point, she felt "vital, healthy, and in control."

In her mid-30s, she had a major depressive episode that lasted 2 years. She had a severely depressed mood, did not talk, "closed down," stayed in bed, was very fatigued, slept more than usual, and was unable to function. This was one of the few times in her life that the binge eating stopped and she lost weight. She denied a history of hypomanic or manic episodes. Although she lived with frequent sadness, she denied other serious depressive episodes until the past year. She denied a history of suicidal ideation, suicide attempts, and any significant use of alcohol, tobacco, or illicit substances.

The evaluation revealed a well-nourished, well-developed female who was coherent and cooperative. Her speech was fluent and not pressured. She had a mildly depressed mood but had a reactive affect with appropriate smiles. She denied guilt, suicidality, and hopelessness. She said her energy was normal except for post-binge fatigue. She denied psychosis and confusion. Her cognition was normal. Her medical history was unremarkable, and physical examination and basic laboratory test results provided by her internist were within normal limits.

Discussion

Ms. Isherwood describes overeating episodes that are marked by a sense of being out of control. She eats rapidly and until overly full. She eats alone and feels disgusted and distressed afterward. These episodes occur several times per week and do not involve inappropriate compensatory behaviors such as vomiting or use of laxatives. Therefore, she meets criteria for the DSM-5 binge-eating disorder (BED).

Although BED shares features with bulimia nervosa (BN) and obesity, it is distinguishable from both conditions. Compared with obese individuals without binge eating, obese individuals with BED have greater weight concerns and higher rates of mood, anxiety, and substance use disorders. Compared with individuals with BN, individuals with BED have lower weight concerns, greater rates of obesity, and lower rates of associated mood, anxiety, and substance use disorders. DSM-5 criteria for BED were broadened from the DSM-IV research criteria that appeared in Appendix B ("Criteria Sets and Axes Provided for Further Study"). Instead of a requirement of 2 binge days per week for 6 months (a binge day is a day in which at least one binge-eating episode occurs), DSM-5 requires one episode per week for 3 months. This shift represents an example of the sort of research that examines symptomatic clustering. In this case, it became apparent that individuals with less frequent and less persistent binge episodes were similar to people with slightly more frequent and more persistent episodes. Ms. Isherwood reports two or three episodes per week, which would put her in the mild category.

Although a diagnosis of BED should not be given in the presence of either BN or AN, patients with BED can have past histories of other eating disorders as well as infrequent inappropriate compensatory behaviors. For example, Ms. Isherwood described a time in her late 20s when she was running 35 miles per week with a chronic foot ailment. Even though she recalls feeling "vital, healthy, and in control" during this time, she may also have had BN if she was binge eating, and the running was intended to compensate for the bingeing.

BED patients often seek treatment initially for obesity (BMI ≥30) or weight gain, but clinical samples indicate that up to one-third of patients with BED are not obese. Nonobese patients with BED—like Ms. Isherwood—are more likely than their obese counterparts to engage in both healthy and unhealthy weight loss behaviors. For example, Ms. Isherwood's regular exercise regimen may have helped her maintain a normal weight despite her extensive binge-eating history. It is also possible that Ms. Isherwood's excessive running was spurred by an episode of hypomania; about 15% of patients with bipolar II disorder have an eating disorder, and BED is the most common.

All patients with BED are at risk for comorbid mood, anxiety, substance use, and impulse-control disorders. Although Ms. Isherwood denies any history of alcohol or drug misuse, she has a history of recurrent major depressive disorder. Although the case does not go into detail, it would be useful to explore the connection between Ms. Isherwood's eating habits and her depressive symptoms. Major depressive disorder can itself lead to excessive eating, but if both BED and major depressive disorder are present, both disorders should be diagnosed. Finally, the patient's history does not mention personality, but bingeing is included in the impulse-control criterion for borderline personality disorder. Again, if full criteria for both disorders are met, then both should be diagnosed.

Diagnoses

- Binge-eating disorder, mild
- Major depressive disorder, recurrent, in remission

Suggested Readings

Masheb RM, White MA, Grilo CM: Substantial weight gains are common prior to treatment-seeking in obese patients with binge eating disorder. Compr Psychiatry 54(7):880–884, 2013

Smith KE, Mason TB, Johnson JS, et al: A systematic review of reviews of neurocognitive functioning in eating disorders: the state-of-the-literature and future directions. Int J Eat Disord 51(8):798–821, 2018

Udo T, Grilo CM: Prevalence and correlates of DSM-5-defined eating disorders in a nationally representative sample of U.S. adults. Biol Psychiatry 84(5):345–354, 2018

Udo T, Grilo CM: Psychiatric and medical correlates of DSM-5 eating disorders in a nationally representative sample of adults in the United States. Int J Eat Disord 52(1):42–50, 2019

CHAPTER 11

Elimination Disorders

INTRODUCTION

John W. Barnhill, M.D.

The chapter on elimination disorders is the second of four consecutive DSM-5 chapters that explicitly deal with variations of normal bodily processes. These normal bodily processes can go awry in multiple ways, but from a diagnostic perspective, the distress and/or dysfunction can emerge as a symptomatic part of another disorder or as a relatively autonomous elimination disorder (with or without comorbidities).

Enuresis and encopresis are the two primary elimination disorders. Each is subdivided in ways that are both logical and clinically relevant. The diagnostic criteria for each disorder specify the developmental age at which the diagnosis becomes applicable. For example, enuresis—the repeated voiding of urine into bed and clothes—is not a diagnosis until the child has reached a developmental age of 5 years. A significant number of younger children simply are not yet ready to reliably use the bathroom.

DSM-5 does not require that the clinician ascertain the degree to which voluntary control plays a role; for example, a psychiatric diagnosis of nighttime bed-wetting (nocturnal enuresis) need not depend on whether the parent indicates that "he is doing it for attention." Similarly, a young boy who refuses to defecate in the bathroom at school and then is regularly and embarrassingly incontinent warrants a diagnosis (encopresis with constipation and overflow incontinence) that does not demand that the clinician delve deeply into the child's views on kindergarten, separation, and bodily control. The clinician may choose to make those assessments, but the diagnostic process does not require such a pursuit.

Instead, the focus is on more readily ascertainable measures. Is the enuresis clinically significant? Is it persistent? Is it causing distress? DSM-5 also encourages the clinician to make an effort to evaluate for physiological causes of enuresis and encopresis, because such common and readily treatable conditions as a urinary tract infection or dehydration can cause highly upsetting symptoms.

Abnormalities of elimination are also seen as secondary to many medical and nonmedical psychiatric conditions. The link between depression and constipation is common, for example, as is the link between gastrointestinal distress and a wide range of medications. These comorbidities should be actively considered. At the same time, it is important to tactfully consider whether an autonomous elimination disorder should be the focus of clinical attention.

Suggested Readings

Irwin GM: Urinary incontinence. Prim Care 46(2):233–242, 2019

Tai TT, Tai BT, Chang YJ, Huang KH: Parents have different perceptions of bed-wetting than children from six to 15 years of age. Acta Paediatr 104(10):e466–e472, 2015

von Gontard A: Wetting in Children and Adolescents: A Practical Guide for Parents, Teachers, and Caregivers. Boston, Hogrefe Publishing, 2017

CASE 11.1

Temper Tantrums and Somatic Complaints

David H. Rubin, M.D.

Zack was an 8-year-old boy brought to the outpatient child psychiatry clinic by his mother because of increasing tantrums and somatic complaints without an apparent cause. The mother reported that the symptoms appeared related to the nights that he spent with his aunt, another single mom with a boy similar in age to Zack. He had been close to this aunt since birth but had only recently begun to spend every Friday night with her when the mother took on a night shift at work.

For 2 months prior to the consultation, Zack would report nausea and headaches on Fridays and complain that his aunt's house was "creepy." He continued to visit, with reluctance, although he did once call his mother at work demanding that she pick him up, saying, "Other kids live in their own home every day of the week."

In recent weeks, Zack screamed and hid when it came time to go to his aunt's home. His mother became concerned that something could have "happened" to Zack during a visit. The mother struggled to reconcile this with the fact that Zack had no objections to seeing the aunt and cousin anywhere else, and he had no objection to the cousin sleeping at their home. Her sister had always been "a good mom" and was always home during the sleepovers. She did have a boyfriend, but Zack seemed to like him. In fact, Zack seemed especially excited to go to the park or ball games with his cousin and the boyfriend.

Zack had never previously had particularly significant separation, behavioral, or emotional issues. He achieved all developmental milestones on time. He had never seen a doctor aside from routine visits and one bad cold when he was age 3. Zack had yet to achieve consistent overnight continence, however, and did wet the bed approximately twice weekly. He had no daytime voiding symptoms or constipation. The pediatrician had told them that this was "normal" at Zack's age. The mother had never made a big deal about the bed-wetting, and Zack had never expressed significant distress about it.

Family history was negative for all psychiatric illness on the mother's side, and the mother said her own developmental landmarks were normal as far as she had been told. The mother knew little about Zack's father's developmental or family history, and she had not seen him since before Zack was born.

On mental status examination, Zack was cooperative and appeared well nourished and well cared for. He had little difficulty separating from his mother. After an initial period of warming up to the interviewer, his speech was spontaneous with a vocabulary appropriate for his age. He maintained age-appropriate eye contact. His affect was initially mildly anxious, but he rapidly calmed. Anxiety only reappeared upon discussing his sleepovers, when Zack demonstrated some fidgeting, decreased eye contact, and mild irritability directed toward his mother. When asked about the bed-wetting, Zack appeared embarrassed. He said he had wet the bed at his aunt's house a few times and that both his cousin and his aunt's boyfriend teased him about it. His aunt had intervened, but he described being "scared" that he would do it again.

Discussion

Zack presents with uncharacteristic temper tantrums, somatic complaints, and persistent refusal to spend the night at his aunt's home. By the end of the interview, the focus of clinical concern had shifted to Zack's enuresis, a disorder that is generally benign but can lead to significant psychosocial distress and behavioral change.

A DSM-5 enuresis diagnosis does not require that the clinician assess motivation (i.e., the urination can be voluntary or involuntary). Instead, the behavior should be clinically significant as defined by frequency (e.g., twice weekly for 3 months) or by its impact (e.g., distress or functional change). Enuresis can develop at any age, although there is a lower age limit of 5 years for the diagnosis. For patients with a neurodevelopmental disorder, that age restriction applies to their developmental, not their chronological, age. Finally, the disorder should not be caused by a substance or medical condition.

The enuresis diagnosis also includes a number of subtypes. Because Zack's enuresis seems to occur only at night, his would be described as "nocturnal only." He has never achieved a 6-month period of consistent overnight dryness, so his enuresis is characterized as primary. Primary nocturnal enuresis is common in children ages 5–10 and is especially common in boys. Although Zack's mother does not know when Zack's father achieved nighttime continence, a family history of enuresis is very common, and a number of genetic factors have been identified as contributory to the disorder. Secondary enuresis, in which incontinence returns after the child has already achieved at least 6 months of consistent dryness, demands a careful consideration of many medical etiologies, including diabetes, seizure disorder, obstructive sleep apnea, neurogenic bladder, constipation, and urethral obstruction. In rare cases, these conditions can be responsible for primary enuresis as well, so Zack's presentation should prompt a coordinated effort with the pediatrician to rule them out.

Any distress associated with the condition is usually dependent on others' reactions to the bed-wetting; however, distress is not necessary for the diagnosis of enuresis. In Zack's case, he became ashamed only after he was teased by his cousin and his aunt's boyfriend. Given that his development has been otherwise normal, Zack most likely has enuresis without any other psychiatric diagnosis.

Enuresis is commonly comorbid with other emotional and behavioral disorders of childhood, however, and Zack should be considered for several specific psychiatric disorders. Zack's anxiety and somatic complaints developed in the context of separation from a primary caregiver. This should lead to an exploration of an anxiety disorder such as separation anxiety. Zack separates easily from his mother in other contexts, such as school and the psychiatric evaluation, making separation anxiety an unlikely explanation for his presenting symptoms.

Zack was brought for evaluation because of defiance, somatic complaints, and temper tantrums. Disorders of behavior, mood, and impulse control—such as oppositional defiant disorder, conduct disorder, and disruptive mood dysregulation disorder—might all be considered. Zack's symptoms have lasted only 2 months, however, and he is generally doing fine. Because the changes appear to be specifically focused on a single context with an understandable trigger, Zack is unlikely to have any of these diagnoses.

It is no surprise that Zack's mother is concerned that the specificity of the trigger might be related to some sort of abuse. Although he has obvious trouble on Friday nights, Zack's general well-being and the ease with which he usually interacts with his cousin, his aunt, and his aunt's boyfriend make it unlikely that he has been abused. His mother is right, however, that something did happen: he was teased by his cousin and his aunt's boyfriend, two people he seems to especially trust, so their words would likely be felt as especially traumatic by this 8-year-old boy.

Diagnosis

- Enuresis, nocturnal only

Suggested Readings

Hussong J, Rosenthal A, Bernhardt A, et al: State and trait anxiety in children with incontinence and their parents. Clin Child Psychol Psychiatry 26(4):1243–1256, 2021

Walker RA: Nocturnal enuresis. Prim Care 46(2):243–248, 2019

CHAPTER 12

Sleep-Wake Disorders

INTRODUCTION

John W. Barnhill, M.D.

The pursuit of restful sleep is bedeviled by work and family pressures, long-distance travel, and the ubiquitous presence of stimulants (e.g., coffee) and electronics (e.g., e-mail). A good night's sleep can be a casualty of a host of psychiatric disorders, including anxiety, depression, and bipolar and psychotic disorders, as well as a variety of nonpsychiatric medical conditions. Sleep problems may not simply be epiphenomena but can precipitate, prolong, and intensify these other psychiatric and medical conditions. All too often, however, sleep-wake disorders exist as silent and undiagnosed contributors to distress and dysfunction.

DSM-5 made use of both a "lumping" and a "splitting" approach to the sleep disorders, thus moving away from making causal attributions (e.g., depression inevitably causes insomnia) and instead acknowledging the bidirectional interactions between sleep and other disorders. Insomnia disorder can exist autonomously, but clinicians are encouraged to consider insomnia's frequent comorbidity with both psychiatric and nonpsychiatric medical conditions. Clarification of an independent sleep disorder can serve as a reminder to the clinician that the sleep problem may not resolve spontaneously but instead may warrant independent psychiatric attention.

In addition to a broad clinical approach, DSM-5 features sleep disorders that require very specific physiological findings. For example, a patient may present with restless sleep and daytime fatigue. If the patient's bed partner identifies unusually loud snoring, sleep apnea would likely be considered. A DSM-5 diagnosis of obstructive sleep apnea hypopnea requires not only clinical evidence but also a polysomnogram that reveals at least five obstructive apneas or hypopneas per hour of sleep (or, if there is no evidence of nocturnal breathing difficulties, 15 or more such apneic events per hour).

Advances in epidemiological, neurobiological, and interventions research have allowed some sleep disorders to be increasingly "split." For example, narcolepsy is defined by two required criteria. The first is clinical: the patient must experience recurrent, persistent episodes marked by irrepressible sleep or an irrepressible need for sleep. The second criterion can be met in three ways: by recurrent episodes of cataplexy (defined clinically); hypocretin deficiency (defined via cerebrospinal fluid levels obtained through lumbar puncture); or specifically abnormal rapid eye movement (REM) sleep latency as determined by nocturnal sleep polysomnography or a multiple sleep latency test. These results led to four separately coded subtypes of DSM-5-TR narcolepsy: 1) with cataplexy or hypocretin deficiency (type 1), 2) without cataplexy and either without hypocretin deficiency or hypocretin unmeasured (type 2), 3) with cataplexy or hypocretin deficiency due to a medical condition, and 4) without cataplexy and without hypocretin deficiency due to a medical condition.

REM sleep behavior disorder and restless legs syndrome were new disorders in DSM-5. For each, substantial evidence had clarified the physiological basis, prevalence, and clinical relevance. Both are often comorbid with other psychiatric and non-psychiatric medical conditions (e.g., REM sleep behavior disorder is often comorbid with narcolepsy and neurodegenerative disorders such as Parkinson's disease; restless legs syndrome is often comorbid with depression, cardiovascular disease, and end-stage renal disease).

The initial sleep assessment generally involves a retrospective patient report. Clinicians are accustomed to working with subjective reports, but a sleep complaint that is impossible ("I haven't slept in weeks") can lead the clinician to think "insomnia" and move on with other aspects of the evaluation. Increasingly robust diagnostic criteria for the sleep-wake disorders are helpful for a variety of reasons, but they are especially helpful as a reminder to the general clinician to explore common complaints that are often underdiagnosed and that contribute to significant distress and dysfunction.

Suggested Readings

American Academy of Sleep Medicine: International Classification of Sleep Disorders, 3rd Edition (ICSD-3). Darien, IL, American Academy of Sleep Medicine, 2014

During EH, Kushida CA (eds): Clinical Sleep Medicine: A Comprehensive Guide for Mental Health and Other Medical Professionals. Washington, DC, American Psychiatric Association Publishing, 2021

Edinger JD, Ulmer CS, Means MK: Sensitivity and specificity of polysomnographic criteria for defining insomnia. J Clin Sleep Med 9(5):481–491, 2013

Hertenstein E, Feige B, Gmeiner T, et al: Insomnia as a predictor of mental disorders: a systematic review and meta-analysis. Sleep Med Rev 43:96–105, 2019

Ohayon M, Wickwire EM, Hirshkowitz M, et al: National Sleep Foundation's sleep quality recommendations: first report. Sleep Health 3(1):6–19, 2017

Poon SH, Quek SY, Lee TS: Insomnia disorders: nosology and classification past, present, and future. J Neuropsychiatry Clin Neurosci 33(3):194–200, 2021

CASE 12.1

Difficulty Staying Asleep

Charles F. Reynolds III, M.D.

Aidan Johns, a 30-year-old graduate student in English, visited a psychiatrist to discuss his difficulty staying asleep. The trouble began 4 months earlier, when he started to wake up at 3:00 every morning, no matter when he went to bed, and then was unable to fall back to sleep. As a result, he felt "out of it" during the day. This led him to feel increasingly worried about how he was going to finish his doctoral dissertation when he was unable to concentrate owing to exhaustion. When his sleep difficulties began, he woke with nothing particular on his mind. As the trouble persisted, he found himself dreading the upcoming day and wondering how he would teach his classes or focus on his writing if he was getting only a few hours of sleep. Some mornings he lay awake in the dark next to his fiancée, who was sleeping soundly. On other mornings he would cut his losses, rise from bed, and go very early to his office on campus.

After a month of interrupted sleep, Mr. Johns visited a physician's assistant at the university's student health services, where he customarily got his medical care. (He suffered from asthma, for which he occasionally took inhaled β_2-adrenergic receptor agonists, and a year earlier he had had mononucleosis.) The physician's assistant prescribed a sedative-hypnotic, which did not help. "Falling asleep was never the problem," Mr. Johns explained. Meanwhile, he heeded some of the advice he read online. Although he felt reliant on coffee during the day, he never drank it after 2:00 P.M. An avid tennis player, he restricted his court time to the early morning. He did have a glass or two of wine every night at dinner with his fiancée, however. "By dinnertime I start to worry about whether I'll be able to sleep," he said, "and, to be honest, the wine helps."

The patient, a slender and fit-appearing young man looking very much the part of the young academic in a tweed jacket and tortoise-rimmed glasses, was pleasant and open in his storytelling. Mr. Johns did not appear tired but told the evaluating psychiatrist, "I made a point to see you in the morning, before I hit the wall." He did not look sad or on edge and was not sure if he had ever felt depressed. But he was certain of the nagging, low-level anxiety that was currently oppressing him. "This sleep problem has taken over," he explained. "I'm stressed about my work, and my fiancée and I have been arguing. But it's all because I'm so tired."

Although this was his first visit to a psychiatrist, Mr. Johns spoke of a fulfilling 3-year psychodynamic psychotherapy with a social worker while in college. "I was just looking to understand myself better," he explained, adding with a chuckle that as the son of a child psychiatrist, he was accustomed to people assuming he was "crazy." He recalled always being an "easy sleeper" prior to his recent difficulties; as a child he was the first to fall asleep at slumber parties, and as an adult he inspired the envy of his fiancée for the ease with which he could doze off on an airplane.

Discussion

Mr. Johns reports 4 months of feeling dissatisfied with his sleep most nights, with difficulty maintaining sleep and early morning awakening. He describes daytime fatigue, difficulty concentrating, mild symptoms of anxiety, and interpersonal and vocational impairment. He does not appear to qualify for diagnoses of other medical, psychiatric, sleep, or substance use disorders. He meets the clinical criteria for DSM-5 insomnia disorder.

The case history suggests that the patient's sleep disturbance began during a period of heightened stress related to time pressures and that he has developed some behaviors that may worsen or perpetuate his sleep disturbance. He worries about not sleeping and creates a self-fulfilling prophecy. He may also be self-medicating with caffeine to maintain alertness during the day and with wine to dampen arousal during the evening.

Also noted is a medical history of asthma, for which Mr. Johns takes occasional β_2-adrenergic receptor agonists. Because asthma medications may be stimulating, it would be helpful to further explore his use of inhalers and other medications.

Mr. Johns reports a history of participating for 3 years in psychodynamic psychotherapy while in college. He said he went to therapy because he wanted to know himself better, but it would be useful to explore this patient's personal and family psychiatric histories more carefully to determine whether his insomnia might be related to an undiagnosed mood or anxiety disorder. Conversely, insomnia itself increases the risk for either new-onset or recurrent episodes of mood, anxiety, or substance use disorders; even if Mr. Johns appears to have only the single insomnia disorder during the initial evaluation, it would be useful for the clinician to attend to other symptoms that may be developing.

Retrospective histories of insomnia are imperfect, so the psychiatrist might suggest a 2-week sleep-wake diary, which would be helpful in evaluating the amount of time the patient spends in bed, his lifestyle (the timing of physical and mental activities that could increase arousal and interfere with sleep), the timing and use of substances that can act on the central nervous system, and other medical issues (e.g., asthma attacks). A history from Mr. Johns's fiancée could be informative with respect to his sleep-related pathologies, such as apnea, loud snoring, leg jerks, or partial arousals from sleep (non-REM or REM parasomnias).

In addition to having Mr. Johns keep a sleep-wake diary, it would be useful to have him document the severity of his current sleep complaint by use of a self-report inventory such as the Insomnia Severity Index (ISI) or the Pittsburgh Sleep Quality Index (PSQI). These instruments provide useful baselines or benchmarks against which to measure change over time. In addition, the use of brief self-report measures of affective state, such as the Patient Health Questionnaire 9-item depression scale

(PHQ-9) or the Generalized Anxiety Disorder 7-item scale (GAD-7), would allow the clinician to further assess for coexisting or supervening mental disorders.

Formal sleep laboratory testing (polysomnography) does not appear to be indicated for Mr. Johns. However, if further information emerged from the history or diary, it could be appropriate to obtain testing for a breathing-related sleep disorder or for periodic limb movement disorder. Another diagnostic possibility is a circadian rhythm sleep disorder, such as an advanced sleep phase syndrome (unlikely, however, given the relatively young age of the patient).

As illustrated in this case, DSM-5 has moved away from categorizing primary or secondary forms of insomnia disorder. Instead, DSM-5 mandates concurrent specification of coexisting conditions (medical, psychiatric, and other sleep disorders), for two reasons: 1) to underscore that the patient has a sleep disorder warranting independent clinical attention, in addition to the medical or psychiatric disorder also present, and 2) to acknowledge bidirectional and interactive effects between sleep disorders and coexisting medical and psychiatric disorders.

This reconceptualization reflects a paradigm shift in the field of sleep disorders medicine. The shift is away from making causal attributions between coexisting disorders ("a" is due to "b"), both because there are often limited empirical data to support such attribution, and because optimal treatment planning requires attention to each pertinent diagnosis.

Diagnosis

- Insomnia disorder

Suggested Readings

Buysse DJ, Rush AJ, Reynolds CF 3rd: Clinical management of insomnia disorder. JAMA 318(20):1973–1974, 2017

Khachatryan SG: Insomnia burden and future perspectives. Sleep Med Clin 16(3):513–521, 2021

Reynolds CF III: Troubled sleep, troubled minds, and DSM-5. Arch Gen Psychiatry 68(10):990–991, 2011

CASE 12.2

Anxious and Sleepy

Maurice M. Ohayon, M.D., D.Sc., Ph.D.

Bernadette Kleber was a 34-year-old divorced, unemployed white mother of three school-age children. She was living with a new companion. Ms. Kleber presented to a psychiatrist for anxiety and sleepiness.

Ms. Kleber had experienced anxiety much of her life, but she had become much more worried and stressed since the birth of her first child 10 years before. She said she was "okay at home" but anxious in social situations. She avoided having to interact with new people, fearing that she would be embarrassed and judged. For example, she wanted to lose the weight that she had gained since the births of her children (current body mass index [BMI] 27.7) but was afraid of the ridicule that might accompany her efforts at the gym. She had gradually withdrawn from situations in which she might be forced to meet new people, and this made it almost impossible for her to interview for a new job, much less work in one. She had been successfully treated for social anxiety disorder 5 years earlier with psychotherapy, a selective serotonin reuptake inhibitor [SSRI] antidepressant, and clonazepam 0.25 mg twice daily, but her symptoms had returned over the prior year. She denied increasing the dose of either medication or taking any other medication (prescribed or over the counter) for anxiety. Although excited about her new relationship, she was worried her new girlfriend would leave her if she did not "tune up my act."

She denied periods of significant depression, although she said she had experienced multiple periods of feeling frustrated with her limited effectiveness. She also denied all manic symptoms.

The psychiatrist then asked Ms. Kleber about her "sleepiness." She said she slept more than anyone she knew. She said she typically slept at least 9 hours per night but then took two naps for 5 additional hours during the day. She did not recall a problem until the end of high school, when she started falling asleep around 8:00 or 9:00 P.M. and dozing every afternoon. When she tried to go to college, she realized how much more sleep she needed than her friends and eventually dropped out because she could not stay awake in class. Despite the naps, she typically fell asleep when visiting friends or family and when reading or watching TV. She quit driving alone for fear of falling asleep at the wheel. Late afternoon naps were not restorative and had no apparent impact on her falling asleep at night.

Raising a family was difficult, especially because mornings were Ms. Kleber's worst period. For at least half an hour after waking, she was disoriented and confused, making it difficult to get her children to school. Throughout the day, she said she felt "scattered and inattentive."

Snoring had appeared 5 years earlier. Her companion was unsure whether Ms. Kleber also had breathing pauses during her sleep. Ms. Kleber denied having ever experienced sleep paralysis or abruptly falling asleep in the middle of a sentence. Although she would fall asleep while socializing, it would generally occur during a lull in the conversation while she was in a quiet spot in the corner of a couch. She denied falling down when she fell asleep. She reported experiencing hypnopompic hallucinations several times per year since she was a teenager.

On examination, Ms. Kleber was an overweight woman who was cooperative and coherent. She was concerned about her anxiety but preoccupied with her sleep problem. She denied depression, suicidality, psychosis, and memory complaints. Her insight and judgment appeared intact.

Her physical examination was essentially noncontributory. Her medical history was significant only for hypercholesterolemia and occasional migraine headaches. Ms. Kleber did have some muscular complaints, such as weakness in her legs and pain in her left arm; these were related to exertion. She has smoked marijuana occasionally to help with her pain but denied that the marijuana was an important contributor to her sleepiness. She denied a history of head trauma and unusual illnesses. She denied a family history of sleep or mood problems, although multiple relatives were "anxious."

Ms. Kleber was referred for sleep studies. Polysomnography showed an apnea hypopnea index of 3 events per hour. The next day, she underwent a multiple sleep latency test (MSLT), which indicated a mean sleep latency of 7 minutes with one sleep-onset REM period during the testing. A lumbar puncture was done to assess cerebrospinal fluid (CSF) levels of hypocretin-1; the level appeared in the normal range.

Discussion

Ms. Kleber appears to have several DSM-5 diagnoses that warrant clinical attention. She has been diagnosed with social anxiety disorder in the past, and its recurrence seems to have led to this psychiatric consultation. She has gained weight since the birth of her children, and her obesity exacerbates her social avoidance and puts her at risk for sleep disturbances and medical complications. Obesity is not a diagnosis in the main text of DSM-5, but it is listed in the DSM-5 chapter "Other Conditions That May Be a Focus of Clinical Attention." Ms. Kleber's anxiety and weight issues might both warrant independent clinical attention, but it is her sleep problems that appear to most profoundly affect her life.

Ms. Kleber sleeps too much. The sleep is not restful or restorative. Because of the sleep problems, she can barely function as a mother and she indicates that she cannot keep or maintain a job, drive independently, or socialize with friends. She is worried she will lose her new romantic partner. The excess sleep and sleepiness have apparently occurred daily since she neared the end of high school. Ms. Kleber's symptoms are indicative of DSM-5 hypersomnolence disorder. Criteria include symptoms at least 3 days per week for at least 3 months (Ms. Kleber has had symptoms almost daily for over 15 years). The nocturnal sleep duration (9 hours) alone might not suggest a problem, but her total daily sleep duration of 14 hours is typical of hypersomnolence, as are her inertia upon awakening and her unexpected lapses into sleep.

It is important to rule out other explanations for her somnolence. Ms. Kleber smokes marijuana and uses a benzodiazepine for anxiety. She insists that her use is either occasional (the marijuana) or at a low, stable dose (the clonazepam), and that her symptoms predated her use of either. Although both agents can be sedating, and she may be underreporting her use, the marijuana and clonazepam do not appear to be causative agents. Ms. Kleber has pain and headaches, so it would be useful to tactfully inquire further about her possible use of pain medications, which can be sedating. She also describes demoralization about her lack of effectiveness, which should prompt a consideration of depression, which can lead to excessive amounts of nonrestorative sleep. At the moment, none of these possibilities seems likely.

There are multiple sleep disorders that can lead to excessive sleep and/or daytime somnolence. Ms. Kleber's obesity, excessive sleepiness, and snoring should prompt a consideration of sleep apnea, and a sleep study was certainly indicated. Polysomnography yielded an apnea hypopnea index of 3 events per hour, a result that is in the normal range and indicates that Ms. Kleber does not have a sleep-related breathing disorder.

Ms. Kleber should also be evaluated for narcolepsy, which is characterized by recurrent periods of an irrepressible need to sleep, lapsing into sleep, or napping within the same day. Ms. Kleber's clinical picture is suggestive. Not only does she fall asleep abruptly, but she has relatively frequent hypnopompic hallucinations. Although generally considered normal, hypnopompic hallucinations can reflect sleep-onset REM intrusions and therefore are suggestive of narcolepsy. To satisfy requirements for DSM-5-TR narcolepsy, the individual should demonstrate cataplexy, CSF hypocretin deficiency, or a reduction of REM sleep latency during nocturnal polysomnography or an MSLT. Ms. Kleber's MSLT showed a mean sleep latency of 7 minutes with only one sleep-onset REM period during the testing. The sleep latency is brief, but to qualify for narcolepsy, she would need at least two early REM periods during the study. Levels of CSF hypocretin-1 appeared in the normal range, which rules out narcolepsy-cataplexy/hypocretin deficiency syndrome. Unless her episodes of falling asleep are viewed as cataplexy, Ms. Kleber would not qualify for a narcolepsy diagnosis. At this point, then, Ms. Kleber qualifies only for DSM-5 hypersomnolence disorder in addition to social anxiety disorder.

Diagnoses

- Social anxiety disorder
- Hypersomnolence disorder

Suggested Readings

Karasu SR, Karasu TB: The Gravity of Weight: A Clinical Guide to Weight Loss and Maintenance. Washington, DC, American Psychiatric Publishing, 2010

Murray BJ: Subjective and objective assessment of hypersomnolence. Sleep Med Clin 15(2):167–176, 2020

Ohayon MM, Reynolds CF 3rd: Epidemiological and clinical relevance of insomnia diagnosis algorithms according to the DSM-IV and the International Classification of Sleep Disorders (ICSD). Sleep Med 10(9):952–960, 2009

Ohayon MM, Dauvilliers Y, Reynolds CF 3rd: Operational definitions and algorithms for excessive sleepiness in the general population: implications for DSM-5 nosology. Arch Gen Psychiatry 69(1):71–79, 2012

CASE 12.3

Sleepiness

Brian Palen, M.D.

Vishesh K. Kapur, M.D., M.P.H.

César Linares, a 57-year-old married Hispanic man, presented for reevaluation of his antidepressant medication. He described several years of worsening fatigue, daytime sleepiness, and generally "not feeling good." He lacked the energy to do his usual activities, but he still enjoyed them when he did participate. He had been having some trouble focusing on his work as an information technology consultant and was worried that he would lose his job. A selective serotonin reuptake inhibitor (SSRI) antidepressant had been started 6 months earlier, resulting in some improvement of symptoms, and Mr. Linares reported that he was adherent to this medication.

He denied recent stressors. In addition to having been diagnosed with depression, he had received diagnoses of hypertension, diabetes, and coronary artery disease. He complained of heartburn as well as erectile dysfunction, for which he had not been medically evaluated.

Mr. Linares was born in Venezuela. He had two grown children. He did not consume tobacco or alcohol but did drink several servings of coffee each day to help maintain alertness.

On physical examination, the patient was 5 feet 10 inches tall, weighed 235 pounds, and had a BMI of 34. His neck circumference was 20 inches. His respiratory rate was 15, and his blood pressure was 155/90. No other abnormalities were present.

On mental status examination, the patient was a cooperative man who appeared tired but was without depressed mood, anxiety, psychosis, or cognitive decline.

More focused questioning revealed that Mr. Linares not only had trouble staying awake at work but also occasionally nodded off while driving. He slept 8–10 hours nightly but had frequent awakenings, made nightly trips to the bathroom (nocturia), and often woke with a choking sensation and sometimes with a headache. He had snored since childhood, and he added, "All the men in my family are snorers." Before she elected to sleep nightly in their guest bedroom, his wife said he snored very loudly and intermittently stopped breathing and gasped for air.

Mr. Linares was referred for a sleep study (polysomnography). Results included the following:

- Apnea hypopnea index: 25 events per hour
- Oxygen desaturation index: 20 events per hour
- Nadir oxygen saturation: 82%
- % Time with oxygen saturation <90%: 10%
- Arousal index: 35 events per hour
- Sleep stage (%):

    % Time in stage N1 sleep: 20%
    % Time in stage N2 sleep: 65%
    % Time in stage N3 sleep: 5%
    % Time in REM sleep: 10%

Discussion

Mr. Linares presents for a reevaluation of his treatment for depression, but his presenting symptoms are much more notable for fatigue and sleepiness than for a mood disorder. The patient's history of loud snoring and episodes of choking and gasping suggest that his most likely underlying disorder is obstructive sleep apnea hypopnea (OSAH), also known as obstructive sleep apnea hypopnea syndrome (OSAHS).

OSAH is a common condition, with up to 13% of men and 6% of women in the United States meeting DSM-5-TR diagnostic criteria based on polysomnography findings. Mr. Linares has additional risk for OSAHS based on age greater than 50 years, obesity with a large neck circumference, and family history notable for "all the men" being snorers. Snoring is a particularly sensitive indicator for OSAH syndrome, especially snoring that is loud and occurs more than 3 days per week. Choking and gasping episodes are likewise very specific indicators. As seen in Mr. Linares, patients with OSAH syndrome also frequently report nocturia, heartburn, sexual dysfunction, and morning headaches, reflecting the multisystem effects of this disorder.

OSAH is characterized by the repetitive collapse or partial collapse of the pharyngeal airway during sleep. Relaxation of the pharyngeal muscles during sleep allows soft tissue in the back of the throat to block the pharyngeal airway. The resultant decrease in airflow can cause significant reductions in blood oxygen saturation. The increased work of breathing through an occluded airway stimulates brief arousals to allow resumption of normal breathing. This pattern can repeat itself hundreds of times throughout the night, resulting in significantly fragmented sleep patterns.

Sleep studies (polysomnography and out-of-center/home sleep apnea testing) measure sleep physiology in multiple ways, but DSM-5-TR severity specifications are based on the apnea hypopnea index (AHI), which is a measure of the number of episodes of complete absence of airflow (apneas) and of reduced airflow (hypopneas) that last for at least 10 seconds per hour of sleep. If patients have at least 15 obstructive apneas or hypopneas per hour of sleep (i.e., an AHI of 15), they meet diagnostic criteria regardless of associated symptoms. If patients have an AHI of 5–15, they must also have associated nocturnal breathing disturbances (i.e., snoring, snorting/gasping, breathing pauses during sleep) or daytime sleepiness, fatigue, or nonrefreshing sleep to meet diagnostic criteria.

The AHI is also used to categorize OSAH severity, with values less than 15 often considered mild and values greater than 30 considered severe. That said, there are limitations to this metric, and it is important to also consider other indices of disease, such as the frequency of oxygen desaturations or the time spent with low oxygen saturations (both abnormal on Mr. Linares's polysomnography), which are more closely tied to long-term negative outcomes. Furthermore, Mr. Linares's polysomnography is notable for abnormal sleep architecture, with a reduction of the percentage of time spent in REM and stage N3 sleep, and his arousal index, which measures cortical arousals per hour, is also elevated. Finally, the severity of symptom burden, such as sleepiness and disrupted sleep, must also be considered, given that these measures may not align with AHI or other sleep study indices.

OSAH is similar to many DSM-5 diagnoses in that if untreated, it can have a seriously negative impact on quality of life. The syndrome is unusual within DSM-5-TR, however, in that its diagnosis is heavily based on the results of a test rather than on clinical observation. OSAH and mental disorders are often intertwined, and both can affect sleep quality. As exemplified in the case of Mr. Linares, many patients with OSAH syndrome experience delayed diagnosis, leading to extended periods of untreated symptoms.

Diagnosis

• Obstructive sleep apnea hypopnea

Suggested Readings

Gottlieb DJ, Punjabi NM: Diagnosis and management of obstructive sleep apnea: a review. JAMA 323(14):1389–1400, 2020
Malhotra A, Ayappa I, Ayas N, et al: Metrics of sleep apnea severity: beyond the apnea-hypopnea index. Sleep 44(7):zsab030, 2021
Peppard PE, Young T, Barnet JH, et al: Increased prevalence of sleep-disordered breathing in adults. Am J Epidemiol 177(9):1006–1014, 2013
Sharafkhaneh A, Giray N, Richardson P, et al: Association of psychiatric disorders and sleep apnea in a large cohort. Sleep 28(11):1405–1411, 2005

CASE 12.4

Feeling Itchy, Creepy, and Crawly

Kathy P. Parker, Ph.D., R.N.

Dingxiang Meng was a 63-year-old Chinese-born man who was referred for a psychiatric consultation for depression and excessive somatic complaints. He had a history of psychotic depression, for which he had been admitted twice in the prior decade. He was evaluated as an outpatient in the renal unit of a small hospital during his routine hemodialysis.

Mr. Meng had been diagnosed with diabetes soon after his immigration to the United States 15 years earlier. He developed progressive renal insufficiency and had begun hemodialysis 7 years earlier. He was divorced, with two adult children and three young grandchildren. He currently lived with one of his children. Before starting on dialysis, Mr. Meng had worked episodically in a local grocery store owned by friends. Prior to emigrating from China, he had enjoyed a career as a pharmacist. He spoke little English; all interviews were conducted with a Mandarin interpreter.

At the time of the evaluation, Mr. Meng said he felt "itchy, creepy, and crawly," like "worms were crawling underneath his skin." These symptoms had fluctuated over the past few years but had worsened in recent weeks, and he felt like he was "going crazy." He described being worried and often tired, but noted that he always cheered up when playing with his grandchildren or when visiting with old friends from his hometown. He did not display a thought disorder. A review of the chart indicated that Mr. Meng's physical complaints had been conceptualized at various times as akathisia, peripheral neuropathy, and "psychosomatic" and "psychotically ruminative" symptoms. He had been euthymic and off all psychiatric medications for 2 years at the time of this evaluation.

Mr. Meng noted that his physical symptoms were worse at night, when he tried to sit still or lie down. The discomfort was only in his legs. Rubbing them helped, but the greatest relief came from standing up and pacing. Dialysis was especially difficult because of "being strapped to a machine for hours." He also complained of daytime sleepiness and fatigue. In the course of the interview, Mr. Meng twice jumped up during the dialysis. One of the nurses mentioned that he often asked them to cut short his dialysis, generally looked tired, and always seemed to be "jumping around." The staff wondered whether he might be nonadherent to his medications as well as being uncooperative at times during the dialysis.

Discussion

Mr. Meng presents with depression, fatigue, a creepy sensation of "worms" crawling under his skin, and an intense urge to move. It was not clear to earlier examiners whether his hospitalizations for psychotic depression were related to these physical sensations. These sensations had been diagnosed in multiple ways over the years: as akathisia, peripheral neuropathy, and "psychosomatic" and "psychotically ruminative" symptoms.

Instead of these diagnoses, Mr. Meng most likely has restless legs syndrome (RLS). RLS is characterized by an urge to move the legs, usually accompanied by disagreeable sensations. Mr. Meng's symptoms are typical. The symptoms are improved by movement and are most intense in the evening or when the person is in some sort of sedentary situation (such as dialysis). The symptoms are frequent, chronic, and distressing.

RLS is a particularly common problem for people with end-stage renal disease (ESRD) who are undergoing dialysis. Usually, but not always, the condition is associated with periodic limb movements: stereotypical movements involving extension of the big toe with partial flexing of the ankle, knee, and sometimes hip. Mr. Meng's daytime sleepiness could be related to a delayed sleep onset but also to a reduction in the quality of his sleep; RLS is associated with both problems. ESRD and dialysis are adequate explanations for the RLS (which often has no explanation), but a search should be made for such contributors as anemia, folate deficiency, and uremia. Although obviously not applicable to Mr. Meng, pregnancy is also associated with RLS.

It is not clear why the RLS diagnosis was delayed, especially since RLS is such a common finding in dialysis units. Mr. Meng's history of psychotic depression might have led the treating team to assume that his complaints were psychological. Such an understanding might have led to the diagnosis of "psychosomatic" symptoms, implying that his physical symptoms were attributable to some sort of psychological disorder or conflict. Not only does that appear to be a misunderstanding of Mr. Meng's complaints, it is a misuse of the term *psychosomatic*, which is better conceptualized as the branch of psychiatry that focuses on comorbidity between psychiatric and medical illnesses; using that definition, it is meaningless to describe someone as "psychosomatic." Because Mr. Meng was taking antipsychotic medication for at least some of the time that he was also symptomatic, it does make some sense that akathisia was considered. Newer antipsychotic medications (i.e., the atypical antipsychotics) are rarely implicated in akathisia, however, and his symptoms persisted 2 years after the discontinuation of all psychiatric medication. Peripheral neuropathy tends to cause pain, burning, and numbness in the extremities, which is not exactly Mr. Meng's actual complaint.

Perhaps of most concern are the chart notes that indicate that Mr. Meng's restless legs were a manifestation of "psychotic rumination." Communication difficulties may have contributed to this understanding, but it is possible that Mr. Meng's two psychiatric admissions for "psychotic depression" might have actually been precipitated by the somatic preoccupations, anxiety, and dysphoria caused by an undiagnosed case of RLS, a condition that has long been known to be comorbid with a number of medical illnesses.

Diagnoses

- Major depressive disorder, in remission
- Restless legs syndrome

Suggested Readings

Araujo SM, de Bruin VM, Nepomuceno LA, et al: Restless legs syndrome in end-stage renal disease: clinical characteristics and associated comorbidities. Sleep Med 11(8):785–790, 2010

Trenkwalder C, Allen R, Högl B, et al: Restless legs syndrome associated with major diseases: a systematic review and new concept. Neurology 86(14):1336–1343, 2016

Trenkwalder C, Tinelli M, Sakkas GK, et al: Socioeconomic impact of restless legs syndrome and inadequate restless legs syndrome management across European settings. Eur J Neurol 28(2):691–706, 2021

CHAPTER 13

Sexual Dysfunctions

INTRODUCTION

John W. Barnhill, M.D.

Although the criteria for the sexual disorders are relatively straightforward, they hint at the challenge of categorizing sexual problems. For example, a diagnostic system that intends to meaningfully describe sexual dysfunction must take into consideration the broad range of normal sexual response. The system must take into account the fact that dysfunction and distress depend heavily on the individual's expectations, wishes, and opportunities regarding sexual activity (as well as those of his or her partner). It should consider the effects of aging. It should consider the effects of proscriptive societal and religious norms on sexual behavior as well as take into account what it means to sexually function as a man or woman (or elsewhere on the modern gender continuum). The system should also take into account medications and illnesses that predictably reduce sexual desire and/or function, as well as those that predictably intensify desire and/or function, in addition to the reality that most assessments of sexual function and dysfunction are incomplete without an understanding that although sexual response has a biological underpinning, it is experienced from intrapersonal, interpersonal, and cultural perspectives.

In that biopsychosocial context, making a diagnosis of, for example, male hypoactive sexual desire disorder is potentially more complicated than briefly exploring whether the patient is interested in having sex.

DSM-5 identifies eight sexual dysfunctions, four specific to men, three specific to women, and one that can apply to either gender (substance/medication-induced sexual dysfunction). DSM-5 terminology and criteria vary somewhat between the genders. For example, men may have erectile disorder and/or male hypoactive sexual desire disorder, but for women, the somewhat comparable condition is merged into female sexual interest/arousal disorder.

DSM-5-TR addresses the fact that both men and women can have difficulties with orgasm. Whereas women may meet criteria for female orgasmic disorder, men may be diagnosed with either delayed ejaculation or premature (early) ejaculation. Women can also have genito-pelvic pain/penetration disorder, a diagnosis that is new to DSM-5 and that was developed in response to the increasing recognition that the prior diagnoses of vaginismus and dyspareunia were highly comorbid and difficult to distinguish. In addition, as is generally the case in DSM-5, there are categories for clinical presentations that either do not quite meet criteria or are incomplete (i.e., other specified or unspecified sexual dysfunction).

Except for substance/medication-induced sexual dysfunction, all of the sexual dysfunctions require a minimum duration of 6 months. In addition, each disorder can be noted to be lifelong versus acquired and generalized versus situational. If a medical condition is deemed pertinent, it can be listed as a specifier, but DSM-5 has specifically excluded the previous diagnosis of sexual dysfunction due to a medical condition because of the view that most of the sexual dysfunctions can be attributable to both psychological and biological factors.

The sexual dysfunction diagnoses are applicable to gender-diverse individuals. In particular, DSM-5-TR encourages clinician judgment when assessing sexual dysfunctions among transgender, nonbinary, agender, and other individuals who may not appear to fit this chapter's categories. When the diagnosis is based on anatomy (e.g., erectile dysfunction), DSM-5-TR guides the clinician to base the diagnosis on the person's current anatomy rather than on the sex assigned at birth.

Suggested Readings

Balon R, Briken P (eds): Compulsive Sexual Behavior Disorder: Understanding, Assessment, and Treatment. Washington, DC, American Psychiatric Association Publishing, 2021
Hall KSK, Binik YM (eds): Principles and Practice of Sex Therapy, 6th Edition. New York, Guilford, 2020

CASE 13.1

Sexual Dysfunction

Cynthia A. Graham, Ph.D.

Elizabeth Olsen and Finn Nelson presented for couples counseling in the context of increased arguments prior to their upcoming wedding. They were both successful attorneys in their late 30s. They had known each other since high school, had been dating for about 2 years, and planned to get married in about 6 months. Both denied ever having previously seen a therapist or received a psychiatric diagnosis.

The couples therapist met with them together for one session. Both Ms. Olsen and Mr. Nelson reported being very much in love and wanting the marriage to work out, but they also said that they were fighting much of the time. Ms. Olsen said she admired Mr. Nelson's intelligence and steadiness and did not know why they fought. He, on the other hand, said he was still "totally infatuated" but upset about Ms. Olsen's overall lack of interest in him. As the session neared a close, Mr. Nelson asked Ms. Olsen whether she wanted to bring up "the schedule, the alcohol, or the sex thing," at which she smiled and said, "I'm afraid we're out of time for today."

The therapist met with each of them separately. At his meeting, Mr. Nelson said his biggest concern with Ms. Olsen was her lack of interest in sex. She seemed to go through the motions, he said, and always relied on alcohol. He worried that he was a "7 trying to date a 10" and that she just did not find him attractive. He was distressed about the fact that, try as he might, he was unable to bring her to orgasm or even to get her significantly aroused. This was, in turn, leading him to initiate sex less frequently, and even when he tried, he would "often just give up half-way through." He had brought it up with her several times, but she had insisted that there was no problem. The therapist asked what he had meant by "the schedule thing." He explained that since they had begun dating, she had limited their time together to one "school night," usually a Tuesday, and then either a Friday or Saturday night. She had insisted that the schedule was necessary for her to complete her work and see her best girlfriends, but he had increasingly come to believe it was to avoid him.

In her individual session, Ms. Olsen said she was most frustrated by Mr. Nelson's intensity and high desire for sex. She had set up their weekly schedule because otherwise he would want to constantly have sex with her. As it was, he wanted sex every time they got together, often twice in the same night. She readily admitted that she got drunk to tolerate intercourse. She added that she had used alcohol to numb herself since she began dating while in her teens. Until she had started dating Mr. Nelson, most of her sexual experiences had been "while drunk with strangers." She had had a couple of boyfriends, but one was secretly gay and the other was "happy to get a blow job every now and then." She had not told Mr. Nelson about these misadventures because she preferred that he continue to see her as "the near-virginal beauty queen." Although alcohol made intercourse acceptable, "sexual arousal was almost never tolerable" and made her want to pass out. In recent months, Mr. Nelson had increasingly "forced the orgasm issue." In the past, she would simply have broken up with any boyfriend who acted that way, but she believed she needed to stick it out because she was nearing 40 and this would be her "last chance to have a baby." When asked why she thought she had these issues with sex, Ms. Olsen looked out the window for almost a minute and then answered, "I'm not going to tell you."

Discussion

Ms. Olsen and Mr. Nelson present for counseling because of increased arguments prior to their upcoming wedding. Sexual and relationship problems frequently co-occur, and it will be important to assess whether their relationship difficulties preclude their working together to resolve their sexual problems.

From a diagnostic perspective, the most obvious issues surround Ms. Olsen, who reports that she is able to tolerate intercourse only when aided by alcohol intoxication and that most of her sexual experiences had been "while drunk with strangers." She says that actual sexual arousal is "almost never tolerable" and makes her want to pass out. Ms. Olsen would ordinarily have broken up with any man who "forced the orgasm issue," but she is approaching 40, is desperate for a child, admires Mr. Nelson, and is trying to forge a workable compromise.

Looking at her issues from a DSM-5 perspective, Ms. Olsen has diminished interest in sexual activity and reduced enjoyment of sex, which indicates the possibility of female sexual interest/arousal disorder. She also does not experience orgasm during sexual activity, which could indicate female orgasmic disorder. Although she does not mention it, Ms. Olsen might experience pain during intercourse. If so, she might have genito-pelvic pain/penetration disorder. It appears that Ms. Olsen's sexual issues have been lifelong, as opposed to acquired. All of these diagnoses, however, require distress in Ms. Olsen. From the case report, it appears that her concern is not with her own sexuality but rather with Mr. Nelson's insistence on making sex part of the relationship.

Another important disqualifier for all of these DSM-5 diagnoses would be the presence of a nonsexual psychiatric diagnosis that could explain the symptoms. Ms. Olsen says sexual arousal makes her want to pass out and then tells the therapist that she is not going to reveal why she has these issues with sex. These statements suggest the possibility of traumatic sexual experience(s) or early sexual abuse. It would be useful to explore further whether she has symptoms of posttraumatic stress disorder, depression, anxiety, or some other nonsexual psychiatric disorder that could be contributing to her sexual issues. If any of these other disorders are deemed causative, then Ms. Olsen would not warrant a separate DSM-5 diagnosis focused on her sexual issues.

Ms. Olsen also indicates a need to use alcohol to "numb herself" before engaging in sexual activity. The alcohol use appears to be directly related to her more primary sexual issues, but the role of alcohol in her life should still be explored. If, for example, she has a history of "sex with strangers" that put her at physical risk and led to recurrent social problems, then she would probably be diagnosed with alcohol use disorder. Her alcohol use may be contributing to their relationship problems and may have other ramifications in her life.

Given the many potential diagnostic issues for this couple, it might be useful to employ Bancroft's "three windows approach" to assessment of sexual dysfunctions. Through the first "window," the clinician explores aspects of the current situation that would affect their sexual relationship. Examples might be the arguing, Mr. Nelson's insecurity, and Ms. Olsen's rigid schedule imposed to limit sexual activity. The second window—vulnerability of the individual—encourages an exploration of past difficulties. Ms. Olsen's sexual issues are most obvious and warrant further exploration, but it would also be important to understand Mr. Nelson's sexual and relationship history. The third window—health-related factors that alter sexual function—emphasizes the importance of exploring potentially pertinent physical, pharmacological, or hormonal factors that might be affecting the couple's sexual life together.

The couple seems to focus very much on Ms. Olsen's sexual problems, but the couple also appears to have a sexual desire discrepancy which, while not a diagnosis in DSM-5, is nevertheless one of the main reasons that couples seek therapy and can inform strategies for therapy.

Although both partners focus on sexual problems, it would be useful to broaden the evaluation to include nonsexual issues that might be pertinent to their relationship. It is also notable that both Mr. Nelson and Ms. Olsen disclosed much more in their individual sessions than during their joint session. Although this is a common occurrence, it is important for the clinician to clarify what can and cannot be shared as well as to explore some of the reasons for each individual's reluctance to talk openly in front of the other.

Diagnosis

- Female sexual interest/arousal disorder

Suggested Readings

Bancroft J: Human Sexuality and Its Problems, 3rd Edition. Edinburgh, Churchill Livingstone/Elsevier, 2009

Bancroft J, Loftus J, Long JS: Distress about sex: a national survey of women in heterosexual relationships. Arch Sex Behav 32(3):193–208, 2003

Brotto LA, Velten J: Sexual interest/arousal disorder in women, in Principles and Practices of Sex Therapy, 6th Edition. Edited by Hall KSK, Binik YM. New York, Guilford, 2020, pp 13–40

Mitchell K, Graham CA: Two challenges for the classification of sexual dysfunction. J Sex Med 5(7):1552–1558, 2008

Rosen NO, Corsini-Munt S, Dubé JP, et al: Partner responses to low desire: associations with sexual, relational, and psychological well-being among couples coping with female sexual interest/arousal disorder. J Sex Med 17(11):2168–2180, 2020

Vowels LM, Mark KP: Strategies for mitigating sexual desire discrepancy in relationships. Arch Sex Behav 49(3):1017–1028, 2020

CASE 13.2

Sexual Problems

Richard Balon, M.D.

Gerhard Palmer, a 55-year-old married accountant, presented to a psychiatrist for a second opinion in the context of recurrent major depressive disorder. He had not responded to two 3-month antidepressant trials, one with fluoxetine and another with sertraline, both at high dosages. At the time of his presentation, he had not taken any antidepressant medication since the trial with sertraline (about a month earlier).

The evaluation revealed a severely depressed man with profound psychomotor retardation, poor concentration, early insomnia, mildly diminished libido, and anhedonia. Mr. Palmer denied a substance use disorder, drank minimally, and did not smoke. He had started taking propranolol for hypertension about 6 months previously. His physical examination was unremarkable. Basic laboratory tests were within normal limits. His blood pressure was 135/85.

Treatment with clomipramine was initiated and was quickly increased, as tolerated, to the recommended maximum dosage of 250 mg/day. Buspirone 30 mg/day was added. After 5 weeks of treatment, Mr. Palmer reported feeling much improved. He was sleeping and eating well, was participating in enjoyable activities with increasing enthusiasm, and, for the first time in many months, felt a return of his sexual interest.

After not having had sexual intercourse in months, Mr. Palmer tried unsuccessfully to have sex several times. He was distressed to find that for the first time in his life, he was unable to maintain an erection during intercourse and was unable to ejaculate, even during masturbation. These problems persisted for a month. He recalled having had slightly delayed ejaculation while taking fluoxetine. He did not recall sexual problems during a prior trial of bupropion.

Discussion

Mr. Palmer complains of sexual problems that partially fulfill the requirements for two DSM-5 diagnoses: erectile disorder and delayed ejaculation. His problems do not fulfill criteria for either of these disorders, however, for two reasons: the duration is less than 6 months, and there is a strong possibility that both of these conditions can be attributed to either medications or medical-psychiatric comorbidity.

Mr. Palmer's erectile and ejaculation difficulties appear to have begun directly after the initiation of clomipramine, a tricyclic antidepressant with strong serotonergic properties. Tricyclic antidepressants are associated with various impairments of sexual function, most frequently erectile dysfunction. Clomipramine's sexual side effects also include delayed or inhibited ejaculation, reflecting its effects as a strong serotonin reuptake inhibitor. Mr. Palmer has also been started on buspirone, a partial serotonin and dopamine agonist that is usually not associated with sexual dysfunction and which is sometimes actually used to ameliorate the sexual dysfunction associated with antidepressants.

If clomipramine is the offending agent, then Mr. Palmer's sexual dysfunction would best fit DSM-5 medication-induced sexual dysfunction. The criteria for this disorder include evidence that the sexual dysfunction was temporally related to the initiation, dosage change, or withdrawal of a specific medication capable of producing such dysfunction. The association of erectile disorder and delayed ejaculation with clomipramine in this case seems to be clear.

DSM-5 also requires an assessment that the sexual dysfunction is not better accounted for by some other mechanism. For example, major depressive disorder is frequently associated with sexual dysfunction, primarily decreased libido, which Mr. Palmer did have prior to taking clomipramine. His decreased libido actually improved with improvement of depression. In addition, various substances of abuse (e.g., alcohol, nicotine, heroin) can also be associated with impairment of sexual function. Mr. Palmer denies misuse of substances, does not smoke, and drinks infrequently. Thus, substance use disorder appears an unlikely cause of his sexual problems.

Various medical illnesses (e.g., diabetes mellitus, cardiovascular disease) are also associated with sexual problems. In fact, sexual dysfunction is sometimes the sentinel of physical illness. In regard to Mr. Palmer, he was diagnosed with high blood pressure and started taking propranolol 6 months earlier. Both hypertension and this medication can impair sexual functioning. However, Mr. Palmer did not report sexual dysfunction until after he started taking the clomipramine, months after starting the propranolol. Such a self-report would seem to rule out both hypertension and propranolol as the cause for the sexual difficulty, but it is also possible that Mr. Palmer's depression led to sexual inactivity, so that the sexual dysfunction simply went unnoticed. Nevertheless, the most likely culprit for his sexual dysfunction remains the clomipramine, the same medication that has significantly improved the quality of his life.

Diagnoses

- Medication-induced sexual dysfunction
- Major depressive disorder, in full remission

Suggested Readings

Balon R: SSRI-associated sexual dysfunction. Am J Psychiatry 163(9):1504–1509, 2006
Goldberg JF, Ernst CL: Managing the Side Effects of Psychotropic Medications, 2nd Edition. Washington, DC, American Psychiatric Association Publishing, 2019

CHAPTER 14

Gender Dysphoria

INTRODUCTION

John W. Barnhill, M.D.

Psychiatrists study, categorize, and treat all manners of mental illness. Although there is a fringe perspective that all mental illness is "myth," almost no one within psychiatry doubts the distress and dysfunction that accompany such mental illnesses as schizophrenia, psychotic depression, and bipolar mania. There is more debate, however, about symptom clusters that blend subtly into variations on normal. When is shyness an anxiety disorder? When does quirkiness become high-functioning autism spectrum disorder? At what point do disagreeable behaviors become a personality disorder? When do "senior moments" become mild neurocognitive disorder? These debates are inevitable and are akin to similar debates about such nonpsychiatric medical diagnoses as diabetes and hypertension.

Definitions of normalcy directly affect psychiatric research funding and clinical insurance coverage, and they affect how society views atypical feelings, behaviors, and thoughts. To deal with this issue, DSM-5-TR focuses heavily on distress and dysfunction and, throughout the text, advises clinicians to make diagnoses only when symptoms are both enduring and significant. This mandate seems clinically and ethically satisfying: if no one is suffering or being negatively affected, there is no disorder.

A heated debate remains, however, in regard to clusters of behaviors, cognitions, and feelings that are not intrinsically pathological but are problematic because they exist within a certain social structure. Perhaps nowhere is this debate more heated than in the discussion of sexual behavior. Historically, for example, homosexuality was classified as a psychiatric disorder. At least partly in response to political pressure, the diagnosis of homosexuality was changed in DSM-III to a diagnosis of unhappiness over being homosexual (ego-dystonic homosexuality). DSM-IV included persistent and marked distress about sexual orientation as a "sexual disorder not otherwise specified." DSM-5 has moved further away from pathologizing homosexuality by eliminating all specific references to sexual orientation as a cause of psychiatric disturbance. Obviously, people who engage in or fantasize about sex with people of the same gender can have any of the DSM-5 diagnoses—and they can also be unhappy about their sexuality—but their sexual orientation is not viewed as a contributor privileged over any other characteristic.

Historically, gender identity referred to an individual's identification as a male or female. Typically, gender identity was viewed as binary and consistent with biological markers such as chromosomes and external genitalia. Some well-known clinics provided evaluations and treatment to assist people with discordant gender identities in their efforts to develop a body that matched their internal identities; however, for most psychiatrists, gender identity was rarely much of an issue.

Societal shifts have muddied these waters, and there are increasing numbers of people who do not see themselves as falling into traditional dichotomies (male/female; heterosexual/homosexual) and instead connect best with identities such as transgender, queer, and gender-fluid.

DSM-III and DSM-IV entered these complex and largely uncharted waters with diagnoses (transsexualism and gender identity disorder, respectively) that indicated that the clinical problem was the discordant gender identity. DSM-5 moved further in the direction of depathologizing discordant gender identity by introducing a new diagnosis, gender dysphoria, that emphasizes clinically significant distress or dysfunction along with the discordance.

The diagnosis of gender dysphoria may reflect a compromise between conflicting, pragmatic goals. For example, having a diagnosis that specifically references gender identity issues might be important for people who seek insurance coverage for gender reassignment surgery and hormonal therapy, as well as for transgender people who seek legal protection when they have experienced discrimination based on gender identity. On the other hand, it might be possible for a diagnosis related to gender identity to be used in legal settings as an indicator of some sort of pathology.

DSM-5-TR is not, however, most concerned with the financial and legal ramifications of its nomenclature. It also seems unlikely that DSM-5 intends the term *gender dysphoria* to refer primarily to psychological reactions to societal prejudice; discrimination comes in many forms, and no other triggers for discrimination are privileged with their own diagnosis. DSM-5 also clarifies that the diagnosis does not refer simply to gender nonconformity or transvestism.

Instead, the DSM-5-TR diagnosis of gender dysphoria reflects a clinical reality: a subset of patients present with unhappiness that seems bound up with the discordance between their bodies and their sense of self as well as the reality that surgical and hormonal interventions are far from perfected. Although perhaps an imperfect label, *gender dysphoria* is intended to improve the likelihood that these patients' specific issues will be the subject of effective clinical attention.

Suggested Readings

Bränström R, Pachankis JE: Reduction in mental health treatment utilization among transgender individuals after gender-affirming surgeries: a total population study. Am J Psychiatry 177(8):727–734, 2020

Kreukels BPC, Köhler B, Nordenström A, et al; dsd-LIFE Group: Gender dysphoria and gender change in disorders of sex development/intersex conditions: results from the dsd-LIFE study. J Sex Med 15(5):777–785, 2018

Leibowitz S, de Vries ALC: Gender dysphoria in adolescence. International Review of Psychiatry 28(1):21–35, 2016

Mueller SC, De Cuypere G, T'Sjoen G: Transgender research in the 21st century: a selective critical review from a neurocognitive perspective. Am J Psychiatry 174(12):1155–1162, 2017

Staub ME: Madness Is Civilization: When the Diagnosis Was Social. Chicago, IL, University of Chicago, 2011

CASE 14.1

Gender Reassignment

Sofia E. Matta, M.D.

John W. Barnhill, M.D.

Irene Rohmer, a 25-year-old salesperson, presented to a psychiatrist because of anxiety and depression. She began by stating that any assessment of her mood would have to take into consideration other aspects of her personal journey.

Ms. Rohmer had been born without complications, assigned male at birth, and raised as a boy. As long as she could remember, she had been teased and called a "sissy" by neighborhood boys. She had generally preferred the company of girls throughout childhood. During her teen years, she continued to have many female friends but considered herself a gay male and dated a few other gay teens. She recalled trying her best to "fit in" but noted that she had always felt like an outsider.

At age 19, during a romantic relationship with a man, she become aware of an intense desire to be a woman. That relationship ended, but Ms. Rohmer's desire to be a woman evolved into a strong sense that she had been born as the wrong gender. She tried to figure out whether this sense had existed earlier, but all she could recall was occasionally wishing she were a girl to fit in more comfortably with her friends.

By age 20, Ms. Rohmer was very unhappy about being seen as a man. She viewed her genitalia as "repugnant" and a "mistake of nature." Her family and some of her friends had not supported her developing sense of herself, and she recalled feeling increasingly hopeless, with episodic suicidal ideation and one nonlethal suicide attempt by overdose at age 21.

Beginning at age 22, Ms. Rohmer lived as a female, including changing her name and exclusively wearing women's clothes. She struggled to access appropriate health services and encountered multiple barriers to obtaining appropriate treatments, but, at the age of 24, Ms. Rohmer was evaluated by two psychiatrists skilled in transgender health, who agreed with her perspective, and she started gender-affirming hormone therapy.

As her transition progressed, she began to feel more comfortable in the female role and pleased with having secondary sexual characteristics that were more consistent with her experienced gender. She explored her sexuality during this time, dating both gay and straight men. Her anxiety diminished, although, as a member of a disenfranchised subgroup, she felt vulnerable to various types of aggression, including potential partner violence.

The following year, at age 25, Ms. Rohmer had the gender on her driver's license and passport changed from male to female (a change of gender markers) and underwent gender-affirming surgeries that included vaginoplasty and breast augmentation. The results of these surgeries were satisfactory, and she was often happy with the transition. She described herself as being "more comfortable in her skin" than she had ever been, and she only infrequently felt hopeless and suicidal. Despite not feeling particularly accepted by her family of origin or by some of her old friends, she found warm support from other friends and colleagues at work. Although she has many friends who are gender nonbinary/gender nonconforming, Ms. Rohmer identifies as a heterosexual female.

She said she tended to worry that people were judging her negatively, but this worry was less intense now than it had been earlier in her transition. She denied any recent suicide attempts, depression, or self-injurious behavior. She said she had "almost" given up on having a successful relationship but was "somehow" still optimistic that something would work out.

Discussion

Ms. Rohmer presents with "anxiety and depression," although most of the initial history focuses on her history of increasing gender incongruence.

Ms. Rohmer was assigned male at birth, and she was raised as a boy. Her childhood behaviors were considered "sissy" and therefore "gender atypical." She would certainly have been aware by adolescence of her "gender-nonconforming" behavior—and if she were not aware, her classmates would no doubt have clarified the point—but she considered herself a homosexual male until age 19. At that point, she became aware of a strong sense of being a woman, although she vaguely recalled childhood memories in which she wished she could have been a girl so that she could more easily play with the girls on the playground.

There is some ambiguity about when Ms. Rohmer first developed the consistent sense that she was female, but it seems most likely to have occurred at about age 19. Gender dissatisfaction that develops in adolescence or adulthood is considered "late-onset," in contrast to gender dissatisfaction that develops during childhood. At the point when Ms. Rohmer first decided to live as a woman, she would have been viewed as "transgender," a term that refers to an individual who seeks or has undergone a social transition between genders (in Ms. Rohmer's case, from male to female). As is generally true of transgender people who were assigned male at birth, Ms. Rohmer is sexually attracted to men. Ms. Rohmer describes herself as having been homosexual in regard to her sexual object choice during adolescence and young adulthood. As an adult transgender/transsexual woman, however, she describes herself as heterosexual.

During that transition phase, Ms. Rohmer might also have met criteria for a DSM-5 diagnosis of gender dysphoria. Gender dysphoria in adolescents and adults is a diagnosis that features a marked incongruence between one's assigned gender and one's experienced/expressed gender. To receive this diagnosis, Ms. Rohmer would also need to meet at least two of six criteria, including a strong desire to be rid of the primary and/or secondary sexual characteristics of the assigned gender; a strong desire to have the primary or secondary sexual characteristics of the other gender; and a strong desire to be of the other gender and/or treated as the other gender. She easily fulfilled these criteria.

Two additional criteria are crucial to the gender dysphoria diagnosis. In the first, Ms. Rohmer's sense of incongruence must have persisted for at least 6 months, a duration intended to specifically exclude transient shifts of identity formation that are commonly seen in children and adolescents. Because her childhood thoughts about being a girl appear to have been transitory and mostly focused on fitting in, Ms. Rohmer would likely not have met criteria for "gender dysphoria in children."

As is true for all DSM diagnoses, the diagnosis of gender dysphoria also requires that the condition be associated with clinically relevant distress or impairment in important areas of functioning. "Gender dysphoria" might have been an applicable term when Ms. Rohmer was ages 19–22; she consistently felt the incongruence between her assigned and experienced gender, and she demonstrated most of the typical criteria. At age 22, she would likely have warranted a specifier, "posttransition," which indicates that the person has begun to live full-time in the experienced gender and has undergone (or is preparing to undergo) medical procedures and/or hormonal treatments.

At the time of the current evaluation, however, Ms. Rohmer appears to be settled into her role as a transgender heterosexual woman. She continues to have lingering mood and anxiety issues, and her family of origin and some of her earlier friends have not been supportive, but she is psychologically much improved and appears to have developed friendships and work environments that are positive and affirming.

The next phase of the evaluation would likely focus on Ms. Rohmer's anxiety and depression (including her episodic suicidal feelings), as well as other life issues that are of importance to her (e.g., relationships and dating, work and social life, life goals).

Diagnosis

- Gender dysphoria, posttransition

Suggested Readings

Claahsen-van der Grinten H, Verhaak C, Steensma T, et al: Gender incongruence and gender dysphoria in childhood and adolescence-current insights in diagnostics, management, and follow-up. Eur J Pediatr 180(5):1349–1357, 2021

Mueller SC, De Cuypere G, T'Sjoen G. Transgender research in the 21st century: a selective critical review from a neurocognitive perspective. Am J Psychiatry 174(12):1155–1162, 2017

Zucker KJ: Epidemiology of gender dysphoria and transgender identity. Sex Health 14(5):404–411, 2017

Disruptive, Impulse-Control, and Conduct Disorders

INTRODUCTION

John W. Barnhill, M.D.

Executive functions help control and regulate attention, memory, and behavior. They are critical to adaptation, to the initiation and completion of tasks, and to the ability to delay gratification. They inhibit inappropriate, dangerous, and hurtful behaviors.

Impaired executive functioning is a key feature of all of the disruptive, impulse-control, and conduct disorders. These conditions include oppositional defiant disorder, intermittent explosive disorder, conduct disorder, antisocial personality disorder, pyromania, and kleptomania, as well as categories for people who have clinically relevant symptoms but do not meet criteria for a named disorder.

Other DSM-5 disorders are associated with impulsivity, poor planning, and interpersonal conflicts, and these other disorders—ranging from attention-deficit/hyperactivity disorder to substance use disorders to some of the personality disorders—are frequently comorbid with the disorders described in this chapter. Furthermore, disruptive impulsivity is associated with substance use, HIV and hepatitis C infections, traumatic brain injury, and all manner of dangerous behavioral patterns that reflect impaired executive functioning and can lead to intensifying cycles of dysfunctional behavior.

All of the disorders in this chapter tend to start early in life, which is unsurprising given the relative immaturity of executive functioning during childhood and adolescence. If the clinical interview indicates that one of the disruptive, impulse-control, or conduct disorders has suddenly sprouted during the adult years, the individual most likely either has developed a serious neuropsychiatric disorder or has not provided an accurate history. On the other hand, children who present with one of these disorders do not inevitably go on to develop pervasively damaging diagnoses such as antisocial personality disorder or lifelong intermittent explosive disorder. However, they are at risk for ongoing problems, including depressive, anxiety, and substance use disorders.

These children are also at risk for encountering a disproportionate amount of societal trouble, and DSM-5 provides a structure for investigating severity. In individuals with oppositional defiant disorder, for example, pervasiveness of symptoms across settings is a useful marker for severity, whereas "limited prosocial emotions" is a specifier for conduct disorder that identifies greater severity and a different treatment response.

Poorly controlled behaviors and emotions lie on a continuum, and most sporadically impulsive behavior and dysregulated emotions do not indicate a DSM-5 disorder but rather immaturity intensified by situational issues such as family and interpersonal strife, substance intoxication, and peer pressure. As is the case throughout DSM-5, the onus is on the clinician to carefully consider the point at which thoughts, feelings, and behaviors cross the line into a level of distress and dysfunction that warrants a diagnosis.

Particularly relevant variables include frequency, setting, and duration of the troublesome episodes. An accurate history is necessary to gather this information. Such an investigation can be stymied by the fact that, as is the case with the personality disorders, people other than the identified patient may be more distressed than the patient. Furthermore, psychiatric history tends to depend on patient honesty, and many of these patients are not spontaneously and transparently forthcoming. For these reasons, evaluations are often initiated by family and institutions (school, work, the legal system) and are unlikely to be complete without collateral information.

Suggested Readings

Buitelaar JK, Smeets KC, Herpers P: Conduct disorders. Eur Child Adolesc Psychiatry 22 (suppl 1):S49–S54, 2013

Coccaro EF, McCloskey MS (eds): Aggression: Clinical Features and Treatment Across the Diagnostic Spectrum. Washington, DC, American Psychiatric Association Publishing, 2019

Matthys W, Lochman JE: Oppositional Defiant Disorder and Conduct Disorder in Childhood, 2nd Edition. West Sussex, UK, Wiley-Blackwell, 2017

CASE 15.1

Doesn't Know the Rules

Juan D. Pedraza, M.D.
Jeffrey H. Newcorn, M.D.

Kyle was a 12-year-old boy who reluctantly agreed to admission to a psychiatric unit after getting arrested for breaking into a grocery store. His mother said she was "exhausted," adding that it was hard to raise a boy who "doesn't know the rules."

Beginning as a young child, Kyle was unusually aggressive, bullying other children and taking their things. When confronted by his mother, stepfather, or a teacher, he had long tended to curse, punch, and show no concern for possible punishment. Disruptive, impulsive, and "fidgety," Kyle was diagnosed with attention-deficit/hyperactivity disorder (ADHD) and placed in a special education program by second grade. He began to see a psychiatrist in fourth grade for weekly psychotherapy and medications (quetiapine and dexmethylphenidate). He was adherent only sporadically with both the medication and the therapy. When asked why this was, he replied that his psychiatrist was "stupid."

During the year prior to the admission, he had been caught stealing from school lockers (a cell phone, a jacket, a laptop computer), disciplined after "mugging" a classmate for his wallet, and suspended after multiple physical fights with classmates. He had been arrested twice for these behaviors. His mother and teachers agreed that although he could be charming to strangers, people quickly caught on to the fact that he was a "con artist." Kyle was consistently unremorseful, externalizing of blame, and uninterested in the feelings of others. He was disorganized, was inattentive and uninterested in following instructions, and constantly lost his possessions. He generally did not do his homework, and when he did, his performance was erratic. When confronted about his poor performance, he tended to say, "And what are you going to do, shoot me?" Kyle, his mother, and his teachers agreed that he was a loner and not well liked by his peers.

Kyle lived with his mother, stepfather, and two younger half-siblings. His stepfather was unemployed, and his mother worked part-time as a cashier in a grocery store. His biological father was in prison for drug possession. Both biological grandfathers had a history of alcohol use disorder.

Kyle's early history was normal. The pregnancy was uneventful, and he reached all of his milestones on time. There was no history of sexual or physical abuse. Kyle had no known medical problems, alcohol or substance abuse, or participation in gang activities. He had not been caught with weapons, had not set fires, and had not been seen as particularly cruel to other children or animals. He had been regularly truant from school but had neither run away nor stayed away from home until late at night.

When interviewed on the psychiatric unit, Kyle was casually groomed and appeared his stated age of 12. He was fidgety and made sporadic eye contact with the interviewer. He said he was "mad" and insisted he would rather be in jail than on a psychiatric unit. His speech was loud but coherent, goal directed, and of normal rate. His affect was irritable and angry. He denied suicidal or homicidal ideation. He denied psychotic symptoms. He denied feeling depressed. He had no obvious cognitive deficits but declined more formal testing. His insight was limited, and his judgment was poor by history.

Discussion

Kyle is a 12-year-old boy who was brought to a psychiatric unit after getting caught breaking into a grocery store. He has a lengthy history of behaviors that violate the rights of others. These behaviors deviate significantly from age-appropriate societal norms and have caused social, academic, and functional impairment. He has a disorder of conduct.

In DSM-5, the criteria for conduct disorder (CD) are organized into four categories of behavior: aggression to people and animals, destruction of property, deceitfulness or theft, and serious violations of rules. A CD diagnosis requires three or more specific behaviors out of the 15 that are listed within these four categories. The behaviors must have been present in the last 12 months, with at least one criterion present in the prior 6 months. Kyle has at least seven of the 15: bullying, fighting, stealing (with and without confrontation), break-ins, lying, and truancy.

Kyle also has a history of comorbid ADHD, as evidenced by persistent symptoms of hyperactivity, restlessness, impulsivity, and inattention. ADHD is found in about 20% of youth with CD. The criteria for the two disorders are relatively distinct, although both entities present with pathological levels of impulsivity.

DSM-5 includes multiple specifiers that allow CD to be further subdivided. Kyle's behavior began before age 10, which places him in the category of childhood-onset type as opposed to adolescent-onset type. There is also an unspecified-onset designation, used when information is inadequate to clarify whether the behaviors began before age 10. When trying to identify the age at onset, the clinician should seek multiple sources of information and recall that estimates are often 2 years later than actual onset. People with an early age at onset—like Kyle—are more likely to be male, to be aggressive, and to have impaired peer relationships. They are also more likely to have comorbid ADHD and to go on to have adulthoods marked by criminal behavior and substance use disorders. In contrast, CD that manifests between ages 10 and 16 (onset is rare after age 16) tends to be milder, and most individuals go on to achieve adequate social and occupational adjustment as adults. Both groups have an elevated risk, however, of many psychiatric disorders.

The second DSM-5 specifier for CD relates to the presence (or absence) of callous and unemotional traits. The "limited prosocial emotions" specifier requires the persistent presence of two or more of the following: lack of remorse or guilt; lack of empathy; lack of concern about performance; and shallow or deficient affect. Kyle has a history of disregard for the feelings of others, appears unconcerned about his performance ("What are you going to do, shoot me?"), and shows no remorse for his actions. This label applies to only a minority of people with CD and is associated with aggression and fearless thrill seeking.

A third specifier for CD relates to the severity of symptoms. Lying and staying out past a curfew might qualify a person for mild CD. Vandalism or stealing without confrontation might lead to a diagnosis of moderate CD. Kyle's behaviors would qualify for the severe subtype.

Multiple other aspects of Kyle's history are useful to understanding his situation. His father is in prison for substance use and/or dealing. Both of his biological grandfathers have a history of alcohol use disorder. His mother and stepfather are underemployed, although details about the stepfather are unknown. In general, CD risk has been found to be increased in families with criminal records, conduct disorder, and substance abuse, as well as mood, anxiety, and schizophrenia spectrum disorders. Environment also contributes, both in regard to chaotic early child-rearing and, later, to living in a dangerous, threatening neighborhood.

Kyle's diagnosis of conduct disorder is an example of how diagnoses can evolve over the course of a lifetime. His earlier behavior would warrant a diagnosis of DSM-5 oppositional defiant disorder (ODD), which is characterized by a pattern of negative, hostile, and defiant behaviors that are usually directed at an authority figure (e.g., parent or teacher) and cause significant distress in social or academic settings. However, ODD cannot be diagnosed if CD is present. As he enters adolescence, Kyle is at risk for many psychiatric disorders, including mood, anxiety, and substance use disorders. Of particular concern is the possibility that his aggression, theft, and rules violations will persist and his diagnosis of conduct disorder will shift in adulthood to antisocial personality disorder.

Diagnoses

- Conduct disorder, childhood-onset type, severe, with limited prosocial emotions
- Attention-deficit/hyperactivity disorder

Suggested Readings

Fairchild G, Hawes DJ, Frick PJ, et al: Conduct disorder. Nat Rev Dis Primers 5(1):43, 2019
Junewicz A, Billick SB: Conduct disorder: biology and developmental trajectories. Psychiatr Q 91(1):77–90, 2020
Rowe R, Maughan B, Moran P, et al: The role of callous and unemotional traits in the diagnosis of conduct disorder. J Child Psychol Psychiatry 51(6):688–695, 2010

CASE 15.2

Impossible to Live With

Emil F. Coccaro, M.D.

Lucas Sandahl, a 32-year-old landscape architect, presented to a psychiatrist for help with anger. He came to the office with his wife, the mother of their two young children. The couple agreed that Mr. Sandahl had become "almost impossible to live with." Mrs. Sandahl reported that although she had always considered her husband "high-strung," his outbursts were increasing in both frequency and intensity, and she worried that he would become violent with her.

Their most recent argument began when Mr. Sandahl came home after a "hard day at work" to find that dinner was not ready. When he entered the kitchen and saw his wife sitting at the table reading the newspaper, he "exploded" and launched into a tirade about how "bad" a wife she was. When Mrs. Sandahl tried to explain her own long day, Mr. Sandahl cursed at her and broke glassware and a kitchen chair. Terrified, she ran out of the kitchen, gathered up the toddlers, and left for her mother's house a few miles away. The next day, she told her husband that he would need to get help immediately or prepare for a divorce.

Mr. Sandahl said his "blowups" began in childhood but did not become "problematic" for him until age 13. At about that time, he started having frequent fights with classmates that would occasionally result in trips to the principal's office. In between the altercations, he was active socially and a solid student.

Mr. Sandahl estimated that he had had approximately four verbal outbursts a week in recent years, generally in response to frustration, unexpected demands, or perceived insults. In addition to these heated verbal tussles, Mr. Sandahl described acts of violence about every 2 months; for example, he threw a computer monitor across the room when it started "acting up," he kicked a hole in a wall when one of his children would not quit crying, and he destroyed his mobile phone during an argument with his mother. He denied physical fights since his adolescence, although he had nearly come to blows with a neighbor as well as an assortment of strangers and employees. The idea that he might physically hurt someone scared Mr. Sandahl "to the core."

These outbursts blighted his relationships with colleagues and romantic partners and led to his decision to start his own landscaping company at age 25. The business had done well, despite his demanding style and "hair-trigger" temper that led to high employee turnover.

Mr. Sandahl described the episodes as short-lived, reaching a peak within seconds and rarely lasting more than a few minutes. Between episodes, he described himself as feeling "fine." He had experienced brief periods of depressed mood and increased anxiety, but these had not impaired him significantly and tended to resolve on their own within a week. Mr. Sandahl drank socially, but neither he nor his wife linked the outbursts to the alcohol. He had a history of experimentation with various drugs of abuse, but not in recent years.

Mr. Sandahl reported at least two other immediate family members with significant "anger issues." His father was emotionally abusive and perfectionistic, expecting "great things" from his only son. Mr. Sandahl's older sister also had problems with her temper; he attributed her three divorces to her emotionally abusive behavior.

On examination, Mr. Sandahl was casually dressed, cooperative, and coherent. He was worried about his behavior and contrite toward his wife. He denied depression, psychosis, and confusion. He denied any thoughts of hurting himself or others. He was cognitively intact. His insight and judgment were good during the course of the interview.

Discussion

Mr. Sandahl reports verbal outbursts four times per week and physically aggressive outbursts every couple of months. This behavior is invariably out of proportion to the provocations, is not planned, and is anger based. It causes impairment and distress, in his personal and work life, and it is not better explained by any other psychiatric disorder or medical illness. He meets all the criteria for intermittent explosive disorder (IED), which is discussed in the DSM-5 chapter on disruptive, impulse-control, and conduct disorders.

Mr. Sandahl also manifests features that are commonly associated with IED but are not part of the core diagnostic criteria. These include hostile attribution bias (e.g., dinner not being ready because his wife is lazy rather than because she had a hard day herself), "trigger points" associated with frustration and/or perceived insults, an immediate family history of problems with anger, a personal history of emotional abuse (from his father), early age at onset, and chronic course. Many or most individuals with IED have traits associated with a personality disorder, even if they do not meet all the criteria for a specific personality disorder (e.g., perfectionism as in obsessive-compulsive personality disorder). This is because the vast majority of individuals with IED have long-standing difficulties with impulse control and interpersonal relationships. When individuals do meet criteria for IED and a personality disorder, both diagnoses should be made.

Individuals with borderline personality disorder and antisocial personality disorder are especially likely to have outbursts that can resemble those of IED. Unless they have a comorbid IED, however, their outbursts are generally less aggressive than those seen in people with IED.

The most common comorbidities with IED are anxiety, depressive, and substance use disorders. Although Mr. Sandahl describes transient periods of depressed mood and anxiety, and he does drink alcohol, none of these appear to fulfill criteria for a DSM-5 diagnosis. Intermittent outbursts are also found in a variety of other psychiatric disorders. If the recurrent explosive episodes were related to traumatic brain injury, delirium, dementia, or recurrent intoxication, then the IED diagnosis would not be applied. None of these appear pertinent to Mr. Sandahl's situation. On the other hand, if Mr. Sandahl had also been diagnosed with attention-deficit/hyperactivity disorder, conduct disorder, oppositional defiant disorder, or autism spectrum disorder, comorbid diagnoses would be appropriate.

In addition to frequent verbal and physical aggression, Mr. Sandahl also engages in intimate partner abuse. This behavior is potentially dangerous, and his wife has finally reached the limit of her tolerance. Treatment is a critical issue not simply for the marriage but also to avoid perpetuating the cycle of violence in his children.

Diagnosis

- Intermittent explosive disorder

Suggested Readings

Coccaro EF, McCloskey MS (eds): Aggression: Clinical Features and Treatment Across the Diagnostic Spectrum. Washington, DC, American Psychiatric Association Publishing, 2019

Coccaro EF, Lee R, McCloskey MS: Relationship between psychopathy, aggression, anger, impulsivity, and intermittent explosive disorder. Aggress Behav 40(6):526–536, 2014

CHAPTER 16

Substance-Related and Addictive Disorders

INTRODUCTION

Jonathan Avery, M.D.

The substance-related and addictive disorders chapter of DSM-5 covers disorders associated with 10 classes of drugs, and also covers gambling disorder.

All of the DSM-5 substance use disorders require clinically significant impairment or distress and the presence of at least two physical, psychological, and social consequences of the drug use. DSM-5 includes several specifiers to further characterize the substance use disorders; these specifiers relate to *course* (e.g., early remission, sustained remission) and *severity* (based on the number of criteria endorsed). Notably, the diagnosis of substance use disorder has replaced the prior categories of substance abuse and dependence.

DSM-5 also provides diagnostic criteria for clinical presentations that are directly related to substance use, such as intoxication and withdrawal, along with descriptive specifiers. For example, if an individual presents with alcohol intoxication, the clinician can add a code indicating the presence or absence of a comorbid alcohol use disorder. For patients who maintain a clear sensorium during alcohol withdrawal but also develop perceptual disturbances, the DSM-5 diagnosis would likely be alcohol withdrawal with perceptual disturbances. In the much more likely event that the perceptual disturbances are accompanied by confusion, the diagnosis would shift to an alcohol withdrawal delirium (a disorder listed in the chapter on neurocognitive disorders rather than the chapter on substance-related disorders).

Substance use can also result in symptom clusters that resemble a broad array of psychiatric diagnoses, including depressive, bipolar, and psychotic disorders. DSM-5 clarifies a diagnostic approach that is based significantly on course and the likely impact of the substance in question. For example, if depressive symptoms occur during acute withdrawal from cocaine, the depressive symptoms would be deemed to be part of the withdrawal. If the clinically significant depressive symptoms begin in the context of cocaine use and then persist after cessation of the cocaine use and beyond the expected duration of withdrawal, the individual would likely qualify for a cocaine-induced depressive disorder. If the significant depressive symptoms persist an appreciable amount of time (e.g., 1 month) following the cessation of cocaine use, then the patient would likely be evaluated as having an independent major depressive disorder. In that event, the cocaine use might be seen as a trigger but would no longer be part of the DSM-5 diagnosis.

Gambling disorder is the only behavioral addiction in the chapter. Evidence indicates that behavioral addictions such as gambling have much in common with substance use disorders, including pattern of use and activation of the same reward system in the brain. Other behavioral addictions are being considered for future editions of DSM.

Suggested Readings

Avery JD, Barnhill JW (eds): Co-Occurring Mental Illness and Substance Use Disorders: A Guide to Diagnosis and Treatment. Arlington, VA, American Psychiatric Association Publishing, 2017

Brady KT, Levin FR, Galanter M, Kleber HD (eds): The American Psychiatric Publishing Textbook of Substance Use Disorder Treatment, 6th Edition. Washington, DC, American Psychiatric Association Publishing, 2021

Hasin DS, O'Brien CP, Auriacombe M, et al: DSM-5 criteria for substance use disorders: recommendations and rationale. Am J Psychiatry 170(8):834–851, 2013

CASE 16.1

Alcohol

Marc A. Schuckit, M.D.

Matthew Tucker, a 45-year-old married European American plumber, was referred for a psychiatric evaluation after his family carried out an intervention to express their concern that his alcohol problems were getting out of control. Mr. Tucker denied having had a drink since making the appointment 3 days earlier.

For 20 years after high school, Mr. Tucker typically drank 3–5 beers per evening, five times per week. Over the last 7 years, he had consumed alcohol almost daily, with an average of 6 beers on weeknights and 12 beers on weekends and holidays. His wife repeatedly voiced her concern that he was "drinking too much," but despite his efforts to limit his alcohol intake, Mr. Tucker continued to spend much of the weekend drinking, sometimes missing family get-togethers, and often passed out while watching TV in the evening. He remained productive at work, however, and never called in sick. In many ways, his history represented what is typically seen in alcohol use disorder. Mr. Tucker had achieved two 30-day periods of abstinence in the previous 4 years. Both times, he said he had quit drinking "cold turkey" in response to his wife's concerns. He denied having had symptoms of alcohol withdrawal either time.

In the 6 months prior to the evaluation, Mr. Tucker had become uncharacteristically irritable, fatigued, dysphoric, and worried. He was unable to enjoy his usual activities, including food and sex, and had difficulty concentrating. He also reacted more emotionally to stresses and expressed unsubstantiated concern about the future of his business. The patient often awoke at 2:00 A.M. and had trouble getting back to sleep.

Mr. Tucker and his wife indicated that although this period of sadness had lasted 6 months, he had experienced several similar episodes in the prior 5 years, lasting 4–6 weeks each. They denied any such episodes earlier in his life.

Mr. Tucker had been married for 18 years, and he and his wife had one 17-year-old daughter. The patient was a high school graduate with 2 years of community college who currently owned a successful plumbing company. He denied any other history of psychiatric or medical problems, as well as any history of mania or suicide attempts. He had never seen a psychiatrist before.

At a recent annual checkup, Mr. Tucker's internist noted a mildly elevated blood pressure (135/92), a γ-glutamyltransferase (GGT) value of 47 IU/L, and a mean corpuscular volume of 92.5 μm^3. All other laboratory results were in the normal range.

At the time of his first visit, Mr. Tucker was neatly dressed, maintained good eye contact, and showed no evidence of confusion or psychotic symptoms. His eyes teared up when he talked about the future, and he admitted to having felt sad for most of the day on a regular basis for the last 6 months, but he denied suicidal ideation or plans. His cognition was within normal limits, and he demonstrated an understanding of the effects that the alcohol was having on him.

A physical examination by the psychiatrist revealed a normal pulse rate, no tremor or sweating, and only a slightly elevated blood pressure.

Discussion

Mr. Tucker meets criteria for two DSM-5 diagnoses. The first is a moderate alcohol use disorder, as indicated by his unsuccessful efforts to cut down, excessive time spent intoxicated or recovering from the effects of alcohol, missed important social activities, and continued use of alcohol despite problems. Mr. Tucker had no clinically significant symptoms of alcohol withdrawal during the evaluation despite having been abstinent for 3 days, and he denied experiencing withdrawal symptoms during prior efforts to stop drinking.

A second diagnosis relates to his mood symptoms. Mr. Tucker meets symptomatic criteria for a major depressive episode with onset about 6 months earlier. He describes a persistently depressed mood, reduced interest in activities, interval insomnia, diminished ability to concentrate, and fatigue. He has experienced "several" such episodes in the past 5 years, all of which had apparently resolved spontaneously with 4–6 weeks of abstinence.

It is important to distinguish between depressive episodes that occur only in the context of heavy alcohol use and those that develop independently of excessive drinking. An independent depressive episode that develops in a person with an alcohol use disorder is likely to run the course of any major depressive episode, with a similar duration and response to usual treatments. Depressive episodes that develop only during periods of heavy drinking—as seen in Mr. Tucker—are different. More properly called an alcohol-induced depressive disorder, these episodes are likely to diminish and disappear within several weeks to a month of abstinence. Few data indicate that these depressive episodes require antidepressant medications, and when the person stops the heavy drinking, the depressive symptoms are likely to diminish in less time than medications would probably take to produce their major effects. Subthreshold symptoms (e.g., sleep impairment) can persist but should improve with ongoing sobriety. If criteria for major depressive disorder were to continue to be met after a month of abstinence, however, Mr. Tucker would be said to have an independent major depressive disorder, although the clinician might view the alcohol use as having been a triggering event.

Diagnoses

- Alcohol use disorder
- Alcohol-induced depressive disorder

Suggested Readings

Farmer RF, Seeley JR, Kosty DB, et al: No reliable evidence that emotional disorders are proximal antecedents, concomitants, or short-term consequences of first episode alcohol use disorders in a representative community sample. J Stud Alcohol Drugs 78(2):222–231, 2017

Grant BF, Chou SP, Saha TD, et al: Prevalence of 12-month alcohol use, high-risk drinking, and DSM-IV alcohol use disorder in the United States, 2001-2002 to 2012-2013: results from the National Epidemiologic Survey on Alcohol and Related Conditions. JAMA Psychiatry 74(9):911–923, 2017

Hasin DS, O'Brien CP, Auriacombe M, et al: DSM-5 criteria for substance use disorders: recommendations and rationale. Am J Psychiatry 170(8):834–851, 2013

Schuckit MA, Smith TL: Endorsement of specific alcohol use disorder criterion items changes with age in individuals with persistent alcohol use disorders in 2 generations of the San Diego Prospective Study. Alcohol Clin Exp Res 45(10):2059–2068, 2021

CASE 16.2

Alcohol Withdrawal

Roger D. Weiss, M.D.

Nicholas Underwood, a 41-year-old married software engineer, entered an alcohol treatment program with this chief complaint: "I need to stop drinking or my wife will divorce me."

At the time of admission, Mr. Underwood stated that he was drinking approximately 1 liter of vodka per day, every day, and had not had an alcohol-free day in over 2 years. For many years, Mr. Underwood had drunk alcohol only after work, but about a year prior to the evaluation he had begun to routinely drink in the morning whenever he had the day off. More recently, he had begun to feel "shaky" every morning and would sometimes treat that sensation with a drink, followed by more alcohol during the day.

Mr. Underwood experienced a number of problems related to drinking. His wife was "at the end of her rope" and considering divorce. His diminished ability to concentrate at work was "sinking" his once-promising career. He was spending more time trying to recover from the effects of drinking and found himself planning strategies both for abstinence and for surreptitiously taking his next drink.

Mr. Underwood first tried alcohol in high school and said that he had always been able to hold his liquor more than his friends could. In college, he was one of the heaviest drinkers in a fraternity known as "Animal House" around campus. Through his 30s, he gradually increased the frequency of his drinking from primarily on weekends to daily. Over the prior year, he had switched from being exclusively a beer drinker to drinking vodka. He had gone to many Alcoholics Anonymous meetings over the years but tended to drink as soon as the meeting ended. He had received no formal treatment.

The patient denied recent use of other substances; he had smoked marijuana and snorted cocaine several times during college but never since. He had used no other illicit drugs and took no medications. He did not smoke cigarettes. He had experienced blackouts on several occasions during college but not since then. He had no history of seizures and no other medical problems. Family history was significant for alcohol use disorder in his father and paternal grandfather.

Mr. Underwood entered the alcohol treatment program at approximately 3:00 P.M., having not had a drink since the evening before. He was diaphoretic and exhibited significant tremulousness in his hands. He complained of anxiety, restlessness, irritability, nausea, and recent insomnia.

Clinical evaluation revealed a casually groomed, diaphoretic man who was cooperative but anxiously pacing and who immediately said, "I'm getting ready to jump out of my skin." Speech was of normal rate, rhythm, and tone. He denied depression. There was no evidence of psychotic thinking, and he denied auditory, visual, or tactile hallucinations. He was alert and oriented to person, place, and date. He had no gross memory deficits, but his attention and concentration were noted to be reduced.

Notable features of his physical examination were marked diaphoresis, a blood pressure of 155/95, a heart rate of 104 beats/minute, severe tremulousness in his upper extremities, and hyperactive deep tendon reflexes throughout. Laboratory test findings were within normal limits except for aspartate aminotransferase and alanine aminotransferase, which were approximately 3 times normal.

Discussion

Mr. Underwood clearly meets the criteria for alcohol withdrawal. In addition to recent cessation of heavy and prolonged alcohol use, Mr. Underwood demonstrates the following symptoms: autonomic hyperactivity, upper-extremity tremor, insomnia, nausea, agitation, and anxiety. In other words, he has six of the eight criteria for alcohol withdrawal, far exceeding the lower required limit of two.

One way to remember the key symptoms of alcohol withdrawal is to think of the so-called four Ss: sleep problems, sweats, stomach problems, and shakes. Notably, a major goal of treatment of alcohol withdrawal is the avoidance of the fifth S—namely, grand mal seizures.

Alcohol withdrawal occurs in the context of physical dependence. Although it can occur upon reduction of drinking in individuals with severe physical dependence, significant withdrawal typically occurs upon sudden, complete cessation of drinking. Symptoms of withdrawal ordinarily can begin 4–12 hours after the last drink, with a peak in intensity 24–48 hours after the last drink.

A major goal in the pharmacological treatment of withdrawal is the avoidance of the two most serious complications of alcohol withdrawal: 1) grand mal seizures and 2) alcohol withdrawal delirium (also known as delirium tremens). Seizures occur in approximately 3% of patients experiencing withdrawal; they typically occur 7–48 hours after the last drink, with the majority of seizures occurring between 17 and 24 hours afterward. In some circumstances, a seizure is followed by alcohol withdrawal delirium, the hallmark of which is disorientation and fluctuation in consciousness, generally with severe autonomic hyperactivity. Patients at greatest risk for delirium are those with serious medical illness and a long-standing history of very heavy drinking. Because alcohol withdrawal delirium is sometimes fatal, it needs to be treated aggressively in a closely monitored medical setting. It is important to note that although seizures are sometimes followed by delirium, the reverse is rarely true. Therefore, if a patient experiences delirium and subsequently has a grand mal seizure, the clinician should look for another cause of the seizure (e.g., a subdural hematoma).

Mr. Underwood also meets symptomatic criteria for alcohol use disorder. He has been drinking large amounts of alcohol despite recurrent efforts to quit. His cravings for alcohol are strong, and he has continued to use despite occupational and marital problems that appear to be exacerbated directly by his alcohol use and by the time necessary to recover from his nightly intoxication. He has also demonstrated both tolerance and withdrawal. Mr. Underwood meets at least eight of the 11 criteria for alcohol use disorder, thereby qualifying for the "severe" specifier.

Diagnoses

- Alcohol withdrawal
- Alcohol use disorder, severe

Suggested Readings

Askgaard G, Hallas J, Fink-Jensen A, et al: Phenobarbital compared to benzodiazepines in alcohol withdrawal treatment: a register-based cohort study of subsequent benzodiazepine use, alcohol recidivism and mortality. Drug Alcohol Depend 161:258–264, 2016
Holleck JL, Merchant N, Gunderson CG: Symptom-triggered therapy for alcohol withdrawal syndrome: a systematic review and meta-analysis of randomized controlled trials. J Gen Intern Med 34(6):1018–1024, 2019

CASE 16.3

Addiction

Petros Levounis, M.D., M.A.

Oliver Vincent had never seen himself as being an addict. He had always been "on top of things." At age 35, he was independently wealthy as the owner of several clothing franchises, lived with an ex-partner in a more-than-comfortable apartment in New York City, worked out every day, enjoyed the company of a group of loving friends, and, although single, had not given up on the idea of someday (preferably soon) finding the perfect man to share his life with. Mr. Vincent came out to his Irish Catholic family when he was 19. His parents had already guessed that Mr. Vincent was gay long before he told them, and they took the non-news fairly well. Their main concern had been that their son might be discriminated against because of his sexuality, get hurt, and live a lonely life. Nothing could be farther from the way things turned out: Mr. Vincent was "out and proud" and living it up.

When Mr. Vincent found himself with a substance use problem, he addressed it the same way he had dealt with pretty much everything else: head on. For the first time in his life, he decided to see a psychiatrist.

Mr. Vincent described a pattern that revolved around weekend "party and play" activities.[1] On Friday and Saturday evenings—and occasionally during the week—he would go out to dinner with friends and then to a club or a private party. He tended to drink two or three cocktails and four to five glasses of wine during the evening. Without the alcohol, he found he could easily say "no" to substances, but "after a good buzz, if someone has coke—and there is always someone around who has coke—I use. And then my heart starts to race, and then I do everything I can to hook up. I used to go online, but these days, it's all on Scruff and good ol' Grindr."[2]

Overall, Mr. Vincent drank alcohol and used cocaine three to four times a week and "occasionally used Tina and bath salts."[3] He could hardly attend Monday morning meetings, much less prepare for them, and had been trying to cut down on his cocaine use for the prior 6 months without success.

Since Mr. Vincent had started using cocaine regularly, he had lost weight and had trouble sleeping. He worried that his effort at the gym was going to waste. His business continued to succeed, but his own effectiveness had decreased. Most importantly, he did not practice safer sex when high on stimulants, and because he did not want to be on a pre-exposure prophylaxis (PrEP) regimen, he worried about HIV seroconversion.

Discussion

Mr. Vincent has a cocaine use disorder. If the use of crystal methamphetamine or bath salts is deemed to be significant, a more accurate diagnosis would be stimulant use disorder. According to DSM-5, a stimulant (specifically cocaine in this case) use disorder involves a pattern of significant impairment and distress accompanied by at least two of 11 criteria. Mr. Vincent has demonstrated a persistent desire to cut down without success, has had recurrent unprotected sex while high, recognizes the attendant risks, and appears to go through withdrawal every Monday. Mr. Vincent's stimulant use disorder manifests at least four of the DSM-5 Criterion A symptoms and would be described as moderate in severity.

Mr. Vincent's situation supports the rationale for the shift in DSM-5 from two separate diagnoses (substance abuse and dependence) to a unified substance use disorder. In the DSM-IV system, *abuse* was meant to signify a less severe disorder than *dependence*, but a case like Mr. Vincent's could be diagnostically challenging. If it were not for using cocaine in physically hazardous situations (unprotected sex with risk of HIV transmission), Mr. Vincent's disorder would fully meet criteria for DSM-IV cocaine dependence but not for abuse—a confusing formulation. DSM-5 unified these two diagnoses and described three levels of severity: mild, moderate, and severe.

---

[1] *Party* and *play* are classic code words for drugs and sex, respectively. The term is sometimes abbreviated PNP.

[2] Scruff and Grindr are smartphone applications that use GPS to identify and connect similarly inclined individuals in a person's geographical vicinity.

[3] *Tina* is slang for crystal methamphetamine (i.e., from *crystal* to *Christina* to *Tina*). *Bath salts* is slang for a powder that contains a variety of synthetic stimulants (e.g., cathinone derivatives).

Mr. Vincent may qualify for several other DSM-5 diagnoses. If evaluated on a Saturday night, he would likely qualify for the diagnosis of cocaine intoxication, as evidenced by tachycardia and poor judgment. If evaluated on Monday morning, he would likely meet criteria for cocaine withdrawal, characterized by dysphoria and fatigue. Mr. Vincent's alcohol use is also problematic. It appears to lead directly to the cocaine use and—depending on additional history that should be elicited—may or may not rise to the level of an alcohol use disorder.

Further investigation might reveal additional symptomatology, but Mr. Vincent does not appear to be suffering from major depressive, anxiety, personality, or trauma-related disorders. His substance use seems to have been fueled primarily by social determinants, specifically a "party and play" subculture of the gay male community, which has accepted, legitimized, and eventually normalized the use of stimulants.

Many substance-using patients have other co-occurring psychiatric disorders, and it is often tempting to assume that substance use must have been caused by (and/or resulted in) some type of major mood disturbance or other psychiatric problem. Nevertheless, a significant number of addicted patients have no comorbidities. Many people—possibly including Mr. Vincent's parents—assume that lesbian, gay, bisexual, transgender, queer, and other sexual and gender minority (LGBTQ+) people live miserable and lonely lives, and that a variety of psychiatric diagnoses are almost inevitable. A different stereotype might suggest that stimulant use and unsafe sex are normative parts of a gay subculture and should simply be accepted as a reasonable part of the "party and play" world. Both of these stereotypes can deskill the clinician, reduce his or her effectiveness, and lead to overestimation or underestimation of psychopathology, respectively.

Furthermore, although dangerous and distressing behavior might sometimes seem like an inherent part of a subculture (e.g., that of young urban gay men), it is useful to recall that most people within that broad category do not routinely use substances or engage in recurrent, risky sexual behavior. By coming for a psychiatric consultation, Mr. Vincent himself has indicated that these aspects of his otherwise terrific life are out of control and in need of professional help.

Diagnosis

- Cocaine use disorder, moderate

Suggested Readings

Levounis P, Ruggiero JS: Outpatient management of crystal methamphetamine dependence among gay and bisexual men: how can it be done? Primary Psychiatry 13(2):75–80, 2006

Levounis P, Yarbrough E (eds): Pocket Guide to LGBTQ Mental Health: Understanding the Spectrum of Gender and Sexuality. Washington, DC, American Psychiatric Association Publishing, 2020

Levounis P, Zerbo EA, Aggarwal R (eds): Pocket Guide to Addiction Assessment and Treatment. Arlington, VA, American Psychiatric Association Publishing, 2016

Levounis P, Arnaout B, Marienfeld CB (eds): Motivational Interviewing for Clinical Practice. Arlington, VA, American Psychiatric Association Publishing, 2017

CASE 16.4

Knee Pain

Jonathan Avery, M.D.
Stephen Ross, M.D.

Peter Winters, a 46-year-old married white minister, was referred to the psychiatry outpatient department by his primary care doctor for depressive symptoms and opioid misuse in the setting of chronic right knee pain.

Mr. Winters injured his right knee playing basketball 17 months earlier. His mother gave him several tablets of hydrocodone-acetaminophen that she had for back pain, and he found this helpful. When he ran out of the pills and his pain persisted, he went to the emergency room. He was told he had a mild sprain. He was given a 1-month supply of hydrocodone-acetaminophen. He took the pills as prescribed for 1 month, and his pain resolved.

After stopping the pills, however, Mr. Winters began to experience a recurrence of the pain in his knee. He saw an orthopedist, who ordered imaging studies and determined that there was no structural damage. Mr. Winters was given another 1-month supply of hydrocodone-acetaminophen. This time, however, he needed to take more than prescribed in order to ease the pain. He also felt dysphoric and "achy" when he abstained from taking the medication, and described a "craving" for more opioids. He returned to the orthopedist, who referred him to a pain specialist.

Mr. Winters was too embarrassed to go to the pain specialist, believing that his faith and strength should help him overcome the pain. He found it impossible to live without the pain medication, however, because of the pain, dysphoria, and muscle aches when he stopped the medication. He also began to "enjoy the high" and experienced intense craving. He began to frequent emergency rooms to receive more opioids, often lying about the timing and nature of his right knee pain, and even stole pills from his mother on two occasions. He became preoccupied with trying to find more opioids, and his work and home life suffered. He endorsed low mood, especially when contemplating the impact of opioids on his life, but denied any other mood or neurovegetative symptoms. Eventually, he told his primary care doctor about his opioid use and low mood, and that doctor referred him to the outpatient psychiatry clinic.

Mr. Winters had a history of two lifetime major depressive episodes that were treated successfully with escitalopram by his primary care doctor. He also had a history of an alcohol use disorder when he was in his 20s. He managed to quit using alcohol on his own after a family intervention. He smoked two packs of cigarettes daily. His father suffered from depression, and "almost everyone" on his mother's side of the family had "issues with addiction." He had been married to his wife for 20 years, and they had two school-age children. He had been a minister in his church for 15 years. Results of a recent physical examination and laboratory testing performed by his primary care physician had been within normal limits.

On mental status examination, Mr. Winters was cooperative and did not exhibit any psychomotor abnormalities. He answered most questions briefly, often simply saying "yes" or "no." Speech was of a normal rate and tone, without tangentiality or circumstantiality. He reported that his mood was "lousy," and his affect was dysphoric and constricted. He denied symptoms of paranoia or hallucinations. He denied any thoughts of harming himself or others. Memory, both recent and remote, was grossly intact.

Discussion

Among substance use disorders, nonmedical misuse of prescription opioids is second in prevalence only to cannabis use. Clinicians often do not screen individuals like Mr. Winters for addiction risk factors before prescribing opioids. The patient not only is a member of the clergy but also has a legitimate reason for taking pain medication. However, Mr. Winters has several risk factors for prescription opioid addiction, including a personal and family history of addiction, current heavy tobacco use, and a history of depression. Whereas at first he was taking the medications as prescribed, his use led to out-of-control compulsive misuse of opioids that ultimately had a negative impact on his life. According to DSM-5, Mr. Winters would be diagnosed with having an opioid use disorder.

In DSM-5, opioid use disorder replaced the DSM-IV categories of opioid abuse and opioid dependence. This change allowed clinicians to better characterize individuals who had a significant opioid use problem but fell outside the definitions of opioid abuse and dependence. Opioid use disorder can be diagnosed when there is a maladaptive pattern of opioid use that leads to clinically significant impairment or distress over a 12-month period, as manifested by at least two of 11 criteria. Mr. Winters exhibits at least six criteria of opioid use disorder: his use has led to a failure to fulfill major role obligations; he demonstrates three different symptoms (tolerance, withdrawal, and craving); he has used larger amounts of opioid over a longer period than were intended; and he spent a great deal of time in activities necessary to obtain, use, or recover from the opioid's effects. Craving, or a strong desire to use substances, is very prominent in Mr. Winters's case. Craving was added to the diagnostic criteria in DSM-5 because it often is a hallmark symptom of addiction.

Mr. Winters's mood symptoms need to be explored further, but they likely represent an exacerbation of his underlying major depressive disorder. An opioid-induced depressive disorder should also be part of the differential diagnosis. Other psychiatric diagnoses that should be considered in an individual with an opioid use disorder include antisocial personality disorder and posttraumatic stress disorder. Mr. Winters was apparently found to be medically healthy by his primary care doctor, but HIV, hepatitis C, and bacterial infections are also common among users of opioids by injection, although less prevalent in individuals who use only prescription opioids.

It may be useful to direct clinical attention to Mr. Winters's depression and use of opioids and tobacco, but it might also be helpful to attend to his seemingly excessive focus on his knee pain. This excessive focus might exacerbate his depression and use of substances, and it might also reduce the overall quality of his life. Although more information would be needed, Mr. Winters might also have DSM-5 somatic symptom disorder (SSD), with predominant pain. SSD is characterized by one or more somatic symptoms that are distressing and/or result in significant disruption of daily activities, as well as excessive thoughts, feelings, and behaviors related to these somatic symptoms or associated health concerns.

Diagnoses

- Opioid use disorder
- Tobacco use disorder
- Alcohol use disorder, in remission
- Major depressive disorder

Suggested Readings

Boscarino JA, Rukstalis MR, Hoffman SN, et al: Prevalence of prescription opioid-use disorder among chronic pain patients: comparison of the DSM-5 vs. DSM-4 diagnostic criteria. J Addict Dis 30(3):185–194, 2011

Cheney B, Galanter M, Dermatis H, Ross S: Medical versus spiritual orientations: differential patient views toward recovery. Am J Drug Alcohol Abuse 35(5):301–304, 2009

Day P, Secrest S, Davis D, et al; ARCHNet Investigators: Prescription opioid use duration and beliefs about pain and pain medication in primary care patients. J Opioid Manag 16(6):425–434, 2020

Wu LT, Woody GE, Yang C, et al: Differences in onset and abuse/dependence episodes between prescription opioids and heroin: results from the National Epidemiologic Survey on Alcohol and Related Conditions. Subst Abuse Rehabil 2011(2):77–88, 2011

CASE 16.5

A Downward Spiral

Charles H. Silberstein, M.D.

Raymond Xavier, a divorced 29-year-old semi-employed landscaper, presented to a private psychiatrist with a complaint that his life was in a downward spiral. At the time of the appointment, he had been without a permanent home for over 6 months. He had lived in various places, including his car and friends' homes. For over 1 month prior to presentation, he had been living in a tent in the woods. He had called his parents on his recent birthday, and they had offered to pay for substance use disorder treatment as long as they could pay directly.

Mr. Xavier reported that his problem started at age 24, when he had a new wife and young child and had taken on two jobs to make ends meet (working in a factory and as a local delivery driver). When he injured his back and could not get to work because of the pain, a friend offered him a few tablets of acetaminophen-oxycodone (Percocet). Not only did his pain disappear, but his energy and mood improved. For the first time in his life, he felt "normal and happy."

Mr. Xavier continued to use one to four Percocet tablets per day for 1½ years. He never took more than one pill at a time. Then, at age 26, he snorted half a bag of heroin (about $5 on the street). "It took about 10 minutes, but I was transported into an indescribable euphoria. Like taking that first Percocet times 10.... You chase that first feeling for the rest of your life. It never repeats." Within months of starting heroin, he began using it intravenously in an effort to glimpse the euphoria again.

After that first experience with heroin, the progression of use was rapid. Within 6 months, Mr. Xavier was unemployed, separated from his family, and homeless. "I was sleeping in my car or on the streets…using up to 30 bags [$300] daily."

Mr. Xavier began to reach out for help. He enrolled in outpatient rehabilitation for opioid users. The cravings to use, even while in treatment, were intense. Mr. Xavier reported multiple relapses. He added cocaine to the heroin injections, and "speedballs" became Mr. Xavier's drug of choice for a while, but he then returned to using only heroin. The first of multiple accidental overdoses occurred in a vacant house when he was 27. He had been admitted to "about 10 detoxes and rehabs" but would typically relapse within hours or weeks of discharge. He had also gone sporadically to Narcotics Anonymous meetings for years.

To acquire money for his habit, he broke into homes, stole from relatives, and wrote bad checks. "Every penny went to drugs. I'm lucky not to be in prison, but not so lucky in that everybody hates me."

He decided to move to Martha's Vineyard a year prior to the consultation because it "sounded like a quiet place." He brought some methadone with him, but the eventual withdrawal was "fierce."

He continued to use heroin and oxycodone when he could easily get them. Otherwise, he drank alcohol heavily, although he said, "I need to stop drinking—that's what really gets me in trouble." He also took diazepam (Valium) sporadically; however, he did not consider that to be a problem but more of a way to get through the day.

He worked occasionally as a landscaper. His boss—someone he had met at a Narcotics Anonymous meeting—had made it clear that he would call when there was extra work to be done, but that until Mr. Xavier got clean, the boss would not actually expect him to show up. He had held a variety of other odd jobs, including office supplies salesman, veterinary assistant, and gas station attendant. He had not seen his daughter in over 2 years.

On examination, Mr. Xavier appeared somewhat unkempt. He was generally cooperative but appeared restless, and at one point he urgently left the room; when he returned, he reported that he was experiencing bouts of diarrhea. His pupils were enlarged and his skin was remarkable for sweating and piloerection. He yawned several times and appeared irritable and unhappy. His arms and legs frequently twitched. He repeatedly blew his nose and appeared tearful. His speech was rapid, and he appeared impatient. He denied psychotic symptoms, suicidality, and homicidality. He said he was hopeful that if he could get some Suboxone (buprenorphine and naloxone), he might be able to keep a job and maybe get to be a real father.

Laboratory studies were negative for HIV and hepatitis A, B, and C.

Discussion

In response to not taking heroin or methadone, Mr. Xavier experiences a cluster of symptoms that are typical of acute opioid withdrawal. These include diarrhea, lacrimation and rhinorrhea, pupillary dilation, sweating, yawning, restlessness, and occasional spasms of his legs (from which the phrase "kicking the habit" is derived). He has a dysphoric, anxious mood.

Symptoms that are attributable to acute opioid withdrawal overlap with a variety of other DSM-5 disorders. For example, Mr. Xavier's anxiety and depression are significant but likely to be directly related to the withdrawal experience; in such a situation, neither warrants a separate diagnosis. If the symptoms extend beyond the immediate withdrawal period (the duration of which varies with the half-life of the particular opioid), then the likely diagnosis would be a substance-induced depressive (or anxiety) disorder. If the symptoms persist 1 month after discontinuation of the substance, then an autonomous disorder could be diagnosed (even if triggered by the substance use).

The patient also reports significant alcohol use as well as sporadic use of diazepam. Both can have intense withdrawal symptoms and could be contributing to the current clinical picture. Neither, however, induces the fairly specific opioid withdrawal symptoms of lacrimation, yawns, and diarrhea. Mr. Xavier does not quantify his alcohol use, but he does say, "I need to stop drinking—that's what really gets me in trouble." Even without much of a clarification of his use, he describes drinking more than he intends and having drinking-related problems; this qualifies him for an alcohol use disorder.

Mr. Xavier has stolen from strangers and family, has abandoned his wife and child, and is apparently an unreliable employee. This might lead to a consideration of antisocial personality disorder. Heroin is illegal and expensive, however, and it is almost impossible for the average user to acquire enough heroin through a legitimate job. For this reason, DSM-5 specifically suggests not diagnosing antisocial personality disorder when the behavior directly stems from efforts to acquire drugs. If, however, the antisocial behavior was evident in childhood or before the onset of the substance abuse, both diagnoses can be made. Without a history of antisocial behavior unrelated to the acquisition of heroin, Mr. Xavier would likely not meet criteria for antisocial personality disorder. He might, however, warrant a diagnosis of adult antisocial behavior, which is listed in the chapter "Other Conditions That May Be a Focus of Clinical Attention." Like other diagnoses that are listed in that chapter but not in the main text of DSM-5, adult antisocial behavior is linked to an ICD-10-CM Z code.

More clear-cut, of course, is Mr. Xavier's severe opioid use disorder, a diagnosis that refers to the compulsive, prolonged self-administered use of opioids without medical supervision. Mr. Xavier's opioid use meets all 11 DSM-5 criteria: taking larger amounts than intended; inability to cut down; excessive time spent obtaining, using, and recovering from the opioid's effects; craving; an inability to fulfill role obligations; persistent social and interpersonal problems; reduced activities; putting oneself at physical risk; continued use despite knowledge of its consequences; tolerance; and withdrawal.

In many ways Mr. Xavier's is a classic presentation. Onset is typically in the late teens and early 20s. The experience of feeling "normal and happy" with first use is common, as is "chasing the high," the relentless pursuit of that initial sense of well-being and euphoria. Some opioid users maintain jobs and families, but many fall into a desperately negative spiral. Mr. Xavier is atypical in one way, however, because he has not been infected with one of the viruses commonly found in intravenous substance users: HIV and hepatitis A, B, and C.

Diagnoses

- Opioid withdrawal
- Opioid use disorder
- Alcohol use disorder

Suggested Reading

Shorter D, Kosten T: The pharmacology of opioids, in The ASAM Principles of Addiction Medicine, 6th Edition. Edited by Miller SC, Fiellin DA, Rosenthal RN, Saitz R. Philadelphia, Wolters Kluwer, 2019, pp 136–149

CASE 16.6

Stress and Substance Abuse

Britney Lambert, M.D.
Coreen Domingo, D.P.H., M.P.H.
Thomas R. Kosten, M.D.
Daryl Shorter, M.D.

Shaun Yates, a 32-year-old married African American information technology (IT) security analyst, presented for treatment with a private psychiatrist because he felt "stressed." He and his wife have two young children, and he reports a stable social life that includes a large extended family. This was his first psychiatric evaluation. He reported no past psychiatric history.

Mr. Yates traced his increased stress to a death in his city 4 months earlier. The death was recorded on video and featured an unarmed Black man being murdered by two white off-duty policemen who had accused him of theft. Like many people, Mr. Yates first saw the video via his social media "timeline," where it was routinely reposted by his friends. Because the murder had occurred in his hometown, it received much local attention.

Mr. Yates's social media timeline began to fill up with other examples of police brutality toward Black men. He said he watched the videos because they were "trending" and appeared on his social media timeline abruptly, unfiltered, and without warning. In addition, he became increasingly aware of news programming, social media posts, and community memorials relating to the deaths and abuse of other Black men. Although he described trying to avoid details about these tragedies, he said that news, images, and videos were unavoidable, and he had become increasingly preoccupied with fears for the safety of his wife, his young sons, his extended family, and himself.

Mr. Yates reported that under normal circumstances, he "didn't like to talk about this stuff," but his wife had insisted that he get treatment because she was concerned that he "didn't seem himself." Mr. Yates wanted the evaluating psychiatrist to understand that he was not paranoid or overly sensitive about racism, and that up until recently, he'd been good about "compartmentalizing." Nevertheless, he admitted that it had become difficult to stop thinking about violence against unarmed Black men. He had recently disabled his social media accounts in a proactive effort to minimize his exposure to images and commentary regarding the incidents. In addition to stopping use of social media, he reported avoidance of newspapers, the internet, and television.

Mr. Yates noted that he had also become edgy, nervous, and always on guard against attack. He had gradually reduced his explorations around the city, preferring to stay close to home. Although he had previously jogged every morning before work, he quit jogging in the local community park because he "didn't want any trouble." Mr. Yates reported his sleep over the past 3 months as being interrupted by vivid, disturbing dreams of being chased by police officers.

For Mr. Yates, evenings were particularly stressful, and he had recently increased his use of alcohol and cannabis to "unwind" at the end of the day. He also had begun to drink a six-pack, or more, of beer after dinner, often "passing out" in the family den. The alcohol helped him to relax, and smoking "a blunt" of marijuana before bedtime improved his sleep and reduced nightmares. He stated that the biggest problem with the cannabis was his wife's complaining that their young children might see him using it or that his use might be detected in a random urine toxicology screen at work. Mr. Yates had been increasingly late to work but had not mentioned to his wife that he had twice been reprimanded by his supervisor for the lateness.

Mr. Yates reported first using both cannabis and alcohol at fraternity parties when he was about 19 years old. Throughout college, he smoked small amounts of marijuana once or twice weekly and rarely drank more than two beers at a time. In the decade since his college graduation, he had smoked marijuana only occasionally and tended to have no more than 1 or 2 beers on the weekend. He had never smoked tobacco or used other substances. His use of alcohol and cannabis had not increased until 3 months prior to the evaluation, after he started seeing the videos.

Mr. Yates denied experiencing feelings of worthlessness, guilt, or hopelessness. He reported no prior history of panic attacks, mania, psychosis, or obsessive-compulsive symptoms, and he had never received psychiatric hospitalization or outpatient treatment. He denied suicidal ideation, suicide attempts, or previous history of suicidality. There was no family psychiatric history aside from his father, who developed post-traumatic stress disorder following military service in Vietnam.

Discussion

Mr. Yates presents for psychiatric evaluation because he has become increasingly stressed and worried about the safety of his loved ones after watching videos of the fatal shootings of unarmed Black men. He describes repetitively watching the video of a nearby killing, and then looking at similar images and videos from around the country. In addition to the threat of physical harm due to "living while Black," Mr. Yates appears to have become further stressed by the psychological fallout of repeatedly witnessing (or hearing about) violence being directed toward people of color, and particularly toward Black men.

Mr. Yates expresses reluctance to talk to the psychiatrist and is at pains to assure the psychiatrist that he "isn't paranoid" and is not "overly sensitive about racism." This may relate to his desire to be seen as "normal," but it might also reflect a mistrust of institutional systems. The clinician will likely get a richer history and a better alliance if he or she recognizes that a mental health evaluation is likely to be challenging for a member of a community that has been historically marginalized and/or underserved by medical institutions. In addition, any trust Mr. Yates may have placed in the protective role of law enforcement institutions is likely to have been severely shaken by the fact that the perpetrators of the violence were off-duty policemen. The case report does not mention anything about the psychiatrist's gender, race, or ethnicity, but these characteristics will have been noticed by Mr. Yates and will affect the nature of the clinician-patient interaction.

In regard to DSM-5 diagnoses, Mr. Yates spontaneously describes a cluster of psychological symptoms as well as excessive use of alcohol and cannabis. His chief complaint of "stress" appears to be clearly related to the traumatic experience of repetitively watching videos of the murders of other Black men. Mr. Yates grew up with a father who suffered from posttraumatic stress disorder (PTSD), and he himself also meets most criteria for PTSD. He reports traumatic exposure to the videos, intrusion symptoms (nightmares, preoccupations), avoidance behaviors (he has stopped jogging), worries about the safety of loved ones and himself, and arousal symptoms (edginess, hypervigilance, and sleep difficulties). These symptoms have persisted for longer than 1 month and are causing significant distress.

It is likely, however, that because of the nature of Mr. Yates's "index trauma," he would not meet criteria for a diagnosis of PTSD. In DSM-5-TR, an adult being evaluated for PTSD must have been exposed to a serious trauma in one of four ways: direct experience, witnessing the event, learning that the trauma occurred to a close family member or close friend, or experiencing repeated or extreme exposure to aversive details of the traumatic event. DSM-5-TR specifically states that exposure "through electronic media, television, movies, or pictures" cannot be counted as traumatic exposure "unless this exposure is work related." Although an extended evaluation might elicit additional information that could lead to a PTSD diagnosis, Mr. Yates would likely receive an initial diagnosis found elsewhere in the chapter on trauma- and stressor-related disorders: adjustment disorder with anxiety. Criteria for adjustment disorder are less specific than those for PTSD and include out-of-proportion distress and functional impairment after a stressor.

Mr. Yates's difficulties with alcohol and marijuana appear to have begun in recent months. Before that time, his use of substances would not have warranted clinical attention. By the time of the evaluation, however, his alcohol and cannabis use are associated with impairment across several domains. His use of alcohol has created conflict with his wife (use despite recurrent interpersonal problems) and resulted in reprimands at work (failure to fulfill work obligations). Although he recognizes these negative consequences, he has not cut back on his use and has continued to engage in heavy consumption (inability to control or cut down use). Mr. Yates meets criteria for alcohol use disorder, mild. Whereas Mr. Yates reports that the cannabis has been helpful with sleep and nightmares, his use has led to marital conflict, escalating use, and craving. Mr. Yates therefore would meet DSM-5 criteria for cannabis use disorder, mild, in addition to the diagnoses of adjustment disorder with anxiety and alcohol use disorder, mild.

Diagnoses

- Adjustment disorder with anxiety
- Alcohol use disorder, mild
- Cannabis use disorder, mild

Suggested Readings

Alcántara C, Casement MD, Lewis-Fernández R: Conditional risk for PTSD among Latinos: a systematic review of racial/ethnic differences and sociocultural explanations. Clin Psychol Rev 33(1):107–119, 2013

Mekawa Y, Carter S, Brown B, et al: Interpersonal trauma and posttraumatic stress disorder among Black women: does racial discrimination matter? J Trauma Dissociation 22(2):154–169, 2021

Motley RO Jr, Chen Y-C, Johnson C, Joe S: Exposure to community-based violence on social media among Black male emerging adults involved with the criminal justice system. Social Work Research 44(22):87–97, 2020

CASE 16.7

Gambling

Silvia Bernardi, M.D.

Carlos Blanco, M.D., Ph.D.

Tomás Zambrano was a 36-year-old married first-generation Hispanic man who presented to the gambling clinic at a major medical center for evaluation and treatment.

A football coach at a suburban high school, Mr. Zambrano had a 5-year-old son. He denied having any prior history of a psychiatric or substance use disorder. He was appropriately dressed and groomed, expressed himself fluently in both English and Spanish, spoke in normal tone and volume, and on examination presented with intact cognitive function and average intelligence.

Mr. Zambrano had been betting on sports and playing cards since childhood, noting in the evaluation that gambling "is part of our culture." His own father's favorite hobby and stress reliever had been to play poker with friends at night, and Mr. Zambrano remembered with affection the father-son camaraderie they shared on these occasions. Poker became for him a familial activity that he increasingly used to relieve work-related stress. He relished the excitement as well as the intellectual challenge and competition.

Card games did not, however, remain a benign pastime for Mr. Zambrano. He had begun to lose more money than he could afford. Over the 2 years prior to his presentation for treatment, he had gradually increased the frequency and stakes of his poker nights. When he lost, he tended to place even larger bets, convinced that the odds would favor him the following time. When he won, he felt great and would continue to play, convinced he was "on a streak." Although losses made him feel unworthy, stupid, and irritable, he believed success would come if he could fine-tune his strategy. He felt a powerful, almost constant impulse to increase the tempo of his gambling and recover the money he had lost. When he tried to cut back on gambling, he felt irritable and preoccupied, and quickly returned to his poker nights.

By the time Mr. Zambrano presented to the gambling clinic, he felt desperate. Nightly poker had led to daytime fatigue and poor performance at his coaching job, which he had previously loved. He was consumed with thoughts about his next poker game. His wife and son had long resented his time away from the family, but his wife had just found out that he had used up his son's college fund plus accumulated $30,000 in credit card debt. When his wife threatened to file for divorce, he felt sad and depressed and decided to seek treatment.

Discussion

Mr. Zambrano is preoccupied with gambling, has a recurrent pattern of chasing his losses, and has been gambling with escalating amounts of money. He lies to his wife about his losses and has jeopardized both his marital relationship and his job. Mr. Zambrano demonstrates at least five of nine criteria for DSM-5 gambling disorder (four of the nine are required for the diagnosis).

If excess gambling is a symptom of a manic episode, the gambling disorder diagnosis is not made. When manic episode is the principal diagnosis, the patient tends to gamble mostly in the context of excitement and grandiosity and will display other symptoms of bipolar disorder, such as increased energy and diminished need for sleep. When gambling is used as a maladaptive coping response, the individual tends to engage in gambling activities mostly during negative mood states, such as anxiety and depression. The clinician should also keep in mind that gambling losses can trigger mood episodes, generally adjustment disorders, although comorbid major depressive disorder and bipolar mania or hypomania may also occur. Assessment of the temporal relationship among symptoms and the intensity of those symptoms helps to establish the principal diagnosis. In this case, Mr. Zambrano specifically denied all manic symptoms.

Mr. Zambrano is somewhat unusual in his denial of all psychiatric comorbidity. A large percentage of people with gambling disorder have a substance use disorder, personality disorder, mood disorder, and/or anxiety disorder. Because accurate assessment of comorbidity is essential for treatment decisions, it would be useful for the clinician to explore the possibility that Mr. Zambrano is minimizing other symptomatology.

Mr. Zambrano is more typical in having a father who was also a gambler. Many people with gambling disorders also report first-degree relatives who gamble, although it is not clear the degree to which the behavior is learned versus genetically inherited.

During the clinical interview, Mr. Zambrano described his gambling behavior in the context of the culture of his family of origin, raising the possibility that cultural factors may have contributed to the manifestation of his gambling disorder. Because Mr. Zambrano's conceptualization of his gambling behavior could profoundly affect the efficacy of different treatment strategies, as well as influencing his own sense of personal identity, a deeper exploration of cultural factors is warranted before implementing comprehensive treatment.

Diagnosis

- Gambling disorder

Suggested Readings

Abbott MW: Gambling and gambling-related harm: recent World Health Organization initiatives. Public Health 184:56–59, 2020

Blanco C, Myers J, Kendler KS: Gambling, disordered gambling and their association with major depression and substance use: a Web-based cohort and twin-sibling study. Psychol Med 42(3): 497–508, 2012

Potenza MN, Balodis IM, Derevensky J, et al: Gambling disorder. Nat Rev Dis Primers 5(1):51, 2019

CHAPTER 17

Neurocognitive Disorders

INTRODUCTION

John W. Barnhill, M.D.

Neurocognitive disorders feature prominent, acquired cognitive deficits. These cognitive disorders can be divided into two broad groups—acute delirium and the more chronic neurocognitive disorders (NCDs)—each of which can be further characterized.

Delirium is characterized as a fluctuating disturbance of attention, awareness, and cognition that develops acutely and in the context of one or more identified physiological precipitants. Delirium can be further characterized in regard to such factors as duration, activity level, and etiology. Most often encountered among medically hospitalized and/or substance-abusing patients, delirium requires a careful search for etiology—which is often multifactorial. If the delirium is caused by substance withdrawal or intoxication, the pertinent diagnosis is delirium, comorbid with possible substance use disorders. For example, a patient might be coded as having alcohol withdrawal delirium, acute, hyperactive, along with an alcohol use disorder.

In addition to describing acute delirium, this chapter of DSM-5-TR also describes chronic neurocognitive disorders. Although acute delirium and the chronic neurocognitive disorders are separated in regard to their diagnostic criteria, DSM-5-TR recognizes that mounting evidence indicates that delirium is significantly associated with long-term cognitive decline.

Two other aspects of the nomenclature may also be confusing. First, most of the chronic neurocognitive disorders have been generally described as dementias. Although still in use, the term *dementia* is sometimes seen as having a pejorative connotation. In addition, this term may better fit the disorders that are progressive and most commonly affect older adults (e.g., Alzheimer's disease) rather than the abrupt and static cognitive decline typically seen in a disorder such as traumatic brain injury (TBI).

A second issue is that the term *neurocognitive* implies an emphasis on cognitive deficits. All of the NCDs involve multiple deficits, however, and DSM-5 suggests that the workup for an NCD include an assessment of executive functions such as complex attention, learning and memory, language, visuoconstructional perceptual ability, and social cognition. Furthermore, all of the NCDs can have prominent personality and behavioral components that may be the most visible and dysfunctional aspect of the clinical presentation.

The neurocognitive disorders are divided into major and mild categories based on the person's cognitive functioning and level of practical independence.

Major neurocognitive disorder conforms to criteria for dementia that have long been used within psychiatry, medicine, and neurology; these criteria identify clusters of people with similar deficits and care needs.

Mild neurocognitive disorder was a new category in DSM-5 and represents an attempt to identify clusters of patients whose impairment may be relatively subtle but still significant. As is true throughout psychiatry, clinical judgment is required to avoid excessive pathologizing. For example, occasional "senior moments" are not mild NCD. Instead, mild NCD is intended to identify people whose deficits are impairing their quality of life to the extent that they warrant clinical attention. A second reason for creating a mild NCD diagnosis is the reality that most of the major neurocognitive disorders are inexorably progressive, and the effort to reduce their catastrophic impact will likely include recognition and treatment at an early stage of disease progression.

Suggested Readings

Arciniegas DB, Yudofsky SC, Hales RE (eds): The American Psychiatric Association Publishing Textbook of Neuropsychiatry and Clinical Neurosciences, 6th Edition. Washington, DC, American Psychiatric Association Publishing, 2018

Goldberg TE, Chen C, Wang Y, et al: Association of delirium with long-term cognitive decline: a meta-analysis. JAMA Neurol 77(11):1373–1381, 2020

Inouye SK, Marcantonio ER, Kosar CM, et al: The short-term and long-term relationship between delirium and cognitive trajectory in older surgical patients. Alzheimers Dement 12(7):766–775, 2016

Steffens DC, Blazer DG, Thakur ME (eds): The American Psychiatric Publishing Textbook of Geriatric Psychiatry, 5th Edition. Arlington, VA, American Psychiatric Publishing, 2015

CASE 17.1

Dysphoria

John W. Barnhill, M.D.

A psychiatric consultant was called to evaluate depression in Victor Alvarez, a 76-year-old widower who appeared dysphoric the day after surgery to repair a broken hip. It was late in the evening, and no one from the admitting team was available, but a social work note in the chart indicated that the patient's fracture appeared to have been the result of his tripping in his messy apartment. The note also stated that the patient had no children or known living family.

The neighbor who had brought Mr. Alvarez to the hospital had stated that the patient had been more reclusive in recent years and that his self-care had worsened after his wife's death 6 months earlier. Up until the day of the surgery, however, he had been able to function independently in his apartment. The neighbor, a nurse, also mentioned that while they were waiting for the ambulance, her husband had sat with Mr. Alvarez while she searched the apartment for pill bottles. She said she had found only an unopened bottle of acetaminophen and a dusty bottle of a medication used for hypertension.

Routine admission laboratory results indicated that Mr. Alvarez had an elevated blood urea nitrogen level, a low albumin level, and a high normal mean corpuscular volume. His blood pressure was 160/110. In addition to medications related to the surgery, the chart indicated that he had received haloperidol 2 mg after a bout of agitation. A nursing note 1 hour after the haloperidol administration indicated that the patient was "worried and stiff."

On mental status examination, Mr. Alvarez was lying at a 45-degree angle in his unkempt bed. He appeared thin and had moderate temporal wasting. His affect was sad, worried, and constricted. He appeared stiff and uncomfortable. He did not immediately respond to the interviewer's questions and comments. His eyes remained generally shut, but they did flicker open a few times, and his body habitus implied that he was awake. After multiple efforts, the psychiatrist was able to get the patient to say "I'm fine" and "Get out." When asked where he was, Mr. Alvarez said, "My apartment." When he did open his eyes, the patient appeared confused. He did not respond to other questions and declined to do a clock drawing test. The surgery team had called in a one-to-one companion earlier in the day, and she said that the patient was generally either asleep or trying to get out of bed and that he had not been making any sense all day.

Discussion

Although information is limited, Mr. Alvarez appears to have developed disturbances in his levels of awareness and attention, and these problems appear acute and directly related to the surgery and hospitalization. A more extensive evaluation would more thoroughly assess his level of awareness and ability to direct, focus, sustain, and shift attention. It would also more carefully document deficits in orientation, executive ability, language, visual perception, learning, and memory. As often happens in acute care settings, however, this psychiatrist must make an initial diagnosis with incomplete information, and Mr. Alvarez does appear to meet DSM-5-TR criteria for delirium.

Delirium is common among hospital inpatients and is especially common among elderly patients following hip surgery. Delirium is often normalized by the treating team (e.g., they might say, "Who wouldn't be a little confused in an intensive care unit?"), and it is generally overlooked unless the quiet confusion is accompanied by agitation. As happened in Mr. Alvarez's case, delirium is often mistaken for depression because hospitalized patients with either disorder can appear sad and worried. As is true for all neurocognitive disorders, however, delirium can affect mood as well as cognition. It is clinically important to identify delirium for a variety of reasons—to reduce falls and treatment delays and to provide an opportunity to reorient the patient and counsel the family about the nature of this acute confusion (delirium can be as scary for the family as it is for the patient).

In addition to documenting a fluctuating course and a set of symptomatic criteria, a diagnosis of delirium requires evidence that directly links the disturbance to a physiological insult. This is an unusual requirement within DSM-5. Although psychiatrists often look for possible causes for a broad array of disorders, diagnoses generally do not require a search for a cause. In Mr. Alvarez's case, the single most likely cause of his delirium is the hip fracture and its surgical treatment. Because they tend to happen to older people and to involve surgery, anesthesia, and pain medications, broken hips are commonly implicated in delirium. Mr. Alvarez's delirium is likely to be multifactorial, however, and the consulting psychiatrist should search the chart for other potential contributors, which might include medications (e.g., anticholinergic medications), laboratory abnormalities (e.g., anemia), and medical comorbidities (e.g., an infection).

In addition to looking for what is most common, the clinician needs to look for what is most dangerous. Perhaps most urgent is the possibility of substance withdrawal. If the neighbor's information is correct—that no pertinent medication bottles were in the apartment—then it is unlikely that Mr. Alvarez is in withdrawal from medications such as benzodiazepines or barbiturates. It is possible, however, that his delirium reflects alcohol withdrawal. The psychiatrist lacks a thorough history, but Mr. Alvarez's lab results indicate a high-normal mean corpuscular volume (MCV), which often reflects chronic alcohol use. His elevated blood pressure could reflect untreated hypertension, which is suggested by the dusty bottle of blood pressure medications found by the patient's neighbor, but the elevated blood pressure could also reflect alcohol withdrawal. Mr. Alvarez has been agitated, a frequent finding in alcohol withdrawal, although he seems to have been generally hypoactive, which is more typical of a postoperative delirium. Such ambiguity should prompt the psychiatrist to seek further clues. For example, after recognizing the elevated MCV, the psychiatrist might look for other objective biomarkers that are often found in people at risk for alcohol withdrawal: aspartate aminotransferase/alanine aminotransferase (AST/ALT) ratio greater than 2:1, low magnesium levels, and elevated vital signs. It might also be useful to directly ask the neighbor if she found discarded alcohol bottles when looking for medication bottles.

This information is critical because delirium secondary to alcohol withdrawal is potentially catastrophic. If the patient turns out to have a significant alcohol use disorder, the treatment plan needs to be adjusted, because the primary treatment for alcohol withdrawal is benzodiazepines, which are generally contraindicated in patients with delirium that is related to surgery and advanced age.

Although not potential emergencies, two other diagnoses should also be considered in Mr. Alvarez. The neighbor notes that he has suffered decline in self-care since his wife died. Whereas the elevated blood urea nitrogen (BUN) suggests acute dehydration, the patient's low albumin and temporal wasting hint at malnutrition, which often accompanies apathy and diminished functionality. As is often the case, Mr. Alvarez may have been primed for the delirium by having had a mild or major neurocognitive disorder (i.e., dementia) in the preceding years.

If he does have a dementia, it is not clear which type is most likely. Alzheimer's disease is the most common type of dementia, but this patient's apparent hypertension also puts him at risk for a vascular etiology as either primary or comorbid with Alzheimer's disease. The patient is also noted to be stiff following the use of haloperidol for agitation, a result that is especially common in cognitive decline related to either Lewy body disease or Parkinson's disease. Accurately clarifying the existence of a dementia is unlikely on the night of the evaluation, but a chronic neurocognitive disorder should be included in the differential diagnosis.

Another diagnosis that should be considered is depression. The patient's wife recently died, and Mr. Alvarez appears to be isolated and poorly functional. Although his chronic decline may be related to a neurocognitive disorder, it would be useful for the psychiatrist to systematically assess the patient for depressive symptoms as the delirium clears.

On the night of the evaluation, however, the psychiatrist would probably limit the diagnosis to unspecified delirium. A more careful search over the next 12–24 hours would be aimed at clarifying potential comorbidities such as alcohol use disorder, depression, and dementia.

Diagnosis

- Unspecified delirium

Suggested Readings

Goldberg TE, Chen C, Wang Y, et al: Association of delirium with long-term cognitive decline: a meta-analysis. JAMA Neurol 77(11):1373–1381, 2020

Inouye SK, Marcantonio ER, Kosar CM, et al: The short-term and long-term relationship between delirium and cognitive trajectory in older surgical patients. Alzheimers Dement 12(7):766–775, 2016

Oh ES, Fong TG, Hshieh TT, Inouye SK: Delirium in older persons: advances in diagnosis and treatment. JAMA 318(12):1161–1174, 2017

Trzepacz PT, Meagher DJ: Delirium, in Clinical Manual of Neuropsychiatry. Edited by Yudofsky SC, Hales RE. Washington, DC, American Psychiatric Publishing, 2012, pp 61–118

CASE 17.2

Agitated and Confused

José R. Maldonado, M.D.

Wesley Brown, a 63-year-old married white businessman, was "found down" in the road by police and brought to the emergency room (ER) of a large university-affiliated hospital. The psychiatry service was consulted for management of "psychotic behavior" in the ER. The patient's family reported that the patient had exhibited an approximately 2-week history of "strange behavior." According to his sister, Mr. Brown had been running around the kitchen with knives, sending paranoid e-mails about the justice system to his friends, showing his guns to the neighbors, seeing people in the walls, having paranoid thoughts that his wife was having an affair, and not sleeping. The patient's wife had reported him missing 3 days prior to admission. Notably, his car was found a few blocks away with a large box in its trunk containing bags filled with numerous medication bottles (both prescribed and over the counter); most of the bottles were partially or completely empty. There were also many items from the patient's extensive gun collection.

Mr. Brown's medical records revealed a history of coronary artery disease and a coronary artery bypass graft 5 years prior to admission, as well as chronic back pain and a history of multiple spinal surgeries, with an associated history of daily opioid use. He had no prior psychiatric history, including any history of depression or antidepressant medications. His outpatient medications included metoprolol, oxycodone, and as-needed doses of cyclobenzaprine and diazepam.

On examination, Mr. Brown was confused and combative, yet somnolent. His skin and oral mucosa were dry, and he manifested mydriasis, hypoactive bowel sounds, urinary retention, epistaxis, and depressed reflexes. His vital signs included a temperature of 39.9°C, a heart rate of 115 bpm, and blood pressure of 172/74, but his breathing rate was normal, and his oxygen saturation was normal on room air. A computed tomography (CT) scan of the head was negative, and a CT of the cervical spine showed degeneration. Mr. Brown's blood alcohol screen was negative, and complete blood count and comprehensive metabolic panel results were within normal limits, as were the electrocardiogram and cerebrospinal fluid from a lumbar puncture. His urine toxicology screen was positive for "benzodiazepines and tricyclics."

Mr. Brown's mental status examination revealed waxing and waning alertness, an unkempt appearance, lack of cooperation with nursing and medical personnel, somewhat slurred speech, and signs of psychomotor retardation. His affect alternated between subdued/somnolent and restless/agitated. He denied suicidal or homicidal ideation but reported significant paranoid ideation that focused on his wife's suspected affair. He also appeared to be suffering from both visual and auditory misperceptions—accusing people of laughing at him and misidentifying hospital staff as acquaintances. His thought process was notably tangential. His judgment and insight were impaired. During his initial evaluation, the patient was noted to have a Mini-Mental State Examination score of 16 of 30 possible points. He lost 7 of 10 points for orientation, 3 for attention and calculation, 2 for recall, and 1 each for sentence writing and copying design.

Discussion

Mr. Brown was "found down" after a 2-week episode of uncharacteristically strange behavior that was of apparently sudden onset. According to his wife and sister, he had become paranoid and threatening, waving knives and showing off his guns. He had been missing for a few days before being brought to the ER. His mental status examination was notable for a marked disturbance in both attention and awareness. His level of attention fluctuated over hours. Various cognitive deficits were new and were seemingly unrelated to another neurocognitive disorder.

Although someone in the ER called this behavior "psychotic," Mr. Brown presents with a fairly classic DSM-5-TR delirium. His fluctuating levels of attention and awareness fulfill Criterion A. The disturbance developed over a short period of time, represents a change from baseline, and fluctuates during the course of the day (Criterion B). The presence of perceptual disturbances and other cognitive deficits meets Criterion C. Mr. Brown has no known relevant preexisting or evolving neuropsychiatric condition (Criterion D). The final set of criteria (Criterion E) requires "evidence from the history, physical examination, or laboratory findings that the disturbance is caused by the physiological consequence of another medical condition, substance intoxication or withdrawal, or a toxin exposure" (or a combination of such factors). This final requirement—linking the psychiatric diagnosis with a physiological trigger—is highly unusual in DSM-5 and can sometimes be difficult to specifically fulfill.

Mr. Brown's initial examination revealed mydriasis, hypoactive bowel sounds, urinary retention, and depressed reflexes, as well as fluctuating levels of sedation, attention, and awareness. These results point toward an anticholinergic delirium. Potential sources of anticholinergic delirium include benzodiazepines and tricyclic antidepressants (TCAs) (as per Mr. Brown's positive toxicology screening test). In addition, opioid agents could be implicated, especially given the patient's history of chronic pain and opioid use. Although Mr. Brown's toxicology screen was negative for opiates, short-acting opioids might have precipitated the delirium but then been out of his system by the time he arrived in the ER. He also has a long-standing history of pain, which itself is associated with both the development and the severity of delirium.

The presence of TCAs in Mr. Brown's toxicology screen is puzzling. His family insisted he had never taken antidepressants, and his records seemed to back them up. However, according to his outpatient records, his medications did include cyclobenzaprine, a centrally acting muscle relaxant often prescribed for patients with chronic pain. Cyclobenzaprine is a tricyclic molecule, closely related to TCAs, that in fact shares many of the pharmacological characteristics and psychoactive effects of TCAs and often cross-reacts with toxicology assays, giving a false positive for benzodiazepines. Mr. Brown's delirium therefore was likely caused by some combination of cyclobenzaprine, opioids, and benzodiazepines. Lack of sleep could have been the result of the delirium that then became a factor in its perpetuation.

Diagnosis

- Delirium

Suggested Readings

Bulbena-Cabre A, Dunn NR, Swift RG: Cyclobenzaprine-induced hallucinosis. Prim Care Companion CNS Disord 17(3):10.4088/PCC.14l01773, 2015

Maldonado JR: Delirium pathophysiology: an updated hypothesis of the etiology of acute brain failure. Int J Geriatr Psychiatry 33(11):1428–1457, 2018

Oh ES, Fong TG, Hshieh TT, Inouye SK: Delirium in older persons: advances in diagnosis and treatment. JAMA 318(12):1161–1174, 2017

Serrano WC, Maldonado J: The use of physostigmine in the diagnosis and treatment of anticholinergic toxicity after olanzapine overdose: literature review and case report. J Acad Consult Liaison Psychiatry 62(3):285–297, 2021

CASE 17.3

Depressed and Withdrawn

Peter V. Rabins, M.D., M.P.H.

Arthur Cullman, a 71-year-old married man, was referred to a psychiatrist by his primary care physician for evaluation of depressive symptoms that had not responded to medication trials. His wife reported that Mr. Cullman had begun to change at age 68, about a year after his retirement. He had gradually stopped playing golf and cards, activities he had enjoyed "for decades." He had explained that seeing his friends was no longer "fun," and he generally refused to socialize. Instead, he sat on the couch all day, worrying about finances and the future. He denied sadness, however, and any suicidal or homicidal ideation. His wife said he was sleeping 10–12 hours a day instead of his customary 7 hours and that he had, uncharacteristically, gained 8 pounds in less than 1 year.

His wife had become worried that retirement had left Mr. Cullman depressed, and she had mentioned her concerns to their primary care physician. Their physician agreed and prescribed sertraline (titrated to 100 mg/day for 8 months) and then sustained-release venlafaxine (titrated to 150 mg twice daily and maintained at that level for over 1 year). Mr. Cullman's symptoms gradually worsened during these medication trials, and the internist ultimately referred him for a psychiatric evaluation.

Mr. Cullman's past psychiatric history was notable for an episode in his 20s when he had difficulty at work, felt apathetic and unconnected, and had difficulty concentrating. These symptoms persisted for several months and resolved without treatment as his work situation improved.

Mr. Cullman's family history was positive for a single major depressive episode in one of his two younger brothers; the depression responded well to psychotherapy and an antidepressant medication. His mother had developed dementia in her 70s.

Mr. Cullman's personal history revealed unremarkable development and childhood, graduation from college with a degree in business, a successful career as a corporate manager, and retirement at age 67. He and his wife had been married for 45 years, denied significant discord, and had three children and four grandchildren who were in good health. Premorbidly, he had been outgoing, energetic, and well organized.

Mr. Cullman's medical history was notable for hypertension, hyperlipidemia, and type 2 diabetes mellitus. He was taking lisinopril, metformin, simvastatin, and venlafaxine.

Mental status examination revealed an alert, cooperative man who was neatly dressed and who had a steady but slow gait and no abnormal movements other than psychomotor slowing. Mr. Cullman's speech was soft in volume but normal in rate and rhythm, without paraphasic errors. He had a limited range of emotional expression, denied feeling sad or guilty, but felt he had retired too early. He denied self-blame, hopelessness, and suicidal thoughts or plans. He was aware that his wife was concerned and acknowledged that he was less energetic and active than in the past. He ascribed these changes to his retirement. He said he was generally satisfied with his life.

On cognitive examination, Mr. Cullman was oriented except for the date. He remembered one of three objects in 2 minutes, performed three of five serial 7 subtractions correctly, named four common objects correctly, and repeated a complex sentence accurately. He was able to draw the face of a clock and place the numbers correctly but was not able to correctly place the hands at 10 minutes after 2. His blood pressure was 142/82, and his pulse was 84 and regular. His physical examination was noncontributory. His neurological examination revealed intact cranial nerves and 1+ symmetric deep tendon reflexes.

Discussion

Mr. Cullman is a 71-year-old man with a 3-year history of gradual social withdrawal. Prominent symptoms on examination are slowness, lack of self-reported sad or dysphoric mood, lack of concern about his decline, increased sleep, and a cognitive examination that indicates impairments in memory, concentration, math, and clock drawing. He has failed to respond to two prolonged trials of antidepressant medication, one of which did not reach the maximum recommended dosage (sertraline) and one of which reached a moderately high dosage (venlafaxine). He has had a successful marriage and career, and the presenting apathy is a significant change from his lifelong baseline. He may have had an episode of depression in his 20s, but this is not well established. He has a family history of depression in a brother and late-life dementia in his mother.

The differential diagnosis in Mr. Cullman's case includes a primary dementia (neurocognitive disorder) and major depressive disorder (MDD) with marked apathy. Favoring MDD is the lack of interest in usually enjoyed activities, hypersomnia, and unhappiness with retirement.

The more likely diagnosis, however, is major neurocognitive disorder due to Alzheimer's disease, with apathy and mood disturbance. Whereas impairments in memory and executive functioning can be seen in both primary neurocognitive disorder and MDD, impairments in visuospatial function (abnormal clock drawing) are not seen in depression. The history of gradual onset and slow progression is also more consistent with a dementia than with MDD, as is the lack of a patient-reported mood change. Although Alzheimer's disease is the most likely cause of the neurocognitive disorder, reversible causes of dementia should be investigated.

DSM-5 improved the diagnostic approach to dementia in several ways. First, it no longer requires that memory be impaired, a requirement that had been appropriate for Alzheimer's disease but not for frontotemporal dementia or vascular dementia. By listing a set of impairments by domain—complex attention, executive functioning, learning and memory, language, perceptual-motor, and social cognition—DSM-5 broadens clinician understanding of the protean manifestations of the neurocognitive disorders. Unfortunately, however, DSM-5 requires impairment in only one domain, a change not only from DSM-IV but also from most conceptualizations of dementia that require multiple impairments. In DSM-IV and ICD, impairments in a single domain, be it language, perception, or memory, were identified as focal impairments and classified separately because the differential diagnosis for them is distinct from that for multiple impairments.

A second major change in DSM-5 was the use of *neurocognitive disorder* as the overarching term. This was presumably done to destigmatize cognitive impairment, because the word *dementia* is thought to be pejorative. The change in terminology has been embraced by clinicians who bill for services, but it has not yet become standard among nonclinician scientists, patients, or caregivers. I find no evidence that it has improved care by breaking down barriers due to stigma. I continue to favor the traditional term *dementia,* because *neurocognitive* implies that the manifestations are cognitive and "neurological," whereas changes in mood, experience (hallucinations and delusions), and behavior (agitation, wandering, apathy) can also be symptoms of dementia.

A third general change in DSM-5 was the division into mild and major neurocognitive disorders. This change acknowledges the recognition in recent years that many neurodegenerative disorders develop so gradually that subtle impairments are present before function is impaired. This demarcation will become clinically relevant in the future when preventive strategies depend on recognizing very mild disorder.

Diagnosis

• Major neurocognitive disorder due to Alzheimer's disease

Suggested Readings

Rabins PV, Lyketsos CG: A commentary on the proposed DSM revision regarding the classification of cognitive disorders. Am J Geriatr Psychiatry 9(3):201–204, 2011

Shin M: Depressive symptoms with cognitive dysfunction increase the risk of cognitive impairment: analysis of the Korean Longitudinal Study of Aging (KLoSA), 2006-2018. Int Psychogeriatr 33(8):791–801, 2021

CASE 17.4

Disheveled and Drained

George S. Alexopoulos, M.D.

Betty Drucker, a 76-year-old white woman, was experiencing sad mood, diminished interest in activities that had given her pleasure in the past, neglect of her personal appearance and household responsibilities, feelings of insecurity when interacting with others, and difficulties in concentration and word finding. She had reduced her social interactions, stopped going to her senior citizens center, and dropped out of her weekly card game because she experienced no pleasure and could not adequately concentrate. She had lost 7 pounds in the prior 2 months, and her sleep was interrupted by periods of insomnia with agonizing ruminations. This was the first time she had experienced any psychiatric symptoms.

Ms. Druker had retired 10 years earlier after a successful career as an attorney. She had been divorced for 30 years. Her two children and three grandchildren lived nearby, and she had been seeing them often before this episode.

Ms. Drucker had hypertension, hyperlipidemia, and a history of coronary occlusion for which she had received a stent. She was taking hydrochlorothiazide, the angiotensin receptor inhibitor olmesartan, atorvastatin, and low-dose aspirin. She had smoked half a pack of cigarettes per day for about 30 years.

On examination, Ms. Drucker was disheveled and appeared drained of energy. She took a long time to respond to questions. She had a depressed, anxious mood and a sad affect, and was preoccupied with her finances but could be temporarily reassured. She complained of forgetfulness; on examination, she was able to recall two out of four objects in 3 minutes and recognized a third when given several choices. She could think of 14 items available in a supermarket over a period of 1 minute. She failed to cluster items of similar kind. Ms. Drucker had difficulty producing a list of vegetables alternating with items of clothing; she produced 12 correct responses and 4 errors. She spaced the hours unequally in drawing a clock but placed the hands correctly. The patient's Mini-Mental State Examination score was 24. She gave 22 correct responses over 1 minute in the Stroop Test, which measures "response inhibition" by asking the person to identify the color of ink in which incongruous words are written (e.g., the word "RED" written in blue ink).

A neurological examination was essentially unremarkable, with the exception of a mild drop on the left side of her mouth. A CT head scan revealed pronounced periventricular and subcortical white matter hyperintensities.

Discussion

Four questions need to be addressed in characterizing Ms. Drucker's syndrome: 1) Are the depressive symptoms and signs a response to chronic stress resulting from increasing social restrictions and functional limitations (DSM-5: adjustment disorder with depressed mood)? 2) Is the cognitive dysfunction a transient aspect of a depressive syndrome (DSM-5: major depressive disorder, single episode)? 3) Is the cognitive impairment an early-stage neurocognitive disorder (DSM-5: mild neurocognitive disorder), possibly unmasked or accentuated by the depressive syndrome (DSM-5: major depressive disorder, single episode)? 4) Are both depressive and cognitive symptoms due to an underlying neurological event, affecting both cognitive and mood networks, that may not progress into dementia (DSM-5: depressive disorder due to another medical condition)? Some of these questions can be addressed by a careful clinical evaluation, but others may be answered only after the depressive symptoms subside or after long-term follow-up.

Increasing functional limitations and the need to adjust to a new, unfamiliar lifestyle often lead to symptoms of depression and anxiety. Most stress-induced reactions consist of low mood, tearfulness, or feelings of hopelessness. However, reactions to chronic stress rarely present with symptoms in all five domains of the depressive syndrome (i.e., mood, motoric activity, cyclic functions, somatic symptoms, and ideational disturbance). When they do involve all domains and cause distress and dysfunction, patients should receive the diagnosis of major depressive disorder (MDD), and chronic stress should be viewed as a triggering factor.

Cognitive dysfunction is an integral part of late-life MDD. Unless there is a coexisting neurological insult such as a neurocognitive disorder, the cognitive dysfunction of late-life depression is mild. Attention, timed tests, and effortful cognitive functions (e.g., verbal free recall) are most impaired. Impairments in executive functioning are also common in late-life depression and include abnormal performance in tasks of semantic fluency, semantic organization, response inhibition, planning, and sequencing. Executive dysfunction occurs in up to 40% of depressed older patients and is a risk factor for poor response to antidepressant medication but not to psychotherapy. Patients with the depression–executive dysfunction syndrome may not develop a major neurocognitive disorder on follow-up, but executive dysfunction often persists even when the depression subsides.

Late-life depression often coexists, however, with major neurocognitive disorders. More than 20% of patients with Alzheimer's disease develop MDD either during the preclinical phase or during the early or middle stages of dementia. Depression is even more common in patients with vascular or mixed-etiology neurocognitive disorder, neurocognitive disorder with Lewy bodies, frontotemporal neurocognitive disorder, and neurocognitive disorder due to Parkinson's disease. As part of a severe depression, some older individuals develop a dementia syndrome whose symptoms and signs subside with improvement of the depression. This syndrome had been viewed as a benign "pseudodementia." However, the symptom improvement generally turns out to be transient. Most cases of late-life depressive pseudodementia evolve into an irreversible neurocognitive disorder that is usually identified during long-term follow-up.

At this point, Ms. Drucker appears to meet DSM-5 criteria for both MDD and mild neurocognitive disorder. Her mild disturbances in memory and her more severe impairment in executive functioning suggest the diagnosis of depression–executive dysfunction syndrome of late life. Her vascular risk factors (hypertension, hyperlipidemia), her history of coronary artery disease, her mouth angle drop, and her white matter hyperintensities suggest a vascular contribution to her depression–executive dysfunction syndrome.

Assuming that Ms. Drucker's syndrome was correctly identified (MDD and mild neurocognitive disorder), the differential diagnosis should focus on the most likely etiological contributors to the syndrome. Clinical examination should focus on common causes of late-life depression and mild cognitive impairment—that is, early-stage Alzheimer's disease, vascular dementia, mixed-etiology dementia, Lewy body disease, Parkinson's disease, and frontotemporal dementia. A history of smoking, hypertension, coronary artery disease, mouth angle drop, and white matter hyperintensities suggest a vascular contribution to both MDD and cognitive symptoms. Psychomotor retardation and executive dysfunction offer further support to this possibility because both symptoms can be caused by compromise of medial frontal and subcortical structures due to small-vessel disease.

Another possibility is that Ms. Drucker has an early-stage mild neurocognitive disorder due to Alzheimer's disease. Cerebrovascular pathology accelerates the clinical expression of the Alzheimer's process. In fact, mixed-etiology cognitive syndromes are more common than cognitive syndromes of exclusively vascular etiology. In Ms. Drucker's case, the diagnoses of neurocognitive disorder due to Lewy body disease or to Parkinson's disease are unlikely because she has no extrapyramidal signs or autonomic instability. Also unlikely is the diagnosis of frontotemporal dementia in a patient with memory disturbance in the absence of emerging personality pathology and behavioral disinhibition.

Diagnoses

- Major depressive disorder
- Mild neurocognitive disorder due to multiple etiologies

Suggested Readings

Alexopoulos GS: "The depression-executive dysfunction syndrome of late life": a specific target for D3 agonists? Am J Geriatr Psychiatry 9(1):22–29, 2001

Alexopoulos GS: Mechanisms and treatment of late-life depression. Transl Psychiatry 9(1):188, 2019

Alexopoulos GS, Meyers BS, Young RC, et al: The course of geriatric depression with "reversible dementia": a controlled study. Am J Psychiatry 150(11):1693–1699, 1993

Alexopoulos GS, Kiosses DN, Klimstra S, et al: Clinical presentation of the "depression-executive dysfunction syndrome" of late life. Am J Geriatr Psychiatry 10(1):98–106, 2002

Alexopoulos GS, Raue PJ, Banerjee S, et al: Comparing the streamlined psychotherapy "Engage" with problem-solving therapy in late-life major depression. A randomized clinical trial. Mol Psychiatry 26(9):5180–5189, 2021

Taylor WD, Aizenstein HJ, Alexopoulos GS: The vascular depression hypothesis: mechanisms linking vascular disease with depression. Mol Psychiatry 18(9):963–974, 2013

CASE 17.5

Stiff and Forgetful

James E. Galvin, M.D., M.P.H.

Carl Estel, a 74-year-old right-handed married man, was brought for a neuropsychiatric evaluation after a multi-year decline marked by stiffness, forgetfulness, and apathy. His wife had been trying to get him in for an evaluation for years and had finally become desperate enough to enlist his brothers to bring him for the evaluation.

Mrs. Estel described her husband's problems as starting when he retired from his job as a plumbing contractor at age 65. He had seemed "out of sorts" almost immediately, and she had wondered at the time whether he was getting depressed. He became uncharacteristically forgetful, misplacing items and neglecting to pay bills. He had trouble with appointments, medications, and calculations. He had refused to see a physician until he was involved in a traffic accident a few years prior to this evaluation. At that time, a physician had found no significant physical injuries but had said that the accident was caused by inattention and diminished depth perception; she had recommended that Mr. Estel stop driving, and suggested that he get a more thorough evaluation for early dementia.

Over the past year, things had gotten worse. Mr. Estel often could not recall the outcome of sporting events that he had just watched on television, although his memory improved with cues. He resisted activities such as travel and socializing that he had previously enjoyed. A former athlete, he stopped taking walks around the neighborhood after several falls. He quit playing cards with neighbors because the rules had become confusing. He looked depressed and acted apathetic but generally said he was fine. His judgment and problem-solving skills appeared to have significantly declined. Despite having completed 4 years of college and worked for many years as a successful professional plumber, Mr. Estel was now periodically unable to operate household appliances.

All of these cognitive problems seemed to fluctuate, so that his wife reported that sometimes he was "almost like his old self," whereas at other times it was "like living with a zombie, a depressed zombie." She also described his frequent exhaustion, daytime drowsiness, and staring spells.

When asked specifically about her husband's sleep, Mrs. Estel reported that in fact neither of them slept well. Mainly, she said, it was because of her husband "acting out his dreams." During these episodes, which occurred several times a month, he would punch and scream, and would occasionally fall out of bed. After sustaining bruises as a result of several of the episodes, Mrs. Estel decided it would be safer to sleep on the couch. She recalled that these sleep episodes began just before her husband retired; she had wondered at the time whether he had posttraumatic stress disorder, but she did not think he had suffered any particular trauma. A few years earlier, a friend had offered her a "sleeping pill" that had helped her own husband with dementia. Mr. Estel had responded to the unknown medication with extreme rigidity and confusion, and his wife had nearly taken him to the emergency room in the middle of the night.

Mrs. Estel denied that her husband had ever had any psychiatric illness. When asked about psychotic symptoms, she said that perhaps every week or so, he swatted at invisible things in the air. She did not think he heard voices or felt suspicious.

Mr. Estel's medical history was notable for hypercholesterolemia, cardiovascular disease with a history of stent placement, and possible transient ischemic attacks. His family history was positive for his mother having developed dementia in her mid-70s.

On examination, Mr. Estel was a stooped, stiff man who shuffled into the office. While listening to his wife present the history, he stared into space, seeming to pay no attention to the content of the conversation. His right hand was tremulous. He appeared depressed, but when asked, he said he felt fine. His voice was so quiet that words were often unintelligible even when the interviewer leaned close. He drooled at times and did not notice until his wife wiped his chin.

When asked to participate in cognitive testing, he shrugged his shoulders and said, "I don't know."

Discussion

Mr. Estel presents with a progressive decline in cognition, particularly in the areas of attention, executive ability, and visuospatial skills. These symptoms are a significant change from his baseline and interfere with his functioning. He therefore meets criteria for major neurocognitive disorder, or dementia.

Mrs. Estel's excellent history allows for a more specific understanding of her husband's neurocognitive disorder. Mr. Estel's first symptom appears to have been a sleep disturbance characterized by a violent enactment of his dreams. His memory and executive functioning have declined significantly, but his overall level of awareness fluctuates during the course of the day. At least a couple of years after the memory decline, he developed parkinsonian symptoms. He appears to have developed periodic visual hallucinations (swatting into the air). He responded to an unknown "sleeping pill" with a severe intensification of his parkinsonian symptoms and apparent "confusion." Mr. Estel likely has DSM-5 major neurocognitive disorder with Lewy bodies (NCDLB).

NCDLB (also known as Lewy body dementia) is characterized by three relatively specific "core" features and two "suggestive" features. A "probable" diagnosis is made if the patient has two core features, or one suggestive feature with one or more core features. For a "possible" diagnosis, the individual should have one core feature, or one or more suggestive features.

The first core feature of NCDLB is a fluctuating cognition with pronounced variations in attention and alertness. Although some variation is seen in other neurocognitive disorders, the fluctuation is more pronounced in NCDLB than in, for example, Alzheimer's dementia. Cognitive fluctuations are not simply variations in memory but instead represent spontaneous alterations in consciousness, attention, or concentration. These may wax and wane over minutes, hours, or days, with symptoms such as excessive daytime sleepiness, including napping for longer than 2 hours daily; illogical or incoherent thinking or conversation; and frequent staring spells. Mrs. Estel reports that Mr. Estel is sometimes almost "his old self" but at other times "a zombie." In addition to fluctuating cognition, Mr. Estel, like other patients with NCDLB, tends to have memory deficits that are improved with cues (as noted in regard to his recollection of sporting events). This contrasts with Alzheimer's disease, in which cues do not generally help in the recollection.

A second core feature is recurrent visual hallucinations. Although Mr. Estel denies having these, his wife reports that he recurrently waves at the air, as if he sees something. Visual hallucinations (which patients commonly describe as small people, children, or animals) may be accompanied by hallucination in other modalities.

Mr. Estel also has the third core feature: his parkinsonian symptoms developed 2 years later than his cognitive impairment. If these symptoms had developed in reverse order, he would be more likely to have Parkinson's disease. Mr. Estel has some of the typical features of spontaneous parkinsonism: bradykinesia, rigidity (with or without the presence of cogwheeling), postural instability, and resting tremor.

Mr. Estel may also meet criteria for both of the suggestive features for NCDLB. He appears to meet criteria for rapid eye movement (REM) sleep behavior disorder, which he developed just before his wife noticed cognitive difficulties. REM sleep disorder is characterized by vocalizations and arm and leg movements during REM sleep. As seen in Mr. Estel, these movements can be violent. REM sleep behavior disorder is a common prodromal symptom of both Parkinson's disease and NCDLB.

A final suggestive criterion is sensitivity to antipsychotic medication. Mr. Estel developed confusion and an exacerbation of his parkinsonian features after taking a "sleeping pill" offered by a friend whose husband took the medication for dementia. Although it is difficult to be sure what the pill was, a likely culprit would be an antipsychotic medication. If so, then Mr. Estel would meet the NCDLB criterion of "severe neuroleptic sensitivity." Neuroleptic sensitivity is characterized by excessive rigidity with exposure to "classic" neuroleptics or other antidopaminergic medications (e.g., antiemetics). Affected patients would also have an increased risk of neuroleptic malignant syndrome.

Although NCDLB is the most likely diagnosis, other possibilities should be considered. Alzheimer's disease is the most common dementia, but the presence of REM sleep behavior disorder points toward a synucleinopathy like NCDLB, as does the fact that his memory improves with cues. Mr. Estel has parkinsonian features, and REM sleep behavior disorder is also associated with Parkinson's disease, but his cognitive symptoms started before his movement disorder, making it unlikely that he has Parkinson's disease. Cerebrovascular disease can cause somewhat similar symptoms, but there should be accompanying focal neurological signs and/or abnormalities on brain imaging. Mr. Estel appears to have no history of psychiatric illness. Although primary psychiatric disorders can emerge in late life, his constellation of symptoms—cognitive, motor, sleep, and behavior—supports a neurocognitive disorder diagnosis rather than a primary psychiatric diagnosis such as a depressive disorder.

Diagnoses

- Major neurocognitive disorder with Lewy bodies
- Rapid eye movement sleep behavior disorder

Suggested Readings

Karantzoulis S, Galvin JE: Distinguishing Alzheimer's disease from other major forms of dementia. Expert Rev Neurother 11(11):1579–1591, 2011

Walaszek A: Behavioral and Psychological Symptoms of Dementia. Washington DC, American Psychiatric Association Publishing, 2020

Walker Z, Possin KL, Boeve BF, Aarsland D: Non-Alzheimer's dementia 2: Lewy body dementias. Lancet 386(10004):1683–1697, 2015

CASE 17.6

Paranoia and Hallucinations

Lorin M. Scher, M.D.

Collin Shumate, M.D.

Barbara J. Kocsis, M.D.

Dorothy Franklin, a 54-year-old married former waitress, was brought into the psychiatric emergency room (ER) by her husband for escalating delusions and visual hallucinations. Her husband reported that she had been episodically agitated for about 10 years, uncharacteristically suspicious for about 6 months, and complaining of daily hallucinations for weeks to months. The patient referred to her experience as "my nightmare." In a terrified voice, she explained, "I see a judge standing in front of me. Plain as day. He is a good judge, but he threatens to kill me, and I can't stop him. I can't believe no one else can see him. Can you help?"

Mr. Franklin reports that his wife had been "completely fine" until about a decade earlier, when she was in her early 40s. At that point, he reports that she had become frequently agitated, paranoid, worried, and occasionally aggressive. He had brought her to psychiatrists and internists, and she had received several diagnoses, including late-onset schizophrenia, bipolar disorder, depression, paranoid personality, and anxiety. She and her husband could not recall the names of all of the many psychiatric medications that she had been prescribed over the years, but they included antidepressant, antipsychotic, antianxiety, and mood-stabilizing medications.

Ms. Franklin had smoked half a pack of cigarettes a day for many years but only rarely drank alcohol and never used recreational drugs. She had worked as a waitress for 20 years but quit 10 years prior to the evaluation because of too many "dropped trays," misremembered customer orders, and uncharacteristic irritability. Around that time, she was arrested for "hitting someone" in a shopping mall, and she and her husband decided she needed to reduce her stress level.

The patient had two healthy adult children in their late 20s. She had one sister with "depression and irritability." The patient's mother had passed away 10 years earlier at age 70. She had been wheelchair bound for years because of severe dementia, postural instability, and involuntary movements. The patient's maternal grandfather "got sick" in his late 50s and completed suicide with a firearm at age 62.

On mental status examination in the ER, Ms. Franklin was frightened but cooperative. She appeared her stated age, with thin body habitus and good grooming and hygiene. She sat next to her husband, holding his hand and often looking to him when asked questions. She had moderate psychomotor slowing, and noticeable involuntary "dancelike" movements of her trunk and upper extremities. Her eye contact was intermittent but intense. Ms. Franklin described her mood as "not well at all," and her affect was blunted and minimally reactive. Her speech was soft and slowed, with minimal spontaneity. Her thought process was linear but slowed. She was preoccupied by paranoid delusions and visual hallucinations. She reported actively hallucinating during the interview. She denied suicidal and homicidal thoughts or plans. On cognitive examination, she was alert and oriented to person, place, and time. She had good attention and concentration, although she had significant impairments in both short- and long-term memory. Her performance on the Mini-Mental State Examination and clock drawing test revealed moderate impairment in planning and visuospatial tasks.

In the ER, results from extensive laboratory testing were normal. The patient was admitted to the inpatient psychiatric unit for safety and for further workup of her psychotic symptoms.

Discussion (Part I)

Ms. Franklin has developed a psychotic disorder with a history and symptomatology that point toward an underlying medical or neuropsychiatric etiology. The onset was relatively late for a psychosis from schizophrenia, for example, and she has visual hallucinations, early-onset cognitive deficits, and a cluster of nonspecific neurological symptoms (clumsiness, choreiform movements, and bradykinesia). Medications and illicit substances do not appear to be implicated.

General medical causes of psychosis are multiple, and include infectious, metabolic, cerebrovascular, epileptic, demyelinating, and degenerative etiologies, as well as substance-induced psychosis and toxidromes.

Potential neuropsychiatric conditions that might explain Ms. Franklin's symptoms include Parkinson's disease, dementia with Lewy bodies, Huntington's disease, epilepsy, and multiple sclerosis.

Parkinson's disease affects 1% of the population older than 50 years and is defined by tremor, bradykinesia, rigidity, and, in some patients, dementia. Depression is widely experienced by patients with Parkinson's disease, and psychosis is not uncommon. While not pertinent to Ms. Franklin, the anticholinergic and dopaminergic drugs used to treat Parkinson's disease are known to precipitate or worsen psychosis.

Neurocognitive disorder with Lewy bodies (NCDLB) is another consideration, given its hallmark symptom of visual hallucinations, coupled with Parkinson's disease–like symptoms.

Huntington's disease is a fatal autosomal dominant disorder that typically manifests in the fourth or fifth decade of life, and is marked by cognitive decline, motor symptoms, and psychiatric disturbance. Psychiatric symptoms are common throughout the disease course and include depression, apathy, irritability, and psychosis.

In patients like Ms. Franklin, epilepsy—particularly complex partial seizures—should always be ruled out with electroencephalography (EEG). Complex partial seizures may present with panic-like symptoms and brief hallucinations, although patients with long-standing epilepsy may develop chronic, unrelenting psychotic symptoms.

Multiple sclerosis, an inflammatory demyelinating disease that most commonly affects women, is often marked by depression, irritability, and cognitive deficits, although hallucinations and delusions are not common manifestations.

While any of the above diagnoses might be possible for Ms. Franklin, her symptoms on admission were nonspecific enough that she would likely be admitted with a diagnosis of unspecified schizophrenia spectrum and other psychotic disorder.

Diagnosis on Admission

• Unspecified schizophrenia spectrum and other psychotic disorder

Case (continued)

After Ms. Franklin was admitted to the psychiatric unit, she received brain magnetic resonance imaging (MRI) to rule out mass lesions (e.g., tumor or stroke) and demyelinating processes (e.g., multiple sclerosis). MRI findings were normal, and the neurology department was consulted for diagnostic assistance and administration of EEG to evaluate for a possible seizure disorder. While she was actively hallucinating, Ms. Franklin's electroencephalogram was negative for seizure activity.

Given the nature and time course of Ms. Franklin's symptoms, coupled with her family history of dementia and delayed-onset psychiatric disturbances, the psychiatry and neurology teams became concerned about the possibility of Huntington's disease. After extensive discussion with the patient and her spouse, she agreed to undergo genetic testing for Huntington's disease, and the test result was positive for 44 trinucleotide (CAG) repeats. After further psychosocial and medication management, she and her husband were referred to a comprehensive outpatient Huntington's disease clinic.

Discussion (Part II)

Given Ms. Franklin's symptomatology and the exclusion of other potential causes, the inpatient team explored the possibility of Huntington's disease. This disease is unusual in that it has a dismal prognosis and is an autosomal dominant disorder that can be identified through genetic testing. It would certainly be important for the team to have "extensive discussions" with Mr. and Ms. Franklin prior to asking for consent to do the genetic testing.

After the couple gets involved in the outpatient Huntington's disease clinic, a similar discussion will likely be offered to their two adult children. While they are currently asymptomatic, each of the children has a 50% chance of having inherited the Huntington's disease gene. The difficult decision for each child is whether they want to know that they are destined to develop Huntington's disease in midlife, and whether they want to know that if in fact they do carry the gene, they would have a 50% chance of passing it on to their own children.

In regard to Ms. Franklin, it appears that she would warrant two DSM-5 diagnoses. Her neurocognitive symptoms are not yet severe, and so she would likely be diagnosed with mild neurocognitive disorder due to Huntington's disease. In addition, she would be diagnosed with psychotic disorder due to Huntington's disease.

Recent research suggests that patients with Huntington's disease and psychosis may have a distinct clinical course from Huntington's disease patients without psychosis. Patients with psychosis appear to demonstrate worse cognition, function, and behavioral disturbances than patients without psychosis, and they tend to function less independently. The outpatient Huntington's disease clinic is likely to follow Ms. Franklin's neurocognitive status closely, since interventions will need to be evaluated and re-evaluated throughout the course of her illness.

Ms. Franklin is at an important phase in her illness. Although she has significant symptoms, it appears that she still understands her situation and maintains the cognition to make many of her own decisions. It becomes important for the treating team to take this opportunity to develop an alliance with the patient, provide the necessary psychological support, and tactfully explore end-of-life issues before her neurocognitive disorder progresses and she develops challenges with medical and legal decision-making capacity. For example, it would be important to help Ms. Franklin (and her husband) clarify her preferences regarding financial issues (e.g., creating a will), caretaking (e.g., long-term care preferences), and advance medical directives (e.g., future code status).

Final Diagnoses

- Mild neurocognitive disorder due to Huntington's disease
- Psychotic disorder due to Huntington's disease

Suggested Readings

Beck BJ, Tompkins KJ: Mental disorders due to another medical condition, in Massachusetts General Hospital Comprehensive Clinical Psychiatry, 2nd Edition. Edited by Stern TA, Fava M, Wilens TE, Rosenbaum JF. Philadelphia, PA, Mosby/Elsevier, 2016, pp 205–228

Connors MH, Teixeira-Pinto A, Loy CT: Psychosis and longitudinal outcomes in Huntington disease: the COHORT Study. J Neurol Neurosurg Psychiatry 91(1):15–20, 2020

Langa KM, Levine DA: The diagnosis and management of mild cognitive impairment: a clinical review. JAMA 312(23):2551–2561, 2014

Scher LM, Kocsis BJ: How to target psychiatric symptoms of Huntington's disease. Current Psychiatry 11(9): 34–39, 2012

CASE 17.7

Suddenly Rebellious

Stuart C. Yudofsky, M.D.
Robert E. Hales, M.D., M.B.A.

Only upon the repeated and fervent insistence of her parents did 19-year-old Emily reluctantly agree to see a psychiatrist. "It's not me you want to see," Emily proclaimed emphatically. "It's my insane parents who need your help." Emily did not offer a chief complaint, aside from the concern that her parents were driving her "crazy." She added, "Everything is going great in my life. I have plenty of friends, go out almost every night, and always have lots of fun."

While Emily was taking some time away from "the so-called real world," her sister was attending Duke University, her younger brother was excelling at a competitive private high school, and both her parents seemed to enjoy their careers as radiologists. She asked, "Don't you think that's enough strivers for one family?"

Emily agreed to have her parents join the session, and they told a different story. They tearfully disclosed that their daughter had become irritable, unproductive, and oppositional. She drank to intoxication almost every night, often not returning home for an entire weekend. In searching her room, they had found small amounts of marijuana, alprazolam (Xanax), cocaine, and prescription stimulants. The parents described the changes in Emily's personality as "an adolescent nightmare" and described her friends as "losers who do nothing but dye their hair, get tattoos, and hate everything." Emily's attitudes and behavior contrasted markedly with those of her parents and siblings. "We don't mind that she is doing her own thing and that she isn't conservative like the rest of us," her father said, "but it's like we don't even recognize who she's become."

According to her parents, Emily's "adolescent nightmare" began 4 years earlier. She had apparently been a studious 15-year-old girl with a lively sense of humor and a wide circle of "terrific friends." "Almost overnight," she began to shun her longtime friends in favor of "dropouts and malcontents" and began to accumulate traffic tickets and school detentions. Instead of her former bright-eyed curiosity, Emily manifested a lack of interest in all her academic subjects, and her grades dropped from As to Ds. The parents were at an absolute loss to explain the sudden and dramatic change.

The abrupt change in performance led the psychiatrist to ask Emily to take a battery of neuropsychological tests so the results could be compared with those of tests that she had taken when she had applied to a private high school several years earlier.

In particular, Emily retook two high school admissions tests: the System for Assessment and Group Evaluation (SAGE), which measures a broad array of academic and perceptual aptitudes, and the Differential Aptitude Tests (DAT), which focus on reasoning, spelling, and perceptual skills.

On the SAGE, her average percentile scores dropped from the upper 10% for a 13-year-old to the bottom 10% for an adult (and the bottom 20% for a 13-year-old). When Emily took the DAT at age 13, she scored in the highest range for ninth graders across almost all measures. Her worst result had been in spelling, where she scored at the second-highest level. Upon repeating the test at age 19, she scored below the high school average in all measures.

EEG, brain CT, and T2-weighted brain MRI scans showed no evidence of structural brain damage. However, fluid-attenuated inversion recovery (FLAIR) T2-weighted MRI displayed a clear lesion in the left frontal cortex, highly suggestive of previous injury to that region.

Upon further questioning about the crucial period in which she seemed to have changed, Emily admitted to being in a traffic accident with her now ex-boyfriend, Mark. Although Emily did not recall much from this episode, she remembered that she hit her head and that she had bad headaches for many weeks thereafter. Because Emily was not bleeding and there was no damage to the car, neither Mark nor Emily reported the incident to anyone. With Emily's permission, the psychiatrist contacted Mark, who was away at college but a willing and excellent historian. He remembered the incident well. "Emily hit her head very, very hard on the dashboard of my car. She was not totally unconscious but very dazed. For about 3 hours, she spoke very slowly, complained that her head hurt badly, and was confused. For about 2 hours she didn't know where she was or what day it was. She also threw up twice. I was really scared, but Emily didn't want me to worry her parents since they're so overprotective. And then she broke up with me, and we've hardly spoken since."

Discussion

Feeling pressured to see a psychiatrist by "overprotective" parents, Emily tries to frame her own story as that of an underachieving young woman who is enjoying her youth and rebelling against her family's academic and social strictures. In contrast, her parents emphasize her "overnight" change from a pleasant, high-achieving 15-year-old girl into a rude, academically failing, substance-abusing "nightmare." The differential diagnosis for such a change is broad but clarified through history, collateral information, and cognitive testing.

Critical to an accurate diagnosis is recognition of change that appears to be somewhat different from what is typically explained by the onset of a mood, anxiety, or substance use disorder. This recognition led to the decision to retest Emily's performance on high school aptitude and achievement examinations, which revealed the dramatic decline in her test scores. Focused historical inquiry led to the discovery of the motor vehicle accident that was pivotal to the development of Emily's symptoms.

In the accident, Emily suffered a traumatic brain injury (TBI). History collected from the car's driver and from Emily indicates that she had two of the four core criteria for a TBI diagnosis: she was disoriented and confused for hours afterward, and she did not recall much about the accident (posttraumatic amnesia). Only one is necessary to make the TBI diagnosis. Emily apparently did not lose consciousness, and no neurological signs were noted in the history. Although routine brain scans were read as normal, a FLAIR T2-weighted MRI done 4 years later revealed a lesion that was "highly suggestive" of trauma to the left frontal cortex.

For a DSM-5 diagnosis of a neurocognitive disorder due to TBI, a person must also have evidence of decline in cognitive functioning. Emily meets this standard; her decline is substantiated by parental observation, school records, and aptitude and achievement tests taken before and after high school. It is less obvious as to whether her neurocognitive disorder is considered mild or major. The more severe category is generally reserved for individuals whose deficits interfere with activities of daily living, such as paying bills and managing medications. The mild category targets people with more modest impairment. Emily's test results reflect a dramatic decline, from the top tenth percentile to the bottom tenth percentile. For Emily and her family, that drop is likely to be viewed as catastrophic. Nevertheless, the fact that she is able to dress, drive, and socialize seems to indicate that the most appropriate diagnosis is mild neurocognitive disorder due to TBI. Although DSM-5 includes a behavioral disturbance specifier for major neurocognitive disorder, it specifically excludes the use of a code for a behavioral disturbance specifier in mild neurocognitive disorder; nevertheless, the behavioral disturbance should still be indicated in writing.

Emily's case reflects two particular challenges in neuropsychiatric diagnosis. First, although some neuropsychiatric disorders have sudden, dramatic onsets, many others are more insidious. In some cases—as with Emily—the insult may have been acute but the link between the underlying neuropsychiatric disorder and the presenting symptoms is obscure. Although the TBI was an acute event with abrupt academic and social sequelae, Emily was not visibly injured, and she maintained many of her verbal skills. Instead of an immediate recognition of deficits, the school and family were left puzzled by Emily's disruptive behavior, academic decline, and personality changes.

Second, it can be difficult to determine whether the presenting symptoms are direct or secondary effects of the brain injury, or a combination of both. The insult to Emily's frontal cortex had a significant cognitive impact, and she is no longer able to achieve to her usual standards. Injury to her prefrontal cortex may also have directly affected her impulse control, executive functioning, social judgment, and capacity to understand and apply abstract concepts.

Resultant academic and interpersonal failures would change how she was seen by her parents, teachers, and classmates, and the failures would change how she saw herself. Unrecognized as suffering from a TBI, Emily was unable to maintain her position among the "strivers" in her family and peer group. Instead, Emily found a fraternity of "dropouts and malcontents," a group that might have helped her regain a sense of belonging. Emily began to use alcohol and illicit substances at about the same time, which leads to other questions: Did she do so to boost her cognition (e.g., with stimulants), to reduce anxiety (e.g., with cannabis), or primarily to get high? Did she use substances to convince herself that her cognition and personality changes were under her control, or to better fit into an outsider subculture that almost requires substance use?

In other words, what is phenomenon and what is epiphenomenon? Were Emily's striking personality changes the direct result of her TBI, or were these changes dysfunctional responses to the psychosocial stresses engendered by her significant cognitive impairment? Or, perhaps, was there a complex interaction between these changes, accompanied by the increasing stresses and opportunities of adolescence?

It may be difficult to elaborate all of the factors that might have contributed to Emily's current situation, but it is important to identify comorbid conditions that can further exacerbate her cognitive deficits and personality issues. Identification of substance use disorders is important, but it will also be crucial to look for disorders across the DSM-5 spectrum, particularly mood and anxiety disorders. Clarifying such issues will likely be important for the development of an eclectic and flexible treatment for this young woman, as well as for her worried family.

Diagnoses

- Mild neurocognitive disorder due to traumatic brain injury, with behavioral disturbance
- Alcohol use disorder

Suggested Readings

McAllister TW: Overview of mild brain injury, in Textbook of Traumatic Brain Injury, 3rd Edition. Edited by Silver JM, McAllister TW, Arciniegas DB. Washington, DC, American Psychiatric Publishing, 2019, pp 583–606

Oldenburg C, Lundin A, Edman G, et al: Cognitive reserve and persistent post-concussion symptoms—a prospective mild traumatic brain injury (mTBI) cohort study. Brain Injury 30(2):146–155, 2016

Silver JM, McAllister TW, Arciniegas DB: Depression and cognitive complaints following mild traumatic brain injury. Am J Psychiatry 166(6):653–661, 2009

Yudofsky SC: Getting help, in Fatal Flaws: Navigating Destructive Relationships With People With Disorders of Personality and Character. Washington, DC, American Psychiatric Publishing, 2005, pp 461–474

Yudofsky SC, Hales RE: Neuropsychiatry: back to the future. J Nerv Ment Dis 200(3):193–196, 2012

CHAPTER 18

Personality Disorders

INTRODUCTION

John W. Barnhill, M.D.

Personality is the enduring pattern of behavior and inner experience. It underlies how we think, feel, and act. It frames how we view ourselves and the people around us. When we think of who we are, we often think of personality as the central defining characteristic.

Psychiatrists and other mental health care practitioners spend considerable time thinking about personality and the ways in which dysfunctional personalities cause distress and dysfunction in individuals and in the people around them. Disorders of personality are, in some ways, as complex as humanity, itself full of idiosyncrasies, half-articulated conflicts, and unknowable complexities.

Like many other complex systems, however, personalities and personality disorders tend to fall into patterns, and, for generations, clinicians and personality researchers from a variety of fields have searched for a holy grail: a nosological system that is both simple to use and sophisticated enough to capture the nuances and paradoxes of human personality.

Traditionally, the field of psychiatry has conceptualized personality disorders categorically, as reflecting distinct clinical syndromes. In another paradigm, personality traits are conceptualized dimensionally, as variants that exist on a gradient from maladaptive to normal. A third model incorporates both paradigms, a hybrid categorical-dimensional model.

Sociocultural contexts add an additional layer of complexity to the identification of personality disorders. DSM-5 takes advantage of continuing research into the ways in which models of mind vary across cultures, as do cognitive and behavioral norms. For example, sociocultural contexts that emphasize individualism and personal autonomy might be more likely to normalize narcissistic traits.

DSM-5 continues to feature the traditional categorical model of personality disorders in the main body of the text. This would generally be seen as the "official" model for personality disorders. In addition, DSM-5 includes an alternative hybrid categorical-dimensional model in Section III (Emerging Measures and Models).

To better understand the similarities and differences of the two models, it may be useful to explore how the two DSM-5 diagnostic systems recommend that a clinician assess a patient with, for example, obsessive-compulsive personality disorder (OCPD). From a categorical perspective, the individual would receive a diagnosis of OCPD when certain criteria were met. First, the clinician should identify a persistent, dysfunctional pattern of, for instance, perfectionism at the expense of flexibility. The clinician would then identify at least four of seven specific symptomatic criteria (e.g., preoccupation with lists, inability to delegate tasks, stubbornness) and search for disorders that might be responsible for the same symptoms. This investigation might lead to the coding of the other diagnosis only, such as when schizophrenia causes symptoms akin to those found in OCPD. That investigation might also lead to the coding of two or more diagnoses, such as when the person meets criteria for OCPD and another personality disorder.

The Alternative DSM-5 Model for Personality Disorders reshapes the 10 DSM-IV personality disorder categories into a roster of six redefined categories (antisocial, avoidant, borderline, narcissistic, obsessive-compulsive, and schizotypal). For each of the six categories, the new model requires two assessments. The first involves a determination that the individual has significant impairment in at least two of four personality functioning areas: identity, self-direction, empathy, and intimacy. For each of the six personality disorders, these personality specifics differ. For example, to qualify for OCPD, an individual must demonstrate multiple specific difficulties in personality functioning (e.g., rigidity and lack of empathy) as well as multiple personality traits (e.g., perfectionism, perseveration, and an avoidance of intimacy).

The alternative hybrid model then requires an assessment of personality traits that are organized under five broad trait domains. As shown in Table 18–1, these traits and trait domains exist on a spectrum; for example, for one of the five trait domains, antagonism lies on one end of the spectrum and agreeableness on the other. These five broad trait domains are new to many psychiatrists, but they have been rigorously studied for several decades within academic psychology under the rubric of the *Five Factor Model*, whose personality dimensions include neuroticism, extraversion, agreeableness, conscientiousness, and openness. For each of these personality dimensions, there are clusters of related personality traits. Applied to a particular person, the Five Factor Model can assign a percentile score for each trait. For example, a theoretical person with OCPD might score in the 95th percentile for conscientiousness and in the 5th percentile for openness. DSM-5 adapted these personality dimensions and traits in order to more specifically focus on psychiatric disorders.

Twenty-five specific pathological personality traits are included under the umbrella of these five negative trait domains. For each of the personality disorders, DSM-5 and DSM-5-TR require that the individual demonstrate most of the typical personality traits. For example, the patient with OCPD must demonstrate the trait of rigid

TABLE 18–1. Alternative DSM-5 model: pathological personality trait domains

Negative trait domain		Positive trait domain
Negative affectivity	vs.	Emotional stability
Detachment	vs.	Extraversion
Antagonism	vs.	Agreeableness
Disinhibition[a]	vs.	Conscientiousness[a]
Psychoticism	vs.	Lucidity

[a]Both poles of this domain are viewed as pathological.

perfectionism (an aspect of the trait domain of conscientiousness) as well as at least two of the following three traits: perseveration (an aspect of negative affectivity), intimacy avoidance (an aspect of detachment), and restricted affectivity (also an aspect of detachment).

The alternative DSM-5 hybrid model also specifies that specific traits can be recorded even if not recognized as part of a diagnosed personality disorder (e.g., hostility, a trait associated with the trait domain of negative affectivity, could be listed alongside any DSM-5 diagnosis and not be considered just a trait associated with, for instance, antisocial personality disorder).

Both of the DSM-5 models have advantages and disadvantages. The new DSM-5 hybrid model might contribute to a more nuanced understanding of patients, and its approach takes advantage of decades' worth of personality research. Its complexity is daunting, however, even to seasoned clinicians, and the use of a new system would potentially reduce the usefulness of existing research data within psychiatry.

The traditional categorical paradigm has been critiqued for excessive comorbidity and intradisorder heterogeneity, as well as for the fact that one of the most common personality disorder diagnoses in the past has been "personality disorder not otherwise specified," which is clarified only marginally by the DSM-5 options of "other specified" and "unspecified" personality disorder. On the other hand, the categorical approach is relatively straightforward to use, is familiar to many mental health care practitioners, and follows the categorical structure used throughout the rest of DSM-5. It is also the personality model included in the main body of the DSM-5 text and, as such, remains the American Psychiatric Association's official perspective on personality disorders.

Suggested Readings

Gore WL, Widiger TA: The DSM-5 dimensional trait model and five-factor models of general personality. J Abnorm Psychol 122(3):816–821, 2013

MacKinnon RA, Michels R, Buckley PJ: The Psychiatric Interview in Clinical Practice, 3rd Edition. Arlington, VA, American Psychiatric Association Publishing, 2015

Michels R: Diagnosing personality disorders. Am J Psychiatry 169(3):241–243, 2012

Ronningstam EF, Keng SL, Ridolfi ME, et al: Cultural aspects in symptomatology, assessment, and treatment of personality disorders. Curr Psychiatry Rep 20(4):22, 2018

Skodol AW, Oldham JM (eds): The American Psychiatric Association Publishing Textbook of Personality Disorders, 3rd Edition. Washington, DC, American Psychiatric Association Publishing, 2021

CASE 18.1

Personality Conflicts

Lauren Z. Rynar, Ph.D.
Larry J. Siever, M.D.[‡]

Frazier Archer was a 34-year-old single white man who called a mood and personality disorders research program because an ex-friend had once said he was "borderline," and Mr. Archer wanted to learn more about his personality.

During his diagnostic research interview, Mr. Archer was initially reluctant to share personal information, citing a concern that his words would be misunderstood, misconstrued, or used against him. When asked about his relationships, he described regular, almost daily situations in which he was sure he was being lied to or deceived. He was particularly wary of people in leadership positions and people who had studied psychology and, therefore, had "training to understand the human mind," which they used to manipulate people. Unlike those around him, Mr. Archer believed he did not "drink the Kool-Aid" and was able to detect manipulation and deceit.

Mr. Archer was employed as an assistant manager for a grocery store chain. He was extremely detail oriented at work, and had trouble delegating and completing tasks. He noted that his coworkers consistently failed to complete tasks the way that he would like. This led him to work routinely long hours "fixing their mistakes." Numerous employers and colleagues had told him that he focused excessively on rules, lists, and small details, and that he needed to be more friendly. He described having held numerous jobs over the years, but he was quick to add, "I've quit as often as I've been fired."

During the interview, he emphasized that unlike many people, he understood the value of quality over productivity. He believed that his "high standards" had contributed to his "bad temper" and emotional "ups and downs." He socialized only "superficially" with a handful of acquaintances and could recall the exact moments when previous "so-called friends and lovers" had betrayed him. He spent most of his time alone.

Mr. Archer denied any significant history of trauma, any current or past problems with substance use, and any history of head trauma or loss of consciousness. He also denied any history of mental health diagnosis or treatment, but he did feel he might have a mental health condition that had not yet been diagnosed. He described some

---

[‡] Dr. Siever passed away in 2021.

social anxiety and difficulties with academic achievement in childhood, which he attributed to his own high standards and "unreliable" childhood friends.

On mental status examination, Mr. Archer appeared well groomed, cooperative, and oriented. His speech varied; at times he would pause thoughtfully prior to answering questions and provide very slow, deliberate responses. At other points in the interview he became angry and offered lengthy and digressive responses. However, he seemed generally coherent and did not evidence any perceptual disturbances. His affect was occasionally inappropriate (e.g., smiling while crying) and generally constricted. He reported apathy as to whether he lived or died but did not report any active suicidal ideation or homicidal ideation.

Notably, Mr. Archer became irritated and argumentative with research staff when he was told that although he could receive verbal feedback on his interviews, he could not receive a copy of the completed questionnaires and diagnostic tools. He commented that he would document in his personal records that research staff were refusing him the forms.

Discussion

Mr. Archer describes a long-standing, inflexible, dysfunctional pattern of dealing with the world. He demonstrates an enduring pattern of distrust and suspiciousness. He believes that others are exploiting or deceiving him, doubts the loyalty of friends, bears grudges, and recurrently mistrusts the fidelity of sexual partners.

A second cluster of personality traits relates to Mr. Archer's preoccupation with perfectionism and control. He is excessively focused on rules, lists, and details. He is inflexible and unable to delegate, resulting in excessive time spent on task completion and perfection at the expense of other, perhaps more leisurely endeavors. Mr. Archer meets criteria for both paranoid personality disorder (PPD) and obsessive-compulsive personality disorder (OCPD).

It is unsurprising that Mr. Archer meets criteria for two personality disorders. An estimated 75% of people with PPD have a comorbid personality disorder. Substance use and panic disorder are also frequently comorbid with PPD, though neither appears to be a problem for Mr. Archer. PPD is often comorbid with schizotypal personality disorder and schizophrenia spectrum disorders, a finding attributable to overlapping paranoia-related criteria. PPD is rarely an "isolated" disorder, and current research is pointing toward the possibility that some personality disorders, including PPD, could be consolidated to create more inclusive diagnoses. Paranoia might then be viewed as a specifier or modifier for other disorders.

PPD and OCPD share symptomatology, including a tendency to be overcontrolled, emotionally constricted, closed to new experience, harshly judgmental of others, and cognitively and behaviorally rigid; individuals may also have low self-esteem and be averse to risk. As was the case for Mr. Archer, individuals with PPD or OCPD are also likely to manifest significant occupational difficulties. Furthermore, whereas rigid perfectionism is a defining trait of OCPD, individuals with PPD may also evidence a tendency toward perfectionism across several domains, including self-oriented perfectionism (requirements of perfection in self) and other-oriented perfectionism (requirements of perfectionism imposed on others).

It is important to distinguish PPD and OCPD from schizophrenia and obsessive-compulsive disorder (OCD). There is genetic, neurobiological, epidemiological, and symptomatic evidence that PPD, like schizotypal personality disorder, is related to schizophrenia and lies on the schizophrenia spectrum. However, PPD is not a precursor to schizophrenia, and its symptoms are not indicative of the prodromal phase of schizophrenia. The prodrome of schizophrenia is best characterized by early psychotic symptoms, including disorganized thoughts and behavior, whereas the thought patterns in PPD are generally more similar to those of delusional disorder and related thought disorders.

Similarly, there has been much debate about the relationship between OCPD and OCD. There is general consensus that OCPD and OCD constitute distinct disorders, although many researchers hypothesize that the conditions are strongly related and may overlap conceptually, with some even suggesting that there may be a severe subtype of OCD in which individuals also meet criteria for OCPD.

Diagnoses

- Paranoid personality disorder
- Obsessive-compulsive personality disorder

Suggested Readings

Diedrich A, Voderholzer U: Obsessive-compulsive personality disorder: a current review. Curr Psychiatry Rep 17(2):2, 2015

Dimaggio G, MacBeth A, Popolo R, et al: The problem of overcontrol: perfectionism, emotional inhibition, and personality disorders. Compr Psychiatry 83:71–78, 2018

Gordon OM, Salkovskis PM, Oldfield VB, Carter N: The association between obsessive compulsive disorder and obsessive compulsive personality disorder: prevalence and clinical presentation. Br J Clin Psychol 52(3):300–315, 2013

Lee R: Mistrustful and misunderstood: a review of paranoid personality disorder. Curr Behav Neurosci Rep 4(2):151–165, 2017

CASE 18.2

Oddly Isolated

Salman Akhtar, M.D.

Grzegorz Buchalski was an 87-year-old white man who was brought to the psychiatric emergency room (ER) by paramedics after they had been called to his apartment by neighbors when they noticed an odd smell. Apparently, his 90-year-old sister had died some days earlier after a lengthy illness. Mr. Buchalski had delayed reporting her death for several reasons. He had become increasingly disorganized as his sister's health had worsened, and he was worried that his landlord would use the apartment's condition as a pretext for eviction. He had tried to clean up, but his attempts consisted mainly of moving items from one place to another. He said he was about to call for help when the police and paramedics showed up.

In the ER, Mr. Buchalski recognized that his actions were odd and that he should have called for help sooner. At times, he became tearful when discussing the situation and his sister's death; at other times, he seemed aloof, speaking about these in a calm, factual way. He also wanted to clarify that his apartment had indeed been a mess but that much of the apparent mess was actually his large collection of articles on bioluminescence, a topic he had been researching for decades.

A licensed plumber, electrician, and locksmith, Mr. Buchalski had worked until age 65. He described his late sister as having been always "a little strange." She had never worked and had been married once, briefly. Aside from the several-month marriage, she and Mr. Buchalski had lived in the family's two-bedroom Manhattan apartment their entire lives. Neither of them had ever seen a psychiatrist.

When questioned, Mr. Buchalski stated that he had never had a romantic or sexual relationship and had never had many friends or social contacts outside his family. He explained that he had been poor and Polish and had had to work all the time. He had taken night classes to better understand "the strange world we live in," and he said his intellectual interests were what he found most gratifying. He said he had been upset as he realized that his sister was dying, but he would call it "numb" rather than depressed. He also denied any history of manic or psychotic symptoms. After an hour with the psychiatric trainee, Mr. Buchalski confided that he hoped the medical school might be interested in some of his papers after his death. He said he believed that bioluminescent and genetic technologies were on the verge of a breakthrough that might allow the skin of animals and then humans to glow in subtle colors that would allow people to more directly recognize emotions. He had written the notes for such technology, but they had grown into a "way-too-long science fiction novel with lots of footnotes."

On examination, Mr. Buchalski was a thin, elderly man dressed neatly in khakis and button-down shirt. He was meticulous and much preferred to discuss his interests in science than his own story. He made appropriate eye contact and had a polite, pleasant demeanor. His speech was coherent and goal directed. His mood was "fine," and his affect was appropriate though perhaps unusually cheerful under the circumstances. He denied all symptoms of psychosis, depression, and mania. Aside from his comments about bioluminescence, he said nothing that sounded delusional. He was cognitively intact, and his insight and judgment were considered generally good, although historically impaired in regard to his delay in calling the police about his sister.

Discussion

Mr. Buchalski's aloof, taciturn, and asexual lifestyle certainly fit the diagnostic criteria for schizoid personality disorder; his explanation that he has been friendless because he is Polish and poor is a weak rationalization for his psychosocial deficits. The eccentricity of his interest in bioluminescence, his exaggerated estimation of the value of his "papers," and his history of having lived essentially all his life in the family's residence with his sister give further evidence of his inward preoccupation and lack of social engagement. The striking poverty of his emotional response at his sister's passing away and his failure to make any sort of funeral arrangements are confirmatory of a flattened affective life and weak ego skills. The fact that he is cognitively intact rules out a gradually occurring, dementing etiology for his withdrawal and "confirms" the diagnosis of schizoid personality disorder.

This diagnosis has a long history in psychiatry and psychoanalysis. In psychiatry, its origins go back to Eugen Bleuler, who coined the term *schizoid* in 1908 to describe a natural component of personality that pulled one's attention toward one's inner life and away from the external world. He labeled a morbid exaggeration of this tendency as "schizoid personality." Such individuals were described as quiet, suspicious, and "comfortably dull." Bleuler's description was elaborated upon over the next century, and many features were added to it. These included solitary lifestyle, love of books, lack of athleticism, tendency toward autistic thinking, poorly developed sexuality, and covert but intense sensitivity to others' emotional responses. This last feature, however, got dropped from the more recent portrayals of schizoid personality, including the ones in DSM-III and DSM-IV. Despite the reservations of many investigators (e.g., Otto Kernberg, John Livesley, and myself), "lacking desire for close relationships" became a prime criterion for the schizoid diagnosis. Among other factors that were emphasized were asexuality, indifference to praise or criticism, anhedonia, and emotional coldness. The hypersensitivity criterion and the ostensible link to schizophrenia were assigned, respectively, to the categories of "avoidant" and "schizotypal" personality disorders.

Within psychoanalysis, the schizoid condition was best described by W.R.D. Fairbairn and Harry Guntrip. According to them, intense sensitivity to both love and rejection and a propensity to readily withdraw from interpersonal relatedness lay at the core of schizoid pathology. The individual thus afflicted oscillated between wanting closeness and dreading it; feared the vigor of his or her own needs and their impact

DSM-5-TR™ Clinical Cases

on others; and was attracted to literary and artistic activities because these were avenues of self-expression without direct human contact. Schizoid personality evolved from one or more of the following scenarios: 1) tantalizing refusal by early caretakers that aroused frightening amounts of emotional hunger; 2) chronic parental rejection, which resulted in compliant apathy and lifelessness; and 3) sustained neglect by parents, which led to retreat into the fantasy world. Working in unison, these variables produced a lifestyle that showed chronic, if subtle and subterranean, conflict between attachment and detachment, elemental curiosity and defensive indifference, and, above all, wishes to die and to be reborn.

The absence of developmental history and of any data about Mr. Buchalski's childhood weakens a psychodynamic understanding of Mr. Buchalski's schizoid personality. However, developmental history is not a required criterion for a descriptive diagnosis; this criterion is primarily utilized by psychodynamically oriented psychiatrists. All in all, the diagnosis of schizoid personality disorder seems reasonable for Mr. Buchalski, although some might argue in favor of a schizotypal personality disorder diagnosis given the oddity of his interests. If further exploration yields information that qualifies this patient for both personality disorders, then both should be recorded.

In regard to other comorbidities, the most likely appears to be hoarding disorder, a diagnosis new to DSM-5. Mr. Buchalski indicates that he delayed calling the police after his sister died because he was worried that his landlord would use the condition of the apartment as a pretext for eviction. He describes a large collection of bioluminescence papers, for example, a statement that could mean a 2-foot-tall stack of manuscripts or an apartment crammed to the ceiling with decades' worth of newspapers, magazines, and scribbled notes, saved because of their potential usefulness. Clarifying the presence of this (or any other) comorbid condition would be crucial to the development of a treatment plan that tries to maximize the likelihood of independent happiness for this patient.

Diagnosis

- Schizoid personality disorder

Suggested Readings

Akhtar S: Schizoid personality disorder: a synthesis of developmental, dynamic, and descriptive features. Am J Psychother 41(4):499–518, 1987
Akhtar S: The schizoid wish to die and be reborn, in The Damaged Core: Origins, Dynamics, Manifestations, and Treatment. Lanham, MD, Jason Aronson, 2009, pp 49–65
Attademo L, Bernardini F, Spatuzzi R: Suicidality in individuals with schizoid personality disorder or traits: a clinical mini-review of a probably underestimated issue. Psychiatr Danub 33(3):261–265, 2021
Dozier ME, Davidson EJ, Pittman JOE, Ayers CR: Personality traits in adults with hoarding disorder. J Affect Disord 276:191–196, 2020
Triebwasser J, Chemerinski E, Roussos P, Siever LJ: Schizoid personality disorder. J Pers Disord 26(6):919–926, 2012

CASE 18.3

Worried and Oddly Preoccupied

Kristin Cadenhead, M.D.

Henry, a 19-year-old college sophomore, was referred to the student health center by a teaching assistant who noticed that he appeared odd, worried, and preoccupied and that his lab notebook was filled with bizarrely threatening drawings.

Henry appeared on time for the psychiatric consultation. Although suspicious about the reason for the referral, he explained that he generally "followed orders" and would do what he was asked. He agreed that he had been suspicious of some of his classmates, believing they were undermining his abilities. He said they were telling his instructors that he was "a weird guy" and that they did not want him as a lab partner. The referral to the psychiatrist was, he said, confirmation of his perception.

Henry described how he had seen two students "flip a coin" over whether he was gay or straight. Coins, he asserted, could often predict the future. He had once flipped a coin and "heads" had predicted his mother's illness. He believed his thoughts often came true.

Henry had transferred to this out-of-town university after an initial year at his local community college. The transfer was his parents' idea, he said, and was part of their agenda to get him to be like everyone else and go to parties and hang out with girls. He said all such behavior was a waste of time. Although they had tried to push him into moving into the dorms, he had refused, and instead lived by himself in an off-campus apartment.

With Henry's permission, his mother was called for collateral information. She said Henry had been quiet, shy, and reserved since childhood. He had never had close friends, had never dated, and had denied wanting to have friends. He acknowledged feeling depressed and anxious at times, but these feelings did not improve when he was around other people. He was teased by other kids and would come home upset. His mother cried while explaining that she always felt bad for him because he never really "fit in," and that she and her husband had tried to coach him for years without success. She wondered how a person could function without any social life.

She added that ghosts, telepathy, and witchcraft had fascinated Henry since junior high school. He had long thought that he could change the outcome of events like earthquakes and hurricanes by thinking about them. He had consistently denied any substance use disorder, and two drug screens had been negative in the prior 2 years. She mentioned that her grandfather had died in an "insane asylum" many years before Henry was born, but she did not know his diagnosis.

On examination, Henry was tall, thin, and dressed in jeans and a T-shirt. He was alert and wary and, although nonspontaneous, he answered questions directly. He denied feeling depressed or confused. Henry denied any history of suicidal thoughts, plans, or attempts. He denied having any auditory or visual hallucinations, panic attacks, obsessions, compulsions, or phobias. His intellectual skills seemed above average, and his Mini-Mental State Examination score was 30 out of 30.

Discussion

Henry presents with a pattern of social and interpersonal deficits accompanied by eccentricities and cognitive distortions. This pattern includes delusional-like symptoms (magical thinking, suspiciousness, ideas of reference, grandiosity), eccentric interests, evidence of social withdrawal (few friends, avoidance of social contact), and restricted affect (emotional coldness). Therefore, Henry appears to meet criteria for DSM-5 schizotypal personality disorder.

Henry also suspects that others are undermining him, reads hidden meanings into benign activities, bears grudges, and is overly sensitive to perceived attacks on his character. In addition to schizotypal personality disorder, he meets criteria for paranoid personality disorder. If (as often occurs) an individual meets criteria for two personality disorders, both should be recorded.

Henry, however, is only 19 years old, and a personality disorder diagnosis should be made only after exploring other diagnoses that could produce similar symptoms. For example, Henry's deficits in social communication and interaction could be consistent with a diagnosis of autism spectrum disorder (ASD) without intellectual impairment. It is possible that he had unreported symptoms beyond "shyness" in the early developmental period; as was reported about Henry, children with ASD commonly undergo schoolyard teasing. He and his mother do not, however, report the sorts of restricted, repetitive patterns of behavior, interests, or activities since childhood that are also a hallmark of ASD. Without these, Henry would not be diagnosed on the autism spectrum.

Henry also may have a psychiatric disorder that develops in young adulthood, and he is at the peak age for the onset of mood, anxiety, and psychotic disorders. Any of these can exacerbate baseline personality traits and make them appear to be disorders, but Henry does not appear to have significant depressive, manic, or anxiety symptoms.

More likely in this case would be a diagnosis on the schizophrenia spectrum. For Henry to qualify for a schizophreniform or schizophrenia diagnosis, however, he would need to meet two or more of the following five criteria—delusions, hallucinations, disorganized speech, grossly disorganized or catatonic behavior, and negative symptoms—and also manifest a deterioration in functioning. He denies hallucinations, his thoughts are linear, and he does not have either odd behavior or negative symptoms. He may have delusions, and it would be useful to clarify the extent to which he has fixed, false beliefs about predicting and affecting the future as well as the extent of his insight into the plausibility of such beliefs.

Although Henry currently may best fit the two personality disorder diagnoses, he appears to be at risk for progression to schizophrenia (or other psychiatric disorders). If he does go on to develop schizophrenia, these initial symptoms would be considered to be an early phase of the schizophrenia. Such progression is not uncommon but currently is not possible to predict. To encourage greater understanding of this patient population, proposed criteria for "attenuated psychosis syndrome" are provided in the "Conditions for Further Study" chapter in DSM-5-TR Section III. Attenuated psychosis syndrome is characterized by new-onset subsyndromal psychotic symptoms that have not crossed the threshold to full psychosis. The hope is that by encouraging research into this at-risk population, early interventions might reduce the psychological suffering and the long-term functional consequences of a chronic psychotic disorder.

Diagnoses

- Schizotypal personality disorder
- Paranoid personality disorder

Suggested Readings

Boldrini T, Tanzilli A, Pontillo M, et al: Comorbid personality disorders in individuals with an at-risk mental state for psychosis: a meta-analytic review. Front Psychiatry 10:429, 2019

Poletti M, Raballo A: Childhood schizotypal features vs. high-functioning autism spectrum disorder: developmental overlaps and phenomenological differences. Schizophr Res 223:53–58, 2020

Salazar de Pablo G, Radua J, Pereira J, et al: Probability of transition to psychosis in individuals at clinical high risk: an updated meta-analysis. JAMA Psychiatry 78(9):970–978, 2021

CASE 18.4

Unfairness

Charles L. Scott, M.D.

Ike Crocker was a 32-year-old white divorced carpenter referred for a mental health evaluation by the human resources department of a large construction business that had been his employer for 2 weeks. At his initial job interview, Mr. Crocker presented as very motivated and provided two carpentry school certifications that indicated a high level of skill and training. Since his employment began, his supervisors had noted frequent arguments, absenteeism, poor workmanship, and multiple errors that might have been dangerous. When confronted, he was reportedly dismissive, indicating that the problem was "cheap wood" and "bad management" and added that if someone got hurt, "it's because of their own stupidity."

When the head of human resources met with him to discuss termination, Mr. Crocker quickly pointed out that he had both attention-deficit/hyperactivity disorder (ADHD) and bipolar disorder. He said that if not granted an accommodation under the Americans with Disabilities Act, he would sue. He demanded a psychiatric evaluation.

During the mental health evaluation, Mr. Crocker focused on unfairness at the company and on how he was "a hell of a better carpenter than anyone there could ever be." He claimed that his two marriages had ended because of jealousy. He said that his wives were "always thinking I was with other women," which is why "they both lied to judges and got restraining orders saying I'd hit them." As "payback for the jail time," he refused to pay child support for his two children. He had no interest in seeing either of his two boys because they were "little liars" like their mothers.

Mr. Crocker said he "must have been smart" because he had been able to make Cs in school despite showing up only half the time. He spent time in juvenile hall at age 14 for stealing "kid stuff, like tennis shoes and wallets that were practically empty." He left school at age 15 after being "framed for stealing a car" by his principal. Mr. Crocker pointed out these historical facts as evidence that he was able to overcome injustice and adversity. A review of a juvenile probation officer's report indicated that beginning in the first grade, he often bullied children with disabilities, was noted to smile when his victims would cry, and consistently lacked remorse or guilt for his actions.

In regard to substance use, Mr. Crocker said he smoked marijuana as a teenager and started drinking alcohol on a "regular basis" after he first got married at age 22. He denied that use of either substance was a problem.

Mr. Crocker concluded the interview by demanding a note from the examiner that he had "bipolar" and "ADHD." He said that he was "bipolar" because he had "ups and downs" and got "mad real fast." Mr. Crocker denied other symptoms of mania. He said he got down when disappointed, but he had "a short memory" and "could get out of a funk pretty quick." Mr. Crocker reported no difficulties in his sleep, mood, or appetite. He learned about ADHD because "both of my boys got it." He concluded the interview with a request for medications, adding that the only ones that worked were stimulants ("any of them") and a specific short-acting benzodiazepine.

On mental status examination, Mr. Crocker was a casually dressed man who made reasonable eye contact and was without abnormal movements. His speech was coherent, goal directed, and of normal rate. There was no evidence of any thought disorder or hallucinations. He was preoccupied with blaming others, but these comments appeared to represent overvalued ideas rather than delusions. He was cognitively intact. His insight into his situation was poor.

The head of human resources did a background check during the course of the psychiatric evaluation. Phone calls revealed that Mr. Crocker had been expelled from two carpentry training programs and that both of his graduation certificates had been falsified. He had been fired from his job at one local construction company after a fistfight with his supervisor and from another job after abruptly leaving a job site. A quick review of the company's records indicated that Mr. Crocker had provided them with the same false documentation.

Discussion

Mr. Crocker has a pervasive pattern of disregard for and violation of the rights of others, as indicated by many different actions. He has been arrested twice for domestic violence—once each from two separate marriages—and has spent time in jail. He has falsified his carpentry credentials and provides ample evidence of repeated fights and irritability, both at work and within his relationships. He demonstrates little or no regard for how his actions affect the safety of his coworkers. He refuses to see his young sons or to pay child support for them, because they are "little liars." He exhibits no remorse for how his actions negatively affect his family, coworkers, or employers. He routinely quits jobs and fails to plan ahead for his next employment. He meets all seven of the symptomatic criteria for DSM-5 antisocial personality disorder (APD). Because of their rule-violating behavior, individuals with APD are overrepresented in correctional populations.

The diagnosis of APD cannot be made until age 18, but it does require evidence for conduct disorder before age 15. Mr. Crocker's history indicates a history of truancy, adjudication for theft at age 14, and expulsion from school at age 15 for car theft. In addition, the probation officer's report noted that Mr. Crocker's conduct disorder began prior to age 10 (childhood-onset type) and that he exhibited limited prosocial emotions, both of which are ominous risk factors for developing APD in adulthood.

At the end of the evaluation, Mr. Crocker requests two potentially addictive medications. He smoked marijuana in high school and may have begun to drink alcohol heavily in his 20s. Although it might be difficult to elicit an honest account of his substance use, Mr. Crocker may indeed have a comorbid substance use disorder. Such a diagnosis would not affect his diagnosis of APD, however, because his antisocial behavior predates his reported use of substances. In addition, his antisocial attitudes and behaviors are evident in multiple settings and are not simply a result of his substance misuse (e.g., stealing to pay for his drugs).

Mr. Crocker's claim that he has ADHD would require evidence that he had some hyperactive-impulsive or inattentive symptoms that caused impairment before age 12 years. Although ADHD could be a comorbid condition and could account for some of his impulsivity, it would not account for his wide-ranging antisocial behavior.

The APD diagnosis also requires that the behavior not occur only during the course of bipolar disorder or schizophrenia. Although Mr. Crocker states that he has bipolar disorder, he provides no evidence that he has ever had mania (or schizophrenia).

Mr. Crocker's interpersonal style is marked by callous disregard for the feelings of others and an arrogant self-appraisal. Such qualities can be found in other personality disorders, such as narcissistic personality disorder, but they are also common in APD. Although comorbidity is not uncommon, individuals with narcissistic personality disorder do not exhibit the same levels of impulsivity, aggression, and deceit as are present in APD. Individuals with histrionic personality disorder or borderline personality disorder may be manipulative or impulsive, but their behaviors are not characteristically antisocial. Individuals with paranoid personality disorder may demonstrate antisocial behaviors, but their actions tend to stem from a paranoid desire for revenge rather than a desire for personal gain. Finally, people with intermittent explosive disorder also get into fights, but they lack the many exploitive traits that are a pervasive part of APD.

Diagnosis

• Antisocial personality disorder

Suggested Readings

Anderson JL, Kelley SE: Antisocial personality disorder and psychopathy: the AMPD in review. Personal Disord 13(4):397–401, 2022

Baliousis M, Duggan C, McCarthy L, et al: Executive function, attention, and memory deficits in antisocial personality disorder and psychopathy. Psychiatry Res 278:151–161, 2019

Nakic M, Stefanovics EA, Rhee TG, Rosenheck RA: Lifetime risk and correlates of incarceration in a nationally representative sample of U.S. adults with non-substance-related mental illness. Soc Psychiatry Psychiatr Epidemiol Aug 28, 2021 [online ahead of print]

Retz W, Ginsberg Y, Turner D, et al: Attention-deficit/hyperactivity disorder (ADHD), antisociality and delinquent behavior over the lifespan. Neurosci Biobehav Rev 120:236–248, 2021

CASE 18.5

Fragile and Angry

Frank Yeomans, M.D., Ph.D.

Otto Kernberg, M.D.

Juanita Delgado, a single, unemployed Hispanic woman, sought therapy at age 33 for treatment of depressed mood, chronic suicidal thoughts, social isolation, and poor personal hygiene. She had spent the prior 6 months isolated in her apartment, lying in bed, eating junk food, watching television, and doing more online shopping than she could afford. Multiple treatments had yielded little effect.

Ms. Delgado was the middle of three children in an upper-middle-class immigrant family in which the father reportedly valued professional achievement over all else. She felt isolated throughout her school years and experienced recurrent periods of depressed mood. Within her family, she was known for angry outbursts. She had done well academically in high school but dropped out of college because of frustrations with a roommate and a professor.

She had attempted a series of internships and entry-level jobs with the expectation that she would return to college, but she kept quitting because "bosses are idiots. They come across as great and they all turn out to be twisted." These "traumas" always left her feeling terrible about herself ("I can't even succeed as a clerk?") and angry at her bosses ("I could run the place and probably will"). She had dated men when she was younger but never let them get close physically because she became too anxious when any intimacy began to develop. Most of her friends from the neighborhood had "become frauds or losers," while she had stayed "Facebook friends" with some friends from college, and they were all "doing amazing things all over the world. I'll definitely meet up with them if they ever come back to town."

Ms. Delgado said that she was generally "down and depressed" but that she had had dozens of 1- to 2-day "manias" in which she was energized and edgy and pulled all-nighters. She tended to "crash" the next day and sleep for 12 hours.

Ms. Delgado reported that she occasionally cut herself, "but only superficially." She had persistent thoughts that she would be better off dead, and she had been psychiatrically hospitalized three times after overdoses.

She indicated that psychotherapy had never been especially helpful, nor had her medication treatments, which had included mood stabilizers, antidepressants, and low-dose antipsychotic medication.

Mrs. Delgado was a casually groomed and somewhat unkempt woman who was cooperative, coherent, and goal directed during the interview. She was generally dysphoric, with a constricted affect, but did smile appropriately several times. She described shame at her poor performance but also believed she was "on Earth to do something great." She described her father as a spectacular success, but he was also a "Machiavellian loser who was always trying to manipulate people." She described quitting jobs because people were disrespectful. Toward the end of the initial session, she became angry with the interviewer after he glanced at the clock ("Are you bored already?").

Discussion

Ms. Delgado presents with affective instability, difficulty controlling her anger, unstable interpersonal relationships, an identity disturbance, self-mutilating behavior, feelings of emptiness, and transient, stress-related paranoia. She therefore meets criteria for DSM-5 borderline personality disorder (BPD).

Individuals with BPD often present with depressive and/or bipolar symptoms, and Ms. Delgado is no exception. Her presenting symptoms include a predominantly depressed mood, diminished interests, overeating, anergia, and chronic suicidal ideation. Because these symptoms are disabling, persistent, and occur in the absence of substance use or a medical disorder, Ms. Delgado also meets criteria for DSM-5 major depressive disorder. If further evaluation indicates that these depressive symptoms have been consistently experienced for 2 years, she would also meet criteria for persistent depressive disorder.

Such comorbidity between BPD and depression is common. It is interesting to note that Ms. Delgado's preoccupations are accusatory, whereas the typical preoccupations of a depressed person without a personality disorder are guilty and self-accusatory. It would be worth exploring the possibility that Ms. Delgado's depressive symptoms are more episodic and reactive than she initially reports. It also seems possible that she qualifies for lifelong depression, which could suggest persistent depressive disorder but could also point toward a personality disorder.

Ms. Delgado reports "manias" that are not typical of someone with bipolar disorder. For example, she describes having had dozens of 1- to 2-day episodes in which she is energized and edgy, followed by a "crash" and 12 hours of sleep. These do not conform to the symptom or duration criteria for bipolar I or bipolar II disorder. The fact that the emotional instability and affect storms of BPD can look very much like a manic or hypomanic episode can lead to underdiagnosis of BPD. Even in the presence of a significant manic episode, the clinician should explore such historical variables as affective stability, maturity of interpersonal relationships, and stability of work, relationships, and self-assessment. If problems are found, a BPD diagnosis is likely.

Criteria for DSM-5 personality disorders remained unchanged from the previous DSM edition (DSM-IV). However, the Alternative DSM-5 Model for Personality Disorders, presented in DSM-5-TR Section III, suggested a more dimensional approach, one in which the interviewer would explicitly consider personality functioning. The personality trait system used in the alternative DSM-5 model defines five different trait domains that exist on a continuum. "Emotional stability" is contrasted with "negative affectivity," for example, whereas "antagonism" is at the other end of the spectrum from "agreeableness" (see Table 18–1 in the introduction to this chapter).

This dimensional view of personality is compatible with Kernberg's long-standing model of borderline personality organization (BPO). In addition to meeting the DSM-5 criteria for BPD, Ms. Delgado fits the criteria for BPO—a psychological structure conceived as being characterized by 1) lack of a clear and coherent sense of self and others (identity diffusion), 2) frequent use of primitive defense mechanisms based on splitting, and 3) intact but fragile reality testing. The more integrated and realistically complex the individual's representations of self and others are, the more the individual is able to modulate and control his or her emotional states and successfully interact with others.

Ms. Delgado demonstrates identity diffusion in her contradictory views of herself (as both superior and inadequate) and others (her father as both spectacular and a "Machiavellian loser"). Her defensive style is characterized by consistent projection of her hostile feelings and perceiving the hostility as coming from others. The fragility of her reality testing, seen in the slights she felt at work, has led to chronic occupational dysfunction.

Because people with personality disorders often do not present an interpersonal narrative that conforms to the story that would be told by others, it is important to attend to the patient's behavior in relation to the therapist. With Ms. Delgado, evidence of her fragility is seen in her sense that the therapist's glancing at the clock meant he did not like her and wanted to get rid of her.

Suicidal tendencies are part of both depression and BPD. In general, acute or chronic parasuicidal behavior is typical of severe personality disorders. Furthermore, suicidality can develop abruptly during crises among a variety of patients, but it is especially prevalent in people—like Ms. Delgado—with a fragile sense of both the world and themselves.

Diagnosis

- Borderline personality disorder

Suggested Readings

Kernberg OF, Yeomans FE: Borderline personality disorder, bipolar disorder, depression, attention deficit/hyperactivity disorder, and narcissistic personality disorder: practical differential diagnosis. Bull Menninger Clin 77(1):1–22, 2013

Skodol AW, Oldham JM (eds): The American Psychiatric Association Publishing Textbook of Personality Disorders, 3rd Edition. Washington, DC, American Psychiatric Association Publishing, 2021

Yeomans FE, Clarkin JF, Kernberg OF: Transference-Focused Psychotherapy for Borderline Personality Disorder: A Clinical Guide. Arlington, VA, American Psychiatric Association Publishing, 2015

CASE 18.6

Painful Suicidality

Elizabeth L. Auchincloss, M.D.

Karmen Fuentes was a 50-year-old married Hispanic woman who presented to the psychiatric emergency room (ER) at the urging of her outpatient psychiatrist after telling him that she had been thinking about overdosing on Advil.

In the ER, Ms. Fuentes explained that her back had been "killing" her since she fell several days earlier at the family-owned grocery store where she had worked for many years. The fall had left her downcast and depressed, although she denied other depressive symptoms aside from a poor mood. She spoke at length about the fall and about how it reminded her of a fall that she had sustained a few years earlier. At that time, she had gone to see a neurosurgeon, who told her to rest and take nonsteroidal anti-inflammatory drugs. She described feeling "abandoned and not cared about" by him. The pain had diminished her ability to exercise, and she was upset that she had gained weight. While relating the events surrounding the fall, Ms. Fuentes began to cry.

When asked about her suicidal comments, she said they were "no big deal"—they were "just a threat" aimed at her husband to "teach him a lesson" because "he has no compassion for me" and had not been supportive since the fall. She insisted that her comments about overdosing did not have another meaning. When her ER interviewer expressed concern about the possibility that she would kill herself, she exclaimed with a smile, "Oh wow, I didn't realize it's so serious. I guess I shouldn't do that again." She then shrugged and laughed. She went on to talk about how "nice and sweet" it was that so many doctors and social workers wanted to hear her story, calling many of them by their first names. She was also somewhat flirtatious with her male resident interviewer, who had mentioned that she was the "best-dressed woman in the ER."

According to her outpatient psychiatrist of 3 years, she had never before expressed suicidal ideation until this week, and he would be unable to check in on her until after he left on vacation the next day. Ms. Fuentes's husband reported that she talked about suicide "like other people complain about the weather. She's just trying to get me worried, but it doesn't work anymore." He said he would never have suggested she go to the ER and thought the psychiatrist had overreacted.

Ms. Fuentes initially sought outpatient psychotherapy at age 47 because she was feeling depressed and unsupported by her husband. During 3 years of outpatient treatment, Ms. Fuentes had been prescribed adequate trials of sertraline, escitalopram, fluoxetine, and paroxetine. None seemed to help.

Ms. Fuentes described being "an early bloomer." She became sexually active with older men when she was in high school. She said dating had been the most fun thing she had ever done and that she missed seeing men "jump through hoops" to sleep with her. She lived with her 73-year-old husband. Her 25-year-old son lived nearby with his wife and young son. She described her husband as a "very famous" musician. She said that he had never helped around the house or with child-rearing and did not appreciate how much work she put into taking care of their son and grandson.

Discussion

Ms. Fuentes presents to the ER with depression and suicidality, but neither of these symptoms is as prominent as her ongoing pattern of excessive emotionality and attention seeking. Her behavior with the ER staff and perhaps the fall itself appear to serve a need for attention and care, and both Ms. Fuentes and her husband describe her chronic suicidal threats as efforts to punish and elicit concern. For example, the ER visit was precipitated by Ms. Fuentes making her first suicidal threat in treatment just as her doctor was going on vacation, suggesting that she might have felt left out and abandoned.

Ms. Fuentes's emotions shift rapidly between tearful and cheerful, but she consistently dismisses the actual threat of suicide. Instead, Ms. Fuentes focuses on her dramatic fall, and on her perception that neither her husband nor her neurosurgeon appears to be interested in her suffering. Throughout her ER visit, she was seductive with her interviewer and unusually friendly with staff, calling many of them by their first names. Even in a busy ER, filled with sick, injured, and presumably unkempt people, Ms. Fuentes maintains her concern about her physical appearance. She implies that her dress, grooming, and weight are centrally important to her sense of self-esteem, and that she continues to pay close attention to their maintenance.

These observations suggest that her suicidality is not part of a major affective disorder. Instead, she has at least six of the eight symptomatic criteria for a DSM-5 diagnosis of histrionic personality disorder (HPD): discomfort when not the center of attention; seductive behavior; intense but shifting and shallow emotionality; the use of physical appearance to draw attention; self-dramatization and theatricality; and a tendency to consider relationships to be more intimate than they are. While Ms. Fuentes does not show clear evidence of other criteria for HPD, such as impressionistic speech and suggestibility, these may have simply not been included in the case report.

Because patients with HPD often have comorbid somatic symptom disorders, careful attention should be given to evaluating the patient for these disorders. Ms. Fuentes has been episodically preoccupied with physical discomfort, and further evaluation might demonstrate a more pervasive and impairing pattern of physical complaints or concerns. Patients with HPD also have elevated rates of major depressive disorder. Indeed, Ms. Fuentes shows many signs of depressed mood. Furthermore, Ms. Fuentes was referred to the ER because of suicidality. Although she and her husband minimize the seriousness of these threats, HPD does appear to be associated with an elevated risk of suicide attempts. Many of these attempts will be sublethal, but a variety of suicidal "gestures" can lead to serious harm and even semi-accidental death. Clinical work with Ms. Fuentes will involve balancing the recognition that her suicidal ideation serves the need for attention with awareness that it may also lead to actual self-harm.

As in all psychiatric assessments, clinicians must consider whether the personality issues are a problem before making a diagnosis. Norms for emotional expressiveness, interpersonal behavior, and style of dress vary significantly between cultures, genders, and age groups, and it is important not to gratuitously pathologize variations that are not accompanied by dysfunction and distress. As an example of potential bias, women are more frequently diagnosed with HPD despite population studies that indicate that HPD is equally common in men and women.

HPD is often comorbid with other personality disorders. Although Ms. Fuentes has traits that are common to other personality disorders, she does not appear to have a second diagnosis. For example, Ms. Fuentes's suicidal threats and dramatic presentation might lead the examiner to consider borderline personality disorder. Ms. Fuentes does not, however, show the marked instability in interpersonal relationships, extreme self-destructiveness, angry disruptions in interpersonal relationships, and chronic feelings of emptiness that are common in borderline personality disorder. Although Ms. Fuentes complains of not receiving the care that she would like, she does not manifest the fear of separation and the sort of submissive and clingy behavior that are typical of dependent personality disorder. Similarly, although she appears to have an excessive need for admiration, she has not demonstrated the lack of empathy that is a cardinal feature of narcissistic personality disorder. Finally, while she demonstrates some manipulative behavior, as do people with antisocial personality disorder, hers is motivated by a desire for attention rather than some sort of profit.

Diagnosis

• Histrionic personality disorder

Suggested Readings

Gabbard GO: Hysterical and histrionic personality disorders, in Psychodynamic Psychiatry in Clinical Practice, 5th Edition. Arlington, VA, American Psychiatric Association Publishing, 2014, pp 545–576

MacKinnon RA, Michels R, Buckley PJ: The histrionic patient, in The Psychiatric Interview in Clinical Practice, 3rd Edition. Arlington, VA, American Psychiatric Association Publishing, 2016, pp 133–172

Roberts LW (ed): The American Psychiatric Publishing Textbook of Psychiatry, 7th Edition. Arlington, VA, American Psychiatric Association Publishing, 2019

CASE 18.7

Dissatisfaction

Robert Michels, M.D.

Larry Goranov was a 57-year-old man who demanded an expert review of the psychiatric care that he had received for the prior 7 years at a psychiatric clinic connected to a medical school. Mr. Goranov indicated to the clinic's psychiatric director that he had been depressed for many years, but weekly psychotherapy and multiple different psychiatric medications had made no difference.

Mr. Goranov reported feeling sad, tired, and frustrated "for decades." He rarely looked forward to anything. He had lost his last job 3 years earlier, had broken up with a girlfriend slightly later, and doubted that he would ever work or date again. He was embarrassed that he still lived with his mother, who was in her 80s. He denied any immediate intention or plan to kill himself, but stated that if he did not improve by the time his mother died, he did not see what he would have to live for. He denied disturbances in sleep, appetite, or concentration.

Clinic records indicated that Mr. Goranov had been adherent to adequate trials of fluoxetine, escitalopram, sertraline, duloxetine, venlafaxine, and bupropion, as well as augmentation with quetiapine, aripiprazole, lithium, and levothyroxine. He had experienced some improvement in his mood while taking escitalopram but did not have remission of symptoms. He also received a course of cognitive-behavioral therapy early in his treatment, but he had been dismissive of the therapist and treatment, did not do his assigned homework, and appeared to make no effort to use the therapy between sessions.

Mr. Goranov expressed frustration at his lack of improvement, the nature of his treatment, and his specific therapy. He found it "humiliating" that he was forced to see trainees who rotated off his case every year or two. He frequently found that the psychiatry residents were not especially educated, cultured, or sophisticated, and thought that they knew less about psychotherapy than he did. He much preferred to work with female therapists "because at least they're pretty, and men are too competitive and envious."

Mr. Goranov had worked as an insurance broker from age 25 to 40. He explained, "It's ridiculous. I was the best broker they had ever seen, but I still can't get a job. I think the problem is that the profession is filled with big egos, and I can't keep my mouth shut about it." After being "blackballed" by insurance agencies, Mr. Goranov did not work for 5 years, until he was hired by an automobile dealer. He said that although it was beneath him to sell cars, he was successful, and "in no time, I was running the place." He quit within a few months after an argument with the owner. Despite encouragement from several therapists, Mr. Goranov had not applied for a job or pursued employment rehabilitation or volunteer work; he strongly viewed these options as beneath him.

Mr. Goranov has "given up on women." He had many partners as a younger man, but he generally found them to be unappreciative and "only in it for the free meals." Psychotherapy notes from the clinic indicate that he responded to demonstrations of interest with suspicion. This tendency held true in regard to both women who had tried to befriend him and therapists who had taken an interest in his care. Mr. Goranov described himself as someone who had a lot of love to give, but added that the world was full of manipulators. He said he had a few buddies, but his mother was the only one he truly cared about. His parents had emigrated from Eastern Europe when he was a child. He had no siblings, and his father had died when the patient was 41. He had met a few relatives over the years, "but they didn't speak English, so I didn't pay them much attention." He enjoyed fine restaurants and "five-star hotels," but he added that he could no longer afford them. He exercised daily and was concerned about maintaining his body. Most of his time was spent at home watching television or reading novels and biographies.

On examination, the patient was neatly groomed, had slicked-back hair, and wore designer hip-hop-inspired clothing generally favored by men in their 20s. He was coherent, goal directed, and generally cooperative. He said he was sad and angry. His affect was constricted and dismissive. He denied an intention to kill himself but felt hopeless and thought of death fairly often. He was cognitively intact.

Discussion

When a patient presents to a psychiatrist, symptoms are generally those aspects of psychopathology that are easiest to recognize and to diagnose. Anxiety, depression, obsessions, and phobias are seen similarly by patient and doctor and are central defining characteristics of many disorders. Patients with personality disorders are different. Their problems are often more distressing to others than to the patient, and their symptoms are often vague and may seem secondary to their central issue. What determines the diagnosis or defines the focus of treatment is not the anxiety or depression, for example, but rather who the patient is, the life he or she has chosen to lead, and the pattern of his or her human relationships.

A corollary is that the patient's complaints may be less revealing than the way in which they are made. The consultation interview with most patients consists of collecting information and making observations. The consultation with most patients who have personality disorders requires the creation of a relationship, and then the doctor's experiencing and understanding of that relationship. Countertransference responses can be important diagnostic tools, and the way in which the patient relates to the clinician reflects the template that structures how the patient relates to others. For example, Mr. Goranov's primary complaint is his sad mood. Although he could have a depressive disorder, he seems to lack most of the pertinent DSM-5 criteria for any of the depressive disorders. Instead, his low mood appears to be a response to chronic disappointment. Despite his view of himself as talented and attractive, he is unemployed, underappreciated, and alone. Empty demoralization is a common accompaniment to personality disorder and, as with Mr. Goranov, is often unresponsive to pharmacotherapy.

Mr. Goranov appears very concerned with maintaining his appearance, which is not typical of people with serious depression. His grooming, clothes, and manner reflect his underlying conviction that he is special and deserving of the appreciation that he has thus far failed to receive.

This story about Mr. Goranov reflects a typical mild to moderate narcissistic personality disorder. Classic features include grandiosity, a conviction that he deserves special treatment, estrangement from others, a strikingly diminished capacity for empathy, and an attitude of arrogant disdain. The depressed affect is clearly present, but it is secondary to his fundamental personality psychopathology.

These patients are difficult to treat. They see their problem as the failure of the world to recognize their true value, and they often withdraw into sadness. A therapeutic alliance requires making contact with patients around their pain, loneliness, and isolation, and developing a functioning, working connection. Mr. Goranov believes, however, that his therapist has not provided him with what he feels entitled to receive. This is a familiar problem for Mr. Goranov. He is dissatisfied with his friends, his employers, and his significant others. Like his therapists, these people have not been good enough, have not recognized his value, and have failed him.

Diagnosis

- Narcissistic personality disorder

Suggested Readings

Ackerman RA, Donnellan MB, Wright AGC: Current conceptualizations of narcissism. Curr Opin Psychiatry 32(1):32–37, 2019

Akhtar S: The shy narcissist, in Changing Ideas in a Changing World: The Revolution in Psychoanalysis. Essays in Honour of Arnold Cooper. Edited by Sandler J, Michels R, Fonagy P. London, Karnac, 2000, pp 111–119

Cooper AM: Narcissism and masochism. The narcissistic-masochistic character. Psychiatr Clin North Am 12(3):541–542, 1989

Ronningstam E: Introduction to the Special Issue on Narcissistic Personality Disorder. J Pers Disord 34 (suppl):1–5, 2020

CASE 18.8

Shyness

J. Christopher Perry, M.P.H., M.D.

Mathilda Herbert was a 23-year-old woman referred for psychiatric consultation to help her "break out of her shell." She had recently moved to a new city to take classes to become an industrial lab technician and had moved in with an older cousin, who was also a psychotherapist and thought she should "get out and enjoy her youth."

Although she had previously been prescribed medications for anxiety, Ms. Herbert said that her real problem was "shyness." School was difficult because everyone was constantly "criticizing." She avoided being called on in class because she knew she would "say something stupid" and blush and everyone would make fun of her. She avoided speaking up or talking on telephones, worried about how she would sound. She dreaded public speaking.

She was similarly reticent with friends. She said she had always been a people pleaser who preferred to hide her feelings with a cheerful, compliant, attentive demeanor. She had a few friends, whom she described as "warm and lifelong." She felt lonely after her recent move and had not yet met anyone from school or the local community.

She said she had broken up with her first serious boyfriend 2 years earlier. He had initially been "kind and patient." Through him, she had a social life by proxy. Soon after she moved in with him, however, he turned out to be an "angry alcoholic." She had not dated since that experience.

Ms. Herbert grew up in a metropolitan area with her parents and three older siblings. Her brother was "hyperactive and antisocial" and took up everyone's attention, whereas her sisters were "hypercompetitive and perfect." Her mother was anxiously compliant, "like me." Ms. Herbert's father was a very successful investment manager who often pointed out ways in which his children did not live up to his expectations. He could be supportive but tended to disregard emotional uncertainty in favor of a "tough optimism." Teasing and competition "saturated" the household, and "it didn't help that I was forced to go to the same girls' school where my sisters had been stars and where everyone was rich and catty." She developed a keen sensitivity to criticism and failure.

Her parents divorced during her senior year of high school. Her father married another woman soon thereafter. Although she had planned to attend the same elite university as her two sisters, she chose to attend a local community college at the last minute. She explained that it was good to be away from all the competition, and her mother needed the support.

Ms. Herbert's strengths included excellent work in her major, chemistry, especially after one senior professor took a special interest. Family camping trips had led to a mastery of outdoor skills, and she found that she enjoyed being out in the woods, flexing her independence. She also enjoyed babysitting and volunteering in animal shelters, because kids and animals "appreciate everything you do and aren't mean."

During the evaluation, Ms. Herbert was a well-dressed young woman of short stature who was attentive, coherent, and goal directed. She smiled a lot, especially when talking about things that would have made most people angry. When the psychiatrist offered a trial comment, linking Ms. Herbert's current anxiety to experiences with her father, the patient said nothing but was visibly upset. After several such instances, the psychiatrist worried that any interpretive comments might be taken as criticism and had to check a tendency to avoid sensitive subjects. Explicitly discussing his concerns led both the patient and psychiatrist to relax and allowed the conversation to continue more productively.

Discussion

Ms. Herbert's shyness extends into a persistent social avoidance that reduces her ability to enjoy herself. She underperforms academically, and she seems to have chosen her college (a local community college) and career (lab technician) largely to reduce perceived risk and to avoid anxiety. She feels lonely but is unable to make connections with friends. She is stymied in her efforts to date men. She appears to have two psychiatric diagnoses that are so frequently comorbid that they may represent differing conceptualizations of similar conditions: avoidant personality disorder and social anxiety disorder.

Avoidant personality disorder reflects a persistent pattern of social inhibition, feelings of inadequacy, and hypersensitivity to negative evaluation. It also requires four or more of seven criteria, which Ms. Herbert easily meets. She avoids occupational activities that involve significant interpersonal contact. For most of her life, she has been reluctant to speak up, fearing to draw criticism or ridicule, even from family members. She avoids being the center of attention, is self-doubting, and blushes easily. She avoids new situations. She is unwilling to get involved with people unless she is certain that she will be liked. These have had a debilitating effect on all aspects of her life.

Like most people with avoidant personality disorder, Ms. Herbert also qualifies for DSM-5-TR social anxiety disorder. She demonstrates fear of social scrutiny and of being negatively evaluated. Social situations are endured, but barely, and her anxiety is almost always present. She appears shy, selects work where there will be limited social interaction, and prefers to live with family members.

Ms. Herbert describes having these symptoms from a young age. Although shyness is commonly reported in individuals with avoidant personality disorder and social anxiety disorder, most shy children do not go on to report the sorts of issues prevalent in people with these disorders: diminished school performance, employment, productivity, socioeconomic status, quality of life, and overall well-being.

During the interview, the psychiatrist sensed Ms. Herbert's distress and felt uncharacteristically restricted in what he could ask. In other words, he became aware of a countertransference reaction in which he feared hurting her feelings. After he shared his own concerns that she would feel criticized by his comments, both the psychiatrist and the patient were able to more comfortably explore her history and deepen the therapeutic alliance. A strong alliance helps mitigate distress and shame and increases the likelihood of a more thorough exploration for common comorbidities as well as a smoother transition into treatment.

Diagnoses

- Avoidant personality disorder
- Social anxiety disorder

Suggested Readings

Di Giuseppe M, Perry JC, Conversano C, et al: Defense mechanisms, gender, and adaptiveness in emerging personality disorders in adolescent outpatients. J Nerv Ment Dis 208(12):933–941, 2020

Perry JC: Cluster C personality disorders: avoidant, obsessive-compulsive, and dependent, in Gabbard's Treatments of Psychiatric Disorders, 5th Edition. Edited by Gabbard GO. Arlington, VA, American Psychiatric Association Publishing, 2014, pp 1087–1116

Sanislow CA, Bartolini EE, Zoloth EC: Avoidant personality disorder, in Encyclopedia of Human Behavior, 2nd Edition. Edited by Ramachandran VS. San Diego, CA, Academic Press, 2012, pp 257–266

CASE 18.9

Lack of Self-Confidence

Raymond Raad, M.D., M.P.H.
Paul S. Appelbaum, M.D.

Nate Irvin was a 31-year-old single white man who sought outpatient psychiatric services for "lack of self-confidence." He reported lifelong troubles with assertiveness and was specifically upset by having been "stuck" for 2 years at his current "dead-end" job as an administrative assistant. He wished someone would tell him where to go next so that he would not have to face the "burden" of decision. At work, he found it easy to follow his boss's directions but had difficulty making even minor independent decisions. The situation was "depressing," he said, but nothing new.

Mr. Irvin also reported dissatisfaction with his relationships with women. He described a series of several-month-long relationships over the prior 10 years that ended despite his doing "everything I could" and "never getting angry or yelling." His most recent relationship had been with an opera singer. He reported having gone to several operas and taken singing classes to impress her, even though he did not particularly enjoy music. That relationship had recently ended for unclear reasons. He said his mood and self-confidence were tied to his dating. Being single made him feel desperate, but desperation made it even harder to get a girlfriend. He said he felt trapped by that spiral. Since the latest breakup, he had been quite sad, with frequent crying spells. It was this depression that had prompted him to seek treatment. He denied all other symptoms of depression, including problems with sleep, appetite, energy, suicidality, and ability to enjoy things.

Mr. Irvin initially denied taking any medications, but he eventually revealed that 1 year earlier his primary care physician had begun to prescribe alprazolam 0.5 mg/day for "anxiety." His dose had escalated, and at the time of the evaluation, Mr. Irvin was taking 5 mg/day and getting prescriptions from three different physicians. Cutting back led to anxiety and "the shakes."

Mr. Irvin denied any prior personal or family psychiatric history, including outpatient psychiatric appointments.

After hearing this history, the psychiatrist was concerned about Mr. Irvin's escalating alprazolam use and his chronic difficulties with independence. She thought the most accurate diagnosis was benzodiazepine use disorder comorbid with a personality disorder. However, she was concerned about the negative unintended effects that these diagnoses might have on the patient, including his employment and insurance coverage, as well as how he would be dealt with by future clinicians. She typed into the electronic medical record a diagnosis of "adjustment disorder with depressed mood." Two weeks later, Mr. Irvin's insurance company asked her for his diagnosis, and she gave the same diagnosis.

Discussion

Mr. Irvin has an excessive need for someone to take care of him and make decisions for him. He has difficulty making decisions independently and wishes that others would make them for him. He lacks the confidence to initiate projects or do things on his own, he generally feels uncomfortable being alone, and he is reluctant to disagree on even minor matters. He goes to almost desperate lengths to seek and maintain relationships and to obtain support and nurturing from others.

Mr. Irvin, therefore, meets at least six of the eight DSM-5 criteria (only five are required) for dependent personality disorder. To meet the criteria for the diagnosis, these patterns must also fit the general criteria for a personality disorder (i.e., the symptoms must differ from cultural expectations and be enduring, inflexible, pervasive, and associated with distress and/or impairment in functioning). Mr. Irvin's symptoms meet this standard. Furthermore, his symptoms are persistent and debilitating, and lie outside the normal expectations for a healthy adult man of his age.

Many psychiatric diagnoses can intensify dependent personality traits or be co-morbid with dependent personality disorder. In this patient, it is especially important to consider a mood disorder, because he presents with "depression" that has recently worsened. Some patients with mood disorders can present with symptoms that mimic personality disorders, so if this patient is in the midst of a major depressive episode, his dependent symptoms may be confined to that episode. Mr. Irvin, however, denies other symptoms of depression and does not meet criteria for any of the depressive disorders.

Notably, Mr. Irvin is using alprazolam. He has been taking the medication in increasing amounts over a longer period of time than was intended. To obtain an adequate supply, he gets prescriptions from three different physicians. He has developed tolerance (resulting in dose escalation) and withdrawal (as demonstrated by anxiety and shakes). Assuming that further exploration would confirm clinically significant impairment or distress, Mr. Irvin meets criteria for a benzodiazepine use disorder. Given his history of use and his tendency not to be entirely transparent, it would be especially important to tactfully explore the possibility that he is using other substances, including alcohol, tobacco, illicit drugs, and prescription drugs such as opioids.

The psychiatrist in this case faces a conflict common in clinical practice. Documentation of patients' diagnoses in clinical charts—and their release to third parties—can sometimes have downstream effects on patients' insurance coverage or disability status and can lead to stigmatization, both within and outside the health care system. Given this reality, psychiatrists can be tempted to record only the least severe of several diagnoses, or sometimes to report inaccurate but presumably less pejorative disorders. In this case, the psychiatrist does both. Although the patient has depressed mood, he does not meet criteria for the adjustment disorder that is recorded by his psychiatrist. He does, however, appear to meet criteria for both dependent personality disorder and benzodiazepine use disorder, but neither of these more serious and potentially more stigmatizing diagnoses is included in the chart or disclosed to the insurer.

When diagnoses are inaccurately recorded in medical charts, ostensibly for the purpose of protecting patients, this may end up causing harm instead. Subsequent clinicians who review the records may lack critical information regarding patients' presentation and treatment. For example, if Mr. Irvin were to urgently call for a prescription of benzodiazepines, a covering psychiatrist might have no way of knowing from the patient's chart about either the pattern of benzodiazepine abuse or the physiological dependence. As a physician who intends to "do no harm," Mr. Irvin's psychiatrist has tried to shield him from stigma but has instead exposed him to medical risk.

The physician has other responsibilities beyond those to the patient. When the physician and patient agree to accept payment from an insurer, the physician may be obligated to provide to insurers and governmental agencies a reasonable amount of honest clinical information. Lack of disclosure is tantamount to fraud and can be prosecuted. In addition, although being part of the medical profession affords many privileges, it also involves responsibilities. Diagnostic deceit may seem like an innocuous effort to protect the patient, but the dishonesty negatively affects the reputation of the entire profession, a reputation that is integral to the ability to render treatment to future patients.

DSM-5-TR™ Clinical Cases

Diagnoses

- Dependent personality disorder
- Benzodiazepine use disorder

Suggested Readings

Appelbaum PS: Privacy in psychiatric treatment: threats and responses. Am J Psychiatry 159(11):1809–1818, 2002

Beauchamp TL: The philosophical dimension, in Psychiatric Ethics, 5th Edition. Edited by Bloch S, Green SA. Oxford, UK, Oxford University Press, 2021, pp 41–76

Disney KL: Dependent personality disorder: a critical review. Clinical Psychology Review 33(8):1184–1196, 2013

CASE 18.10

Relationship Control

Michael F. Walton, M.D.

Ogden Judd, a 24-year-old attorney, and his boyfriend, Peter Kleinman, a 22-year-old freelance graphic designer, presented for couples therapy to address escalating conflict around the issue of moving in together. Mr. Kleinman described a several-month-long apartment search that was made "agonizing" by Mr. Judd's work schedule and his "endless" list of apartment demands. They were unable to come to a decision, and eventually they decided to just share Mr. Judd's apartment. As Mr. Kleinman concluded, "Ogden won."

Mr. Judd refused to hire movers for his boyfriend's belongings, insisting on personally packing and taking an inventory of every item in his boyfriend's place. What should have taken 2 days took 1 week. Once the items were transported to Mr. Judd's apartment, Mr. Kleinman began to complain about Mr. Judd's "crazy rules" about where items could be placed on the bookshelf, which direction the hangers in the closet faced, and whether their clothes could be intermingled. Moreover, Mr. Kleinman complained that there was hardly any space for his possessions because Mr. Judd never threw anything away. "I'm terrified of losing something important," added Mr. Judd.

Over the ensuing weeks, arguments broke out nightly as they unpacked boxes and settled in. Making matters worse, Mr. Judd would often come home after 9:00 or 10:00 P.M., because he had a personal rule to always have a blank "to-do" list by the end of the day. Mr. Kleinman would often wake early in the morning to find Mr. Judd grimly organizing shelves or closets or cleaning the floor. Throughout this process, Mr. Judd appeared to be working hard at everything while enjoying himself less and getting less done. Mr. Kleinman found himself feeling increasingly detached from his boyfriend the longer they lived together.

Mr. Judd denied symptoms of depression and free-floating anxiety. He said that he had never experimented with cigarettes or alcohol, adding, "I wouldn't want to feel like I was out of control." He denied a family history of mental illness. He was raised in a two-parent household and was an above-average high school and college student. He was an only child and first shared a room as a college freshman. He described that experience as being difficult due to "conflicting styles—he was a mess and I knew that things should be kept neat." He had moved mid-year into a single dorm room and had not lived with anyone until Mr. Kleinman moved in. Mr. Judd was well liked by his boss, earning recognition as "employee of the month" three times in 2 years. Feedback from colleagues and subordinates was less enthusiastic, indicating that he was a micromanager on shared projects, and often critical of his colleagues' efforts. Also, it seemed he had a reputation as a bore, stemming from a happy hour trivia night in which he had repeatedly questioned the answers his coworkers provided.

On examination, Mr. Judd was a thin man with eyeglasses and gelled hair, sitting on a couch next to his boyfriend. He was meticulously dressed. He was cooperative with the interview and sat quietly while his boyfriend spoke, interrupting on a few occasions to contradict. His speech was normal in rate and tone. His affect was irritable. There was no evidence of depression. He denied specific phobias and did not think he had ever experienced a panic attack. At the end of the consultation, Mr. Judd remarked, "I know I'm difficult, but I really do want this to work out."

Discussion

Couples treatment would probably focus on the relationship rather than on either of the two men, but the case report clearly focuses on Mr. Judd's contribution to the difficulties in the relationship. Mr. Judd is viewed as a controlling, perfection-driven, and inflexible "workaholic." He holds on to belongings excessively and finds it difficult to integrate new items into his apartment, spending hours single-handedly organizing books that could otherwise just be placed on a bookshelf. He is driven and unable to delegate, and although those qualities can be adaptive in some circumstances, they are causing him distress and dysfunction in regard to his situation with his boyfriend and with his colleagues at work. Mr. Judd appears to fulfill criteria, therefore, for a DSM-5 diagnosis of obsessive-compulsive personality disorder (OCPD).

OCPD and obsessive-compulsive disorder (OCD) can be comorbid, but the two conditions usually exist separately. The important distinguishing factor is that whereas OCPD is considered a maladaptive pattern of behavior marked by excessive control and inflexibility, OCD is characterized by the presence of true obsessions and compulsions.

There can, however, be significant behavioral overlap between OCD and OCPD. For example, hoarding behaviors can be common to both diagnoses. In OCPD, the cause of the hoarding disorder is the need for order and completeness, and Mr. Judd reports that he is "terrified of losing something important." To compensate for the fact that his apartment is now shared with his boyfriend—and is overfull—Mr. Judd works grimly into the night so that his closets maintain their usual standard of excessive organization. In OCD, the cause of the hoarding tends to be either the avoidance of onerous compulsive rituals or obsessional and often irrational fears of incompleteness, harm, and contamination. The behaviors are typically unwanted and distressing, and are likely to lead to the accumulation of odd debris such as fingernail clippings or rotten food. In hoarding disorder, a new diagnosis in DSM-5, the focus is exclusively on a persistent difficulty discarding or parting with possessions rather than on a need for order or on obsessions and compulsions.

To assess Mr. Judd for possible hoarding, it would be useful to explore the extent of his accumulations and whether his hoarding behavior attenuates a specific, particularly distressing or intrusive thought. For his list-making and rearranging behaviors to meet criteria for the compulsions of OCD, they should be time-consuming, distressing, overly repetitive, and ritualistic and also accompanied by tension and difficulty relaxing. Although DSM-5 encourages an effort to distinguish among OCPD, OCD, and hoarding disorder, these three disorders can co-occur.

As discussed in the introduction to this chapter (see Table 18–1), the Alternative DSM-5 Model for Personality Disorders provided in Section III includes five personality disorder trait domains: negative affectivity, detachment, antagonism, disinhibition (vs. conscientiousness), and psychoticism. Several of these factors are pertinent to a diagnosis of OCPD. For example, Mr. Judd's interpersonal style with both his boyfriend and his coworkers appears to be marked by inflexible detachment and restricted levels of intimacy. He manifests significant amounts of negative affectivity, as reflected in his grim persistence in continuing tasks past the point of usefulness. Finally, Mr. Judd's compulsivity pervades the entire story, as marked by extreme conscientiousness and rigid perfectionism.

Diagnosis

• Obsessive-compulsive personality disorder

Suggested Readings

Cain NM, Ansell EB, Simpson HB, Pinto A: Interpersonal functioning in obsessive-compulsive personality disorder. J Pers Assess 97(1):90–99, 2015

Hays P: Determination of the obsessional personality. Am J Psychiatry 129(2):217–219, 1972

Liggett J, Sellbom M: Examining the DSM-5 alternative model of personality disorders operationalization of obsessive-compulsive personality disorder in a mental health sample. Personal Disord 9(5):397–407, 2018

Pozza A, Starcevic V, Ferretti F, et al: Obsessive-compulsive personality disorder co-occurring in individuals with obsessive-compulsive disorder: a systematic review and meta-analysis. Harv Rev Psychiatry 29(2):95–107, 2021

CHAPTER 19

Paraphilic Disorders

INTRODUCTION

John W. Barnhill, M.D.

Paraphilias are defined as intense and persistent sexual interests outside of foreplay and genital stimulation with phenotypically normal, consenting adults. A paraphilic *disorder* requires both the presence of a paraphilia and the existence of distress, dysfunction, and/or acting on the urges (as described in more detail later in this introduction). The definition of *paraphilia* is broad enough that there are dozens, even hundreds, of identified paraphilias and paraphilic disorders, all of which are replete with ambiguity and controversy, but DSM-5 specifically identifies only eight: voyeuristic, exhibitionistic, frotteuristic, sexual masochism, sexual sadism, pedophilic, fetishistic, and transvestic disorders.

Paraphilias can be divided into those that feature anomalous activities (e.g., sexual masochism) and those that feature anomalous targets (e.g., fetishes). Paraphilias can also be divided into those that are victimless (e.g., transvestism) and those that are defined in such a way that, when enacted, they inevitably include victimization (e.g., sexual sadism and pedophilic disorders).

For example, an individual might indicate that he experiences recurrent and intense sexual arousal from either the use of nonliving objects (e.g., shoes) or a focus on a nongenital body part (e.g., feet). If the associated fantasies, urges, or behaviors transcend his "normophilic" sexual interests and behaviors, then he can be said to have a specific paraphilia—that is, a fetish. If, on the other hand, the fetish is not intense or persistent but is used as an occasional part of a broad sexual repertoire in the pursuit of genital stimulation, then the individual would likely not meet criteria for a paraphilia. If the fetish leads the individual to experience dysfunction (e.g., clinically relevant sexual difficulties with a partner) or distress (e.g., clinically relevant shame), then he—and people with fetishes are almost always men—would warrant a diagnosis of fetishistic disorder.

Some of the paraphilias included in DSM-5 were selected because their enactment inevitably leads to victimization. Voyeurism is the most common of these paraphilias. DSM-5 voyeurism does not refer to someone who casually ogles a passerby or who is sexually excited by "spying" on people at a clothing-optional beach. DSM-5 voyeuristic disorder involves nonconsenting persons and, as such, is a criminal activity. The disorder is diagnosed when voyeuristic urges are recurrently enacted, leading to distress or significant impairment in social, occupational, or other important areas of functioning. As is the case with all the paraphilias associated with criminal activity, a disorder is also diagnosed even if the individual denies distress and dysfunction, as long as there is a pattern of criminally significant paraphilic behavior. Like the other potentially criminal paraphilias, voyeuristic disorder can also be diagnosed in an individual who does not act on his desires but whose urges or fantasies are causing clinically significant distress or impairment in social, occupational, or other areas of functioning.

Some of these paraphilias are associated with particularly heinous crimes. From a forensic perspective, pedophilic disorder identifies people—almost always men—who act on their persistent sexual interest in prepubertal children. From a forensic perspective, the diagnosis is not generally aimed at men who, among their various sexual fantasies, consider teenagers attractive, yet do not break laws or encounter interpersonal difficulty and are not bothered by their fantasies. DSM-5 also clarifies that the child should be less than 13 years old and that the perpetrator should be at least 16 years old and 5 years older than the victim. The primary forensic interest is in behaviors that transcend what is typically meant by sexuality and move into predation and sociopathy. DSM-5 does allow for the pedophilic disorder diagnosis to be made, however, in situations in which the sexual interest in prepubertal children is not enacted but the urges or fantasies cause marked distress or interpersonal difficulty.

Similarly, the diagnosis of sexual sadism disorder appears to identify two different clinical populations. In both groups, the individual experiences recurrent and intense sexual arousal from another's suffering, as manifested by fantasies, urges, or behaviors. The primary forensic interest is in people who force unconsenting children and adults to experience physical and psychological suffering as part of the perpetrator's own pursuit of sexual arousal. In such settings, the sexual sadism disorder is most commonly applied to men with comorbid antisocial personality disorder who are awaiting trial. The diagnosis of sexual sadism disorder can also be used to describe people who do not act on their sadistic urges and/or do not involve unconsenting victims in their behaviors but who experience distress or impairment. Sexual sadism disorder does not apply to the vast majority of people whose sexual behavior and fantasies lie under the broad umbrella of BDSM (bondage, domination/discipline, sadism/submission, and masochism). For the majority of people who engage in practices associated with BDSM, mutual agreement and consent are central. Although the fantasy and the specific behavior may include control, pain, and/or humiliation, the people involved are consenting adults, and most do not appear to suffer associated distress or impairment.

Criteria for a paraphilic diagnosis are somewhat unusual among diagnoses in DSM-5. For example, voyeurism, pedophilia, and sexual sadism can be diagnosed

DSM-5-TR™ Clinical Cases

when the individual denies distress, dysfunction, sexual arousal, or even any involvement in the activity, as long as there is evidence of involvement that indicates a likelihood of persistent sexual arousal related to the paraphilia. This definition is true for all the paraphilias that tend to lead to criminal behavior, including frotteurism (touching or rubbing against a nonconsenting individual) and exhibitionism (exposing the genitals to an unconsenting person). The idea that conclusions can be made based on external evidence regardless of psychiatric assessment (including some combination of patient history, clinical observation, and mental status examination) is typical in the legal system but is not typical of most psychiatric evaluations. The inclusion of external evidence is also not part of the definition for the paraphilias that do not typically involve the criminal justice system.

The paraphilias prompt interesting questions. The first is whether the psychiatric nomenclature should get involved in sexual behaviors that are heavily influenced by cultural norms and may lead to little or no distress and dysfunction in the individual. For example, a diagnosis that identifies a cluster of people who sexually abuse prepubertal children (pedophilia) may be useful both for the legal system and for clinicians who create treatment programs. If expanded to include a focused sexual interest in adolescents (so-called hebephilia, which was considered for inclusion but ultimately not discussed in DSM-5), the paraphilia runs up against the wide variations that exist in regard to human maturation and to what is legally and culturally acceptable in different states, countries, and eras.

Paraphilia nosology prompts the important question of what, exactly, is the key factor that turns a behavior into a disorder. Is it the atypicality? Is it the individual's distress (e.g., guilt if someone has been hurt)? In the case of paraphilias that feature a victim, is it the effect of the actions (e.g., the hurt person), regardless of the perpetrator's reactions or intent? Is it the compulsive, driven nature of the behavior? Historically, the field of psychiatry was fairly confident about the landmarks and behaviors that could be considered part of normal human sexual development. In the twenty-first century, definitions of sexual normalcy are hotly contested. The DSM paraphilias no longer include, for example, homosexuality, but they do include other sexual behaviors that lack both a victim and inevitable dysfunction or distress (e.g., fetishes and transvestism). The boundaries of paraphilic behaviors are shifting, and it remains to be seen how the field will further incorporate the notion that many atypical patterns of sexual development and behavior are being increasingly seen as normal variations both within the profession and throughout the broader culture.

The updated DSM-5-TR made no substantive changes in the criteria for any of the paraphilic disorders. The edits to the discussion section largely involve reminders of cultural variability and updates on evidence.

In regard to cultural relativism, DSM-5-TR reminds the reader to distinguish self-harming behaviors that occur during collectively accepted spiritual and societal practices from sadomasochistic behavior conducted for sexual arousal. As examples, DSM-5-TR points to rituals that include self-flagellation and suspension from hooks.

Research continues to improve our knowledge base. For example, it has long been recognized that of those people incarcerated with a sexual sadism disorder, the large majority are men. More recent population samples appear to indicate, however, that men are only modestly more likely than women to report sexually sadistic behavior (as opposed to a disorder).

Other evidence discussed within DSM-5-TR reflects an expansion of understanding. For example, the group of people with pedophilic disorder is heterogeneous and includes a subset of people who feel particular emotional and cognitive affinity with children, also known as emotional congruence with children. They may prefer the company of children, feel they have more in common with children than adults, and choose jobs or volunteer activities that allow them to spend time with children.

Despite the ongoing flux and debate, the current diagnostic approach to the paraphilic disorders is fairly clear and can be considered from two angles. One angle is predominantly legal. If a victim is harmed because of another person's pattern of non-normative sexual behavior, there is likely an underlying paraphilic disorder (as well as a likely comorbidity such as antisocial personality disorder). The second angle does not involve the legal system. If an individual indicates a persistent, non-normative pattern of sexual behavior, urges, or fantasies, then a paraphilia can likely be identified. If that paraphilia directly causes distress or dysfunction, then a disorder can be diagnosed. And through this complexity, it remains a matter of clinical judgment whether this diagnosis merits professional attention.

Suggested Readings

Balon R: Controversies in the diagnosis and treatment of paraphilias. J Sex Marital Ther 39(1):7–20, 2013

De Block A, Adriaens PR: Pathologizing sexual deviance: a history. J Sex Res 50(3–4):276–298, 2013

Joyal CC: Defining "normophilic" and "paraphilic" sexual fantasies in a population-based sample: on the importance of considering subgroups. Sex Med 3(4):321–330, 2015

Seto MC: The motivation-facilitation model of sexual offending. Sex Abuse 31(1):3–24, 2019

CASE 19.1

Sadomasochism

J. Paul Fedoroff, M.D.

Raven Lundquist (she/her, preferring Raven) was a 24-year-old graduate student in philosophy who presented for a psychiatric evaluation at her brother's insistence. The two siblings lived together, and the brother threatened to withhold her allowance from a small trust if she didn't get "some help."

Raven explained that her brother was worried about her being "sadomasochistic." In public, he might just say that he was worried that she was an alcoholic and out of control, but she thought he just didn't like her interest in "BDSM" (bondage, domination/discipline, sadism/submission, and masochism).

She said that she had been in a relationship with Lilly for about a year. The two of them self-identified as queer, a label they found less stigmatizing than "lesbian." One evening, after an evening of drinking with her brother, Raven told him that she and Lilly enjoyed going to bondage parties, where they would role-play "mistress-slave scenes" in which they would wear tight leather clothing and high heels, and Lilly would whip Raven and call her derogatory or humiliating names. Raven was fine with being seen as a masochist in public, but in private, she generally enjoyed being in charge.

Raven asked the psychiatrist whether he was "the kind of shrink who pathologizes everything? Surely, you're not like my brother, who gets squeamish about anything related to kink. But that's his problem, right doctor? Don't you agree that his concerns are just homophobia?" She asked whether the psychiatrist had read *Justine* by the Marquis de Sade, "which isn't as well written as *Lolita*, but it strikes a chord. By the way, Lilly laughs at my reading choices, calling me an 'old-school perv.'"

On questioning about other BDSM activities, Raven said she sometimes drugged Lilly without Lilly's knowledge. She found the sense of control to be extremely sexually exciting. Raven said she did not think Lilly would mind if she found out, given that Lilly identified as a sadomasochist and would often let Raven tie her up. Raven admitted that she had secretly drugged previous sexual partners, but that only one had complained about it, and "only when she found photos on my camera." That lover had broken off the relationship immediately and claimed that she would have gone to the police if the "photos weren't so embarrassing."

When asked about her brother's concern about her alcohol use, Raven immediately said she did "no illegal drugs, no tobacco, not even weed." Upon further questioning, she did say she might have an alcohol problem. She said she often planned to have a single drink but generally ended up getting significantly intoxicated. She generally got along well with Lilly and her brother, but they often got into verbal fights after everyone had "become really drunk." She said she often enjoyed her "binges," with the only problem being that she often missed early morning classes because of hangovers. She had no criminal history.

Raven's childhood history was notable for having been abandoned by their mother while young. She and her brother had lived with relatives and in foster homes before they had been adopted by a woman whom she referred to as our "intrusive but well-meaning pseudo-mother." That woman had died the year before, leaving behind a small trust fund for the two of them. Raven had memory gaps from her childhood and thought she might have been sexually molested. "The abuse narrative would make sense, wouldn't it? But I really don't remember." Raven's medical history was pertinent for having had scoliosis; as a child, she was treated with insertion of a Harrington rod and an extended hospitalization.

Raven described sexual attraction to both men and women but preferred women because "they are typically more submissive." When she masturbated, and when she drugged sexual partners, she fantasized about "power and control," particularly about molesting unwilling partners.

She said she felt calm when in sexual control, and when intoxicated, but that she otherwise felt "pretty anxious." Previous psychiatrists had diagnosed her with generalized anxiety disorder, for which she had been prescribed a benzodiazepine; these were also the medications she used to drug sexual partners.

Raven said she sometimes felt down and depressed but did not think she had ever had a "clinical depression." While often anxious, she denied ever having phobias or panic. She denied ever feeling suicidal but had sometimes thought about killing the drugged sexual partners, which, "as you surely know, I would never actually do." She denied obsessions, compulsions, delusions, and hallucinations. She was intelligent and cognitively intact.

Discussion

Raven presented for a psychiatric assessment at the insistence of her brother, who was concerned that her sexual activities and alcohol use were out of control and hurtful.

Raven enjoys masochistic role-playing at BDSM parties. Does she meet criteria for DSM-5 sexual masochism disorder? She does seem to get aroused from the act of being humiliated, beaten, bound, and/or made to suffer, and she has done so for at least 6 months. She appears to fulfill the first criterion. As is true for all DSM diagnoses, however, a disorder requires the presence of dysfunction, and her masochistic activities do not appear to cause distress or impairment in regard to social, occupational, or other important areas of functioning. Because she does not meet this second criterion, Raven would not be diagnosed with sexual masochism disorder.

Raven's sadistic activities are a little different. Typically, people who enjoy BDSM emphasize consent. Activities tend to be clearly spelled out in advance, often including a way to immediately end the activity (e.g., safe words). In Raven's case, however, she drugs her partners without telling them, and her behaviors have led to significant repercussions (a former lover found photos, broke off the relationship, and threatened to go to the police).

Does Raven meet criteria for DSM-5 sexual sadism disorder? She meets the first of the two criteria: the person must have experienced sexual arousal from the suffering (psychological or physical) of others for at least 6 months. The second criterion goes past the paraphilic interest (sadism) and focuses on whether the arousal should be considered a psychiatric disorder. DSM-5 clarifies that to meet criteria, the person must have acted on these urges with a nonconsenting person or the urges or fantasies have caused significant impairment or distress. Raven has acted on these urges with an unwilling person, and they have caused distress, both in her former girlfriend and in herself. She therefore meets that second criterion. Notably, most courts consider sexual activity with unconscious victims to be illegal even if the victim agreed in advance; in the eyes of the court, consent must be revocable, and an unconscious victim cannot revoke consent.

It is often difficult to develop a solid understanding of how someone develops sadomasochistic interests. Raven reports surgical treatment for scoliosis, which led to a lengthy hospitalization as a child. Would such an experience contribute to her interest in bondage and/or control? Possibly. Similarly, she moved through multiple households as a child and has wondered whether she has blocked memories of being sexually molested. As she said, "the abuse narrative would make sense, wouldn't it?"

Possibly. In working with all patients—including those with a paraphilic disorder—it can be useful to look for such links but not search exclusively for a simple equation that explains adult complexity.

DSM-5 provides two specifiers for sexual sadism disorder. The first specifier, "in a controlled environment," is applicable to situations in which the individual is living in a setting, such as prison, in which there are limited opportunities to engage in sadistic sexual behavior. The second specifier, "in full remission," refers to situations in which the individual has not met criteria for 5 years while in an uncontrolled environment. In other words, a person in solitary confinement for 5 years could not meet criteria for "full remission" because opportunities for the sadistic behavior would have been limited. Neither of these specifiers applies to Raven.

In regard to other diagnoses, Raven admits to frequently drinking alcohol to excess, being unable to control her intake, missing morning classes because of the aftereffects of alcohol, and having interpersonal conflicts that appear to be directly related to intoxication. She meets DSM-5 diagnostic criteria for alcohol use disorder. She also describes having been diagnosed with generalized anxiety disorder. Earlier physicians have prescribed her benzodiazepines, which she apparently uses for anxiety as well as to sedate sexual partners. Further evaluation would be necessary to clarify the anxiety disorder diagnosis.

Diagnoses

- Sexual sadism disorder
- Alcohol use disorder
- Generalized anxiety disorder (provisional)

Suggested Readings

Fedoroff JP: The Paraphilias: Changing Suits in the Evolution of Sexual Interest Paradigms. Oxford, UK, Oxford University Press, 2019

Nabokov V: Lolita. New York, Knopf, 1992

Rosner J: Looking for Mr. Goodbar. New York, Simon & Schuster, 1975

The Marquis De Sade: The Complete Justine, Philosophy in the Bedroom, and Other Writings. Translated and compiled by Seaver R, Wainhouse A. New York, Grove Press, 1990

CASE 19.2

Relationship Problems

Richard Balon, M.D.

Terry Najarian, a 65-year-old salesman for a large corporation, presented for a psychiatric evaluation after his wife threatened to leave him. Although he said he was embarrassed to discuss his issues with a stranger, he described his sexual interest in women's undergarments in a quite matter-of-fact manner. This interest had surfaced several years earlier and had not been a problem until he was caught masturbating by his wife 6 weeks prior to the evaluation. Upon seeing him dressed in panties and a bra, she initially "went nuts," thinking he was having an affair. After he clarified that he was not seeing anyone else, she "shut him out" and hardly spoke to him. When they argued, she called him a "pervert" and made it clear that she was considering divorce unless he "got help."

Mr. Najarian's habit began in the setting of his wife's severe arthritis and likely depression, both of which significantly reduced her overall activity level and specifically her interest in sex. His "fetish" was the bright spot during his frequent and otherwise dreary business trips. He also masturbated at home but generally waited until his wife was out of the house. His specific pattern was to masturbate about twice weekly, using bras and panties that he had collected over several years. He said that intercourse with his wife had faded to "every month or two" but was mutually satisfying.

The patient had been married for over 30 years, and the couple had two grown children. Mr. Najarian had planned to retire comfortably later that year, but not if the two choices were either "to be poor after we split the assets or to sit around the house all day and be called a pervert."

He became visibly anxious when discussing his marital difficulties. He described some recent difficulty falling asleep and "worried constantly" about his marriage but denied other psychiatric problems. He had made a show of throwing away a half dozen pieces of underwear, which had seemed to reassure his wife, but he had saved his "favorites" and "could always buy more." He said he was of mixed mind. He did not want to end his marriage, but he saw nothing harmful in his new mode of masturbating. "I'm not unfaithful or doing anything bad," he said. "It just excites me, and my wife certainly doesn't want to be having sex a few times a week."

Mr. Najarian denied any difficulties related to sexual functioning, adding that he could maintain erections and achieve orgasm without women's undergarments. He recalled being aroused when he touched women's underwear as a teenager and had masturbated repeatedly to that experience. That fantasy had disappeared when he became sexually active with his wife. He denied any personal or family history of mental illness.

Discussion

Mr. Najarian presents with a several-year history of sexual arousal from women's underwear. His behavior fits the definition of a fetish, which is defined as persistent, intense sexual arousal from either the use of nonliving objects (e.g., women's underwear) or a highly specific focus on a nongenital body part (e.g., a foot). Paraphilias are commonly divided on the basis of the activity or the target of the activity, so that fetishism would be considered an example of an "anomalous target" behavior, along with such paraphilias as pedophilia and transvestism.

However, paraphilias do not qualify for a DSM-5 paraphilic disorder diagnosis until they cause distress, entail risk, or potentially cause harm in others. In the case of Mr. Najarian, his behavior appears to have been ego-syntonic and causing him no difficulty until he was caught wearing women's underwear by his wife. At that point, Mr. Najarian began to experience distress, which led to the psychiatric evaluation and would likely lead to a diagnosis of DSM-5 fetishistic disorder. If his wife were to accept or embrace his fetish and his own distress were to fade, he would likely no longer be considered to have a disorder.

It would be useful to explore more aspects of Mr. Najarian's situation. First, he seems to present to a psychiatrist not because he wants help but because he does not want to get divorced. It is possible, therefore, that he is minimizing his issues. He says his teenage interest in women's underwear returned in the context of his wife's illness, but paraphilias—which usually do start in adolescence, as they did with Mr. Najarian—tend to persist; he may have had a decades-long hiatus, but he may also want to slant the story in a way that might make sense to his wife. In addition, many people with one paraphilia have more than one. Does he choose age-specific underwear (e.g., that worn by young girls or older women)? He was not simply aroused by the underwear but was wearing it. Does he cross-dress or derive arousal from being dressed in female undergarments outside the context of masturbation? If so, his behavior would fit transvestism. It would also be useful to know more about his masturbation fantasies when he uses the women's underwear. For example, he might be imagining having sex with another man. If so, he might be reluctant to discuss his homosexual feelings (or behavior) because of shame or because his wife does not (yet) know about this other aspect of his sexuality.

It is not entirely clear that Mr. Najarian's behavior meets the DSM-5 criterion of recurrent and intense sexual arousal. He implies that he has good sexual experiences with his wife and only became interested in women's underwear after she became more physically debilitated. It would be potentially useful to explore whether his interest in women's underwear is greater than his interest in "normophilic" sexual interests and behaviors.

Mr. Najarian reports long-standing good functioning and an absence of psychiatric disturbance aside from situation-specific anxiety and worries. This implies that he has this single paraphilia without any comorbidity. Even though Mr. Najarian would like to frame his story in that way, it would be useful to explore other possibilities. For example, does he have anxiety, depressive, or substance use disorders that he has not spontaneously mentioned? How does he feel about being in his mid-60s, nearing retirement, and having a wife with a chronic illness? The stress of aging can bring out multiple psychiatric issues, and the paraphilia might be only the most obvious one.

Diagnosis

- Fetishistic disorder

Suggested Readings

Balon R (ed): Practical Guide to Paraphilia and Paraphilic Disorders. Switzerland, Springer International Publishing, 2016

Balon R, Segraves RT (eds): Clinical Manual of Sexual Disorders. Arlington, VA, American Psychiatric Publishing, 2009

Seto MC, Curry S, Dawson SJ, et al: Concordance of paraphilic interests and behaviors. J Sex Res 58(4):424–437, 2021

CASE 19.3

Sexual Offenses

Nancy J. Needell, M.D.

Vance Orren was a 28-year-old self-reported cisgender heterosexual man who was arrested after pushing a stranger in front of an oncoming subway train. He told police that he believed the man was going to "tell everyone that I was a faggot" and that he, Mr. Orren, was trying to protect himself from the "homosexual conspiracy."

Mr. Orren had a history of a psychotic disorder, a cocaine use disorder, and nonadherence to medication and psychotherapy at the time of the incident. He was unemployed. In court, Mr. Orren entered a plea of not guilty by reason of mental disease (the "insanity defense") and underwent a full psychiatric evaluation, including assessment of his sexual history and desires.

As part of his legal case, Mr. Orren underwent a structured sex offender evaluation. He reported that his first sexual contact was at age 12, when his uncle and an 18-year-old male cousin "did things" to him while he was in foster care. They would take him to McDonald's afterward, "so it was fine." By the time he was 14 or 15, he was regularly having sex with males and females who ranged in age "from about ten to in their thirties."

He was unable to answer whether the sexual contact was always consensual, saying, "No one ever called the cops." As an adult, he said that he preferred having sex with "young girls, because they don't fight much." He said that he usually only had sex with adults when he hired prostitutes or prostituted himself in exchange for money or drugs, although he said that sometimes when high, he "might have done stuff that I don't really remember."

The structured sex offender evaluation included penile plethysmography, assessment of visual reaction time using Viewing Time (a measure of the amount of time a person looks at a particular photo or other visual representation of a sexually stimulating situation), and a detailed interview about his sexual practices. This evaluation concluded that his main sexual attraction was to girls between the ages of 8 and 13 years.

Mr. Orren's personal history was significant for multiple childhood disruptions that led to his moving into the foster care system at age 7. At age 9, his first foster mother caught him repeatedly stealing toys and bullying other children. When she reprimanded him, he hit her with a brick, knocking her unconscious. That led to placement in a second foster home. He began using drugs and alcohol at age 11. He was first incarcerated at 13, for shoplifting from an electronics store in order to obtain money for marijuana. At that point, he went back to live with his maternal grandmother, who has episodically provided him a home since then. During those 15 years, he has been arrested at least a dozen times, mostly for drug possession.

Mr. Orren stopped attending school in eighth grade, at about the same time that he was admitted to his first psychiatric inpatient unit. That admission was triggered by his beating his head against a wall "to stop the voices." He was given a DSM-IV diagnosis of psychosis not otherwise specified, treated with risperidone, and discharged after 1 week. Soon after discharge, he discontinued the antipsychotic medication.

Between the ages of 15 and 28, Mr. Orren regularly abused cocaine and alcohol and often used other substances when they were available. By the time of his arrest, he had had at least seven psychiatric admissions, always for auditory hallucinations and persecutory delusions (usually of a sexual nature). It was not clear which substances he was using prior to and during these episodes of psychosis or whether they were implicated in the development of his psychiatric symptoms. He had also been admitted twice for alcohol detoxification after he went into withdrawal while unable to acquire alcohol. He was consistently nonadherent to any type of outpatient treatment. He maintained sobriety only while in hospitals or jails. When contacted by the consulting psychiatrist, his grandmother pointed out that Mr. Orren had always been "reckless, dishonest, and angry. I don't think I've ever heard him apologize. I love him, but he probably belongs in jail for lots of reasons."

Discussion

Although the brief case report does not fully explore Mr. Orren's lengthy history of psychiatric disturbance, he appears to meet criteria for several comorbid DSM-5 disorders. He abuses multiple substances, for example, and almost certainly meets criteria for alcohol and cocaine use disorders. He has a history of psychosis, often labeled "schizoaffective disorder" by prior clinicians. Delusions and auditory hallucinations appear to be the most prominent symptoms, and there is no mention of symptoms of depression and mania. It is unclear whether Mr. Orren met clinical criteria for DSM-IV schizoaffective disorder, much less the tightened criteria in DSM-5. It is also not clear whether his history of hallucinations and delusions might be at least partly attributable to his substance use. Until additional information is elicited, Mr. Orren's psychotic symptoms are probably best conceptualized as an unspecified schizophrenia spectrum and other psychotic disorder.

Mr. Orren also meets criteria for antisocial personality disorder (APD). By his own report and that of his grandmother, he is chronically deceitful, angry, reckless, and lacking in remorse. He also appears to repeatedly break the law in regard to underage sexual behavior, prostitution, and drugs, thereby easily meeting the required three of seven criteria for APD. Mr. Orren also meets the requirement for symptoms of conduct disorder before age 15. Finally, DSM-5 mandates that the antisocial behavior not occur exclusively during the course of schizophrenia or bipolar disorder. Mr. Orren has been previously diagnosed with schizoaffective disorder, but that diagnosis is uncertain, and much of his antisocial behavior appears unrelated to mania or psychosis. DSM-5 also cautions against making the diagnosis of APD when the index behavior is related to the acquisition of illicit drugs. Although some of Mr. Orren's antisocial behavior might be attributable to the acquisition of illicit and often expensive substances, he has multiple other behaviors that have nothing to do with drug acquisition, including the offense that led to his most recent arrest (pushing someone off the subway platform).

In addition to his other psychiatric diagnoses, Mr. Orren has a strong sexual interest in children. As is often the case in pedophilic disorder, he had never identified his persistent sexual interest as a problem until he was arrested, had never sought treatment, and has multiple comorbidities.

The diagnostic evaluation of Mr. Orren's sexual behavior toward children has several components. The first need is to determine whether he has a pedophilic paraphilia, which is defined as a pattern of sexually arousing fantasies, urges, or behaviors involving prepubescent children (Criterion A). Because such information often is not willingly divulged, especially by someone who is in jail, Mr. Orren underwent a structured sex offender evaluation. The focus of this evaluation is to determine the object of a person's fantasies. Tools for this evaluation include penile plethysmography, a technique that measures the changes in penile arousal when a person is exposed to certain visual, auditory, or emotional cues, as well as visual reaction time, which measures how long a person looks at different visual images aimed at providing sexual stimulation. In Mr. Orren's case, these tests showed that he derived the most sexual stimulation when exposed to images of girls between the ages of 8 and 13 years.

The second part of the evaluation focuses on whether Mr. Orren's pedophilic paraphilia meets criteria for pedophilic disorder: he must have either acted on his sexual urges or experienced marked distress or interpersonal difficulty secondary to the sexual urges or fantasies (Criterion B). Although Mr. Orren seems not to feel distress or guilt over his sexual behavior, he does appear to have had sex with underage boys and girls since he himself was a minor. As he said about his adult behavior, he prefers sex with "young girls, because they don't fight much." The case report is unclear whether these "young girls" were actually prepubertal, although that appears to be the implication. Men who act on their urges and feel no remorse or distress tend to be extremely hard to treat, because their only serious concern is often whether they will get in trouble.

The third portion of the evaluation focuses on the exclusionary requirement that the pedophilic disorder diagnosis should not be applied to a person who is under the age of 16 or who is less than 5 years older than the prepubertal child or children (Criterion C). This exception helps to reduce the likelihood of pathologizing relatively common behavior that is considered normal in many parts of the world. Mr. Orren seems to have begun having sex with 10-year-olds when he was 14 or 15. Although problematic, his behavior at that time would not have met criteria for paraphilic disorder. However, if he continued to have sex with prepubertal children after he reached the age of 16, he would then be said to meet criteria.

Arguments are sometimes made that pedophilic disorder should be outside the purview of psychiatry and that sex offenders are best handled by the criminal justice system. One worry is that having recourse to a psychiatric diagnosis will provide an exculpatory explanation for people who rape children and possibly lead to a successful insanity defense (which it does not). As with other diagnoses that are often marked by damaging behavior, pedophilic disorder is intended to systematize the diagnosis of a recognizable cluster of distressed and/or dysfunctional people with similar behaviors, urges, thoughts, and feelings. The societal response to people with pedophilic disorder—including possible treatments and punishments—is not a matter for DSM-5 to decide.

Diagnoses

- Unspecified schizophrenia spectrum and other psychotic disorder
- Cocaine use disorder
- Alcohol use disorder
- Antisocial personality disorder
- Pedophilic disorder, nonexclusive type, sexually attracted to both

Suggested Readings

Blanchard R: The DSM diagnostic criteria for pedophilia. Arch Sex Behav 39(2):304–316, 2010
Gerwinn H, Weiss S, Tenbergen G, et al: Clinical characteristics associated with paedophilia and child sex offending—differentiating sexual preference from offence status. Eur Psychiatry 51:74–85, 2018

CASE 19.4

A Few Kinks

John W. Barnhill, M.D.

Wallace Pickering was a 29-year-old man who presented for outpatient therapy with a chief complaint of "I've never been to a shrink before, but I just read DSM-5, and I have ten diagnoses, including six paraphilias, two personality disorders, a substance use disorder, and maybe something else." The patient described himself as an attorney who is "a run-of-the-mill cisgender gay guy with a few kinks." He had been dating a former college classmate for the prior 2 years. A native of a mid-size city in the Midwest, Mr. Pickering was raised in a politically and religiously conservative household that included his parents and two younger siblings. Mr. Pickering's father and grandfather ran a prosperous business, and his family was very involved in their community. Mr. Pickering attended an elite college and law school. Since graduation, he had worked at a large law firm. He added that he was interested in his diagnoses at least partly because of his boyfriend, who was in his final year of training to be a psychiatrist.

Mr. Pickering described his problems as being about "sex and drugs; I've never cared much for rock and roll." Ever since high school, he described an interest in random sexual encounters. "Not to be narcissistic—though that's one of my diagnoses—but I am kinda hot," he said, "and I play it for what it's worth." This led him to frequent bathhouses and bars, where he could quickly connect to attractive, anonymous partners. He described feeling aroused when watching other people having sex and added that although he had quit the habit when he entered law school, he had previously gotten a thrill out of being watched while having sex. He said he had "hooked up" about once a month since age 20. He said he had never once had unsafe sex with anyone aside from his boyfriend, and this led him to mention another of his "diagnoses": a fetishistic interest in rubber. He said condoms were great: they were virus proof, delayed ejaculation, and had an excellent smell. His interest in condoms had led him to get an outfit made entirely of rubber. He said it had been quite the hit at a bondage club, but it had made him so sweaty that he had worn it only once and had then thrown it away before his boyfriend found it. He mentioned that COVID had been isolating and terrible, but "at least he got a chance to wear latex gloves out in public for a while, which was exciting in its way."

He said he also enjoyed tying up his boyfriend during sex and feeling completely in control. He said he liked being a "sadistic top" every month or two but added that he also sometimes liked being a "bottom" and at other times did not feel sexual at all.

Mr. Pickering said that during his occasional pursuits of anonymous sex, he had a couple of "toxic habits." Whenever he went out partying, he would do a few lines of cocaine and drink about 4–6 beers. He said he always timed these "trips to the underworld" for times when his boyfriend went out of town, and he would have time to recover. He added that withdrawing from cocaine "really sucks" for a day or two, adding that he probably has "a mood disorder related to the cocaine withdrawal."

He added that the planning had become more complicated and that he actually had probably only gone to a club twice in the prior year. Overall, his "social life is pretty boring. We have a lot of friends, but we're kinda like an old married couple. My only real vice is smoking. I have tried for years, but I haven't been able to get down below half a pack a day. Yawn."

When asked to say more about himself, Mr. Pickering answered, "Right… I almost forgot. I am obsessed by the hours that I work. I keep careful track so that I am among the top billers in the firm every month, and I always get my projects done on time, even if it means I don't sleep. My own theory is that it's part of my need to feel invulnerable and perfect despite being a mess on the inside." Mr. Pickering paused, smiled, and continued. "That made me wonder if I'm obsessive-compulsive or narcissistic as well as having all the different paraphilias. Oh, and if hypersexuality is a diagnosis, then I'm really screwed."

Toward the end of the initial interview, the psychiatrist said, "I'm not sure if any of these behaviors are going to make it as a diagnosis, but I am very interested in how you feel." At that, Mr. Pickering welled up in tears and said he had felt sad and lonely all his life. He added that his family knew almost nothing about him, and that only a lesbian cousin—who had also moved to New York—knew that he was gay.

On examination, Mr. Pickering was a well-groomed, attractive young man who was coherent and goal directed. He smiled readily but showed an appropriate affective range. He denied suicidality, confusion, and psychosis. He was cognitively very bright. His insight and judgment were viewed as intact.

Discussion

The presentation of Mr. Pickering prompts as many questions as it answers. He presents for his first psychiatric consultation because he "read DSM-5." Why would that compel him to seek a consultation at this particular time? He freely and amusingly discusses his sexual interests, substance use, and personality style, and he wants them labeled disorders despite the fact that they do not actually bother him. Why would he seek out diagnoses when he is also denying distress and dysfunction? Multiple statements by Mr. Pickering provide some insight, but his presentation lacks both a clear illness and a clear history.

Mr. Pickering does offer some theories about why he might need to see a therapist. He wonders whether he has a "paraphilia," which is defined in DSM-5 as "any sexual interest greater than or equal to normophilic sexual interests." He does have erotic interests that have been linked to paraphilias (rubber, bondage, voyeurism, exhibitionism), and with further history he might be said to have a paraphilia or two. A paraphilia is not, however, a disorder. As is generally true for disorders throughout DSM-5, a paraphilic disorder requires distress or impairment to the individual and/or involves harm to self or others. DSM-5 leaves intact the difference between normative and non-normative sexual behavior, but it underlines that non-normative sexual behavior is not necessarily pathological. Although clinicians might be tempted to insert their own bias into the assessment, DSM-5 makes clear that if the paraphilia is not problematic, it is not a disorder.

Mr. Pickering does use an illicit substance, cocaine, and he possibly binges on alcohol. He reports that he uses both monthly without significant ill effects; on reflection, he reduces the frequency of both his substance use and sexual adventures. Without dysfunction, his use does not qualify for a substance use disorder. Before writing off his substance use as inconsequential, however, the clinician should explore Mr. Pickering's ability to separate his "toxic habits" from the rest of his life. Substance use may get minimized, so follow-up questions should elaborate the extent of his cocaine and alcohol use as well as explore a possible substance-induced mood disorder ("withdrawal from cocaine sucks"). If Mr. Pickering does use cocaine at clubs, it would not be surprising if he also used other "club drugs," such as MDMA (ecstasy), methamphetamine (crystal meth), ketamine (special K), and amyl nitrite (poppers). Alcohol might be used to help him come down from a stimulant, as could benzodiazepines and opiates. Amphetamines might improve the lowered energy, mood, and/or attention that might accompany a cocaine crash, especially for someone with heavy work requirements. He does smoke tobacco and, despite some effort, has been unable to stop. Although details are lacking, and smoking cigarettes is not one of Mr. Pickering's prominent concerns, he does likely meet criteria for a tobacco use disorder.

Mr. Pickering also wonders whether he has a narcissistic or obsessive-compulsive personality disorder. As evidence, he offers up a strong interest in performing well and in keeping track of his rank within his law firm. Assessing psychopathology requires attention to cultural and subcultural norms. Mr. Pickering belongs to several subcultures, one of which is his profession. While he might be excessively dedicated to work compared to the average person, he would be a law firm outlier if he were not somewhat "obsessed" by his monthly billable hours. More information would be useful, but Mr. Pickering does not appear to meet criteria for any of the DSM-5 personality disorders.

Another consideration is whether Mr. Pickering has major depressive disorder. He describes dysphoria but does not mention vegetative depressive symptoms. Mr. Pickering reports frequent all-nighters, which could reflect hypomania, a substance use disorder, and/or a sleep disorder, but long work hours are normative in his work environment. Without further information, none of these diagnoses seems likely.

Despite the absence of a clear-cut DSM-5 diagnosis apart from tobacco use disorder, Mr. Pickering sees himself as flawed, isolated, and sad. One possible clue to this curious situation is that Mr. Pickering has not mentioned his homosexuality to anyone in his "conservative" family of origin aside from a lesbian cousin. This might prompt questions about what his own views are on homosexuality, what progress he has made in regard to coming out as gay, and whether and to what extent he might have incorporated society's negative perspectives on gay men and women. Mr. Pickering wonders whether he might have "hypersexuality disorder," but he does not mention engaging in sexual behavior that is especially frequent, compulsive, or hurtful. Perhaps he views all homosexual behavior as hypersexual and abnormal. If so, he might perpetually feel inadequate regardless of his many accomplishments.

Mr. Pickering's sad mood, sexual behaviors, and almost all of his substance use do not appear to reach a threshold for a diagnosis. His possible ambivalence about his sexual orientation is also not a DSM-5 diagnosis. Mr. Pickering may be making a dramatic case for polydiagnoses in an effort to distract the interviewer from pursuing his lifelong experience of lonely sadness. It would be useful to explore these issues in future sessions. Even if Mr. Pickering's only DSM-5 diagnosis is a mild tobacco use disorder, he would still likely be an excellent candidate for psychotherapy.

Diagnosis

- Tobacco use disorder, mild

Suggested Readings

Goldsmith SJ: Oedipus or Orestes? Homosexual men, their mothers, and other women revisited. J Am Psychoanal Assoc 49(4):1269–1287, 2001

Levounis P, Drescher J, Barber ME: The LGBT Casebook. Washington DC, American Psychiatric Publishing, 2012

Lyonga F: Shades of homophobia: a framework for analyzing negative attitudes toward homosexuality. J Homosex 68(10):1664–1684, 2021

Subject Index

DSM-5-TR Diagnostic Categories are printed in **boldface** type. Entries for Clinical Cases by Diagnostic Categories are printed in *italics*. For detailed information on Clinical Cases of specific disorders and combinations of disorders, refer to the following **Clinical Case Index.**

Behavior. *See also* Aggression; Agitation;
    Apathy; Avoidance; Criminal behavior;
    Preoccupation; Repetitive behaviors;
    Shyness
    ADHD and, 79
    bipolar I disorder and postpartum
        changes in, 69–71
    clusters of symptoms and variations on
        normal, 251
    conduct disorder and, 260
    cyclothymic disorder and, 61
    disinhibited social engagement disorder
        and, 151–153
    disruptive mood dysregulation disorder
        and, 79
    mild neurocognitive disorder and
        disturbance of, 308–311
    schizophrenia and odd, 27–29
Behavioral addiction, and gambling
    disorder, 266
Benzodiazepines
    antisocial personality disorder and, 325
    catatonia and, 68
    delirium and, 291, 293, 294
    hypersomnolence disorder and, 236
    medication-induced anxiety disorder
        and, 130, 131
    sexual sadism disorder and generalized
        anxiety disorder, 350
Benzodiazepine use disorder, 338–341
Bereavement, and depressive disorders, 76,
    84–85.
    See also Grief
Binge eating, and bulimia nervosa, 221
Binge-eating disorder, 195, 209, 210,
    222–224
Biomarkers
    for alcohol withdrawal, 291
    for functional neurological symptom
        disorder, 201
Bipolar disorder. *See also* Bipolar I disorder;
    Bipolar II disorder
    antisocial personality disorder and, 325,
        326
    brief psychotic disorder and, 43
    cannabis-induced psychotic disorder
        and, 40–41
    cycles of depression and, 51–54
    delusional disorder and, 35
    disruptive mood dysregulation disorder
        and, 77

gambling disorder and, 284
major depressive disorder and, 82, 88,
    105, 106
panic attacks and, 120
schizophrenia and, 29
somatic symptom disorder and, 195
Bipolar I disorder
    cyclothymic disorder and development
        of, 62
    emotional disturbance and, 48–51
    postpartum behavior changes and,
        69–71
Bipolar II disorder
    binge-eating disorder and, 224
    cyclothymic disorder and development
        of, 62
    episodic depression in, 57–59
    hypomania in, 46
    preoccupation with suicide and, 54–56
    PTSD and, 160
Bipolar and related disorder due to HIV
    infection, 63–65
Bipolar and related disorders.
    See also Bipolar disorder; Bipolar I
        disorder; Bipolar II disorder;
        Cyclothymic disorder; Other specified
        bipolar and related disorder
    clinical cases of, 48–74
    overview of, 45–47
    suggested readings on, 47, 51, 54, 56–57,
        60, 62, 65, 69, 71, 74
Blood-injection-injury, and specific phobia,
    125
Bleuler, Eugen, 320
Body dysmorphic disorder (BDD), 22, 133,
    134, 141–143, 148
Body image, and anorexia nervosa, 217
Body mass index (BMI), and anorexia
    nervosa, 218
Borderline personality disorder
    antisocial personality disorder and, 326
    binge-eating disorder and, 224
    comorbidity with bipolar disorders, 56,
        62, 73
    histrionic personality disorder and, 332
    intermittent explosive disorder and, 263
Brief Assessment of Cognition in
    Schizophrenia, 26
Brief psychotic disorder, 22, 34, 41, 42–44
Brown Assessment of Beliefs Scale, 140
Bulimia nervosa, 210, 220–222, 223

Bullying
    antisocial personality disorder and, 325
    autism spectrum disorder and, 9
    conduct disorder and, 259, 260
    separation anxiety disorder with panic
        attacks and, 116
    social anxiety disorder and PTSD, 121,
        122
Buprenorphine, 278
Bupropion, 222, 248, 333
Burnout
    in medical professionals, 169–173
    classification as occupational
        phenomenon in ICD-11, 171
Buspirone, 248, 249

Cancer
    adjustment disorder and, 164–166
    steroid-induced bipolar and related
        disorder, 66, 67
Cannabis-induced psychotic disorder, 39–41
Cannabis use disorder, 36–38, 41, 190–192,
    280–282
Cataplexy, 230, 236
Catatonia
    diagnostic criteria for schizophrenia and,
        21–22
    in steroid-induced bipolar and related
        disorder, 66–68
Categorical model of personality disorders,
    314, 315
Cerebrovascular disease, and major
    neurocognitive disorder with Lewy
    bodies, 303
Chemotherapy, and steroid-induced bipolar
    and related disorder, 67, 68
Childhood abuse. See also Sexual abuse
    depersonalization/derealization disorder
        and, 181, 182
    persistent depressive disorder and, 93–94
Childhood-onset schizophrenia, 24, 25
Children. See also Adoption; Age; Childhood
    abuse; Developmental history;
    Parenting style
    anxiety and mood disorders in, 16
    autism spectrum disorder in, 7–9
    avoidant/restrictive food intake disorder
        and, 210, 214–216
    diagnostic thresholds for PTSD in, 150
    disinhibited social engagement disorder
        in, 151–153

disruptive, impulse-control, and conduct
    disorders in, 257–261
disruptive mood dysregulation disorder
    and ADHD in, 78–80
dissociative identity disorder in, 176
enuresis in, 226–228
gender reassignment and, 253, 254, 255
pica in, 211–213
provisional tic disorder and separation
    anxiety disorder in, 18–20
reactive attachment disorder in, 150
separation anxiety disorder with panic
    attacks in, 115–117
shyness in, 337
specific learning disorder and generalized
    anxiety disorder in, 14–17
temper tantrums and affective
    dysregulation in, 76–77
Childhood-onset fluency disorder, 2, 8, 9
Circadian rhythm sleep disorder, 233
Cirrhosis, and medication-induced anxiety
    disorder, 128–131
Citalopram, 93, 135
Clock drawing test, 305
Clomipramine, 248–249
Clonazepam, 51, 53–54, 109, 167, 196, 234, 236
Clozapine, 25, 37
Cocaine-induced depressive disorder, 266
Cocaine use disorder, 97–99, 271–273,
    354–357
Cognitive-behavioral therapy
    for adjustment disorder, 167
    for generalized anxiety disorder, 127
    for narcissistic personality disorder, 333
    for OCD, 138
Cognitive functioning
    alcohol use disorder and medication-
        induced anxiety disorder, 130–131
    delirium and long-term decline in, 287
    depressive disorder due to another
        medical condition and rapid eye
        movement sleep behavior disorder,
        100, 102
    major depressive disorder and mild
        neurocognitive disorder, 297
    major neurocognitive disorder due to
        Alzheimer's disease and, 295, 296
    major neurocognitive disorder with
        Lewy bodies and, 301, 302
    mild neurocognitive disorder due to
        traumatic brain injury and, 310

Cognitive functioning *(continued)*
   reactions to trauma and, 155
   schizophrenia and, 25, 26, 28
   somatic symptom disorder and, 194
Collateral information, and schizotypal
    personality disorder with paranoid
    personality disorder, 322
Columbia Suicide Severity Rating Scale, 167
Communication disorders, 8–9
Comorbidity, of diagnoses.
   See also specific disorders
   ADHD and, 13
   anxiety disorders and, 9, 113, 115, 125
   bipolar disorders and, 56, 59, 73
   borderline personality disorder and,
    328–329
   cocaine use disorder and, 273
   dependent personality disorder and, 340
   disinhibited social engagement disorder
    and, 153
   disruptive, impulse-control, and conduct
    disorders and, 257, 260, 263–264
   disruptive mood dysregulation disorder
    and, 80
   enuresis and, 228
   feeding and eating disorders and, 210,
    212, 224
   gambling disorder and, 284
   histrionic personality disorder and, 332
   obsessive-compulsive personality
    disorder and, 342–343
   panic disorder and, 120
   paranoid personality disorder and, 317
   premenstrual dysphoric disorder and, 96
   PTSD and, 31, 160
   schizophrenia and, 31
   somatic symptom disorders and, 189, 197
   specific learning disorder and, 13
   trauma- and stressor-related disorders
    and, 150
Compulsions, and obsessive-compulsive
    disorder, 133, 136–137, 139, 343
"Conditions for Further Study" (chapter in
   DSM-5/DSM-5-TR Section III)
   attenuated psychosis syndrome in, 23, 324
   nonsuicidal self-injury disorder in, 168
   persistent complex bereavement disorder
    in DSM-5, 76, 85, 149, 171
   suicidal behavior disorder in, 168–169
Conduct disorder, 228, 258, 259–261, 326, 356
Confusion, and delirium, 292–294

Constipation, and pica, 211, 212
Contamination, phobias of, 42, 136
Conversion disorder. *See* Functional
   neurological symptom disorder
Coping skills
   adjustment disorder and, 167
   depressive disorder and rapid eye
    movement sleep behavior disorder,
    102
   gambling disorder and, 284
   psychological factors affecting other
    medical conditions and, 206
Core Cultural Formulation Interview
   (DSM-5-TR), 11, 91, 185
Countertransference.
   See also Therapeutic alliance
   avoidant personality disorder and social
    anxiety disorder and, 336
   factitious disorder and, 203
Couples therapy, 245, 247, 341
COVID-19 pandemic, 43, 135, 138, 139, 170,
   358
Craving, in opioid use disorder, 274, 275, 277
Creatine phosphokinase (CPK), and steroid-
   induced bipolar and related disorder,
   66, 67, 68
Criminal behavior. *See also* Police; Theft
   conduct disorder and, 259
   paraphilic disorders and, 346, 354–357
Crohn's disease, and factitious disorder,
   201–204
Culture. *See also* African Americans; Ethnic
   minorities; Hispanic Americans
   anorexia nervosa and, 217, 218–219
   anxiety and sexual orientation, 11, 12, 13
   dissociative identity disorder and
    "possession," 175–176
   emotional expression and, 332
   gambling disorder and, 283, 284–285
   illness anxiety disorder and, 198
   importance of in DSM-5-TR, 114, 150, 185,
    198, 313–315, 347
   major depressive disorder and prolonged
    grief disorder and, 172
   other specified depressive disorder in
    refugee and, 109–111
   other specified dissociative disorder and,
    185
   psychological factors affecting other
    medical conditions and, 207
   restless legs syndrome and, 240–242

Dexmethylphenidate, 259
Diabetes, and restless legs syndrome, 240
Diagnosis. *See also* Comorbidity; Differential
    diagnosis; Distress; DSM-5; DSM-5-TR;
    Duration; Misdiagnosis; Other specified
    diagnosis; Specifiers; Symptoms;
    Underdiagnosis; *specific disorders*
    of bipolar I and II disorders, 59
    of catatonia, 68
    complicating factors for bipolar and
        related disorders, 45
    conduct disorder and evolution of over
        time, 261
    of dementia in DSM-5, 296
    documentation of in clinical chart, 340
    importance of accurate for bipolar and
        related disorders, 47
    of major depressive disorder, 75–76
    medical illness and inclusive approach to
        depression, 130
    psychotic disorders with atypical or
        incomplete presentations, 23
    threshold for DSM-5, 361
    of "unspecified schizophrenia spectrum
        and other psychotic disorder," 49
Dialysis, and restless legs syndrome, 240, 241
Diary, sleep-wake, 232
Diazepam, 277, 278
Differential Aptitude Tests (DAT), 309
Differential diagnosis
    of autism spectrum disorder, 5
    of avoidant/restrictive food intake
        disorder, 215–216
    bipolar disorder and "mixed features," 53
    of brief psychotic disorder, 43
    of cyclothymic disorder, 62
    of factitious disorder, 201
    of functional neurological symptom
        disorder, 200
    of major depressive disorder and mild
        neurocognitive disorder, 299
    of major neurocognitive disorder due to
        Alzheimer's disease, 296
    of neurodevelopmental disorders, 3
    of opioid use disorder, 275
    of other specified bipolar and related
        disorder, 73
    of pica, 212
    of psychological factors affecting other
        medical conditions, 206
    of schizophrenia, 29

of schizophreniform disorder, 30–31, 32
of separation anxiety disorder, 117
temper tantrums and, 79
Dimensional (versus categorical)
    conceptualization
    of personality traits, 313–315, 329, 343
    of schizophrenia, 28, 29
Diphenhydramine, 48
Disinhibited social engagement disorder
    (DSED), 150, 151–153
**Disruptive, impulse-control, and conduct
    disorders.**
    See also Antisocial personality disorder;
    Conduct disorder; Intermittent
    explosive disorder; Oppositional
    defiant disorder
    clinical cases of, 259–264
    overview of, 257–258
    suggested readings on, 258, 261, 264
Disruptive mood dysregulation disorder
    (DMDD), 77, 78–80, 228
Dissociative amnesia, 176, 177–179, 182
Dissociative disorders.
    See also Depersonalization/
    derealization disorder; Dissociative
    amnesia; Dissociative fugue;
    Dissociative identity disorder; Other
    specified dissociative disorder
    clinical cases of, 177–185
    overview of, 175–176
    suggested readings on, 176, 180, 183,
        185–186
Dissociative fugue, 179
Dissociative identity disorder (DID), 175–176,
    179, 182
Distractibility, in bipolar and related
    disorders, 45, 70, 105
Distress, and impairment as requirements
    for diagnosis
    in avoidant/restrictive food intake
        disorder, 210
    in bipolar II disorder, 55
    in enuresis, 228
    in fetishistic disorder, 353
    in gender dysphoria, 255
    in hoarding disorder, 145
    in OCD, 137
    in paraphilic disorders, 346, 348, 359
    in substance-related and addictive
        disorders, 265
    in trichotillomania, 148

Hip fracture, and unspecified delirium, 289–291

Hispanic Americans, clinical cases involving. *See also* Culture
  borderline personality disorder, 327–329
  gambling disorder, 283–285
  histrionic personality disorder, 330–332
  major depressive disorder with peripartum onset, 81–83
  obstructive sleep apnea hypopnea, 237–239
  other specified dissociative disorder, 183–185

Histrionic personality disorder, 326, 330–332

HIV-associated neurocognitive disorder, 65

HIV infection
  bipolar and related disorder due to, 63–65
  cocaine use disorder and, 272

Hoarding disorder, 134, 144–146, 321, 343

Home visits, and diagnosis of hoarding disorder, 145

Hormone therapy, gender-affirming, 254

Huntington's disease, neurocognitive disorder due to, 304–307

Hybrid categorical-dimensional model of personality disorders, 313–315

Hydrochlorothiazide, 297

Hydrocodone/acetaminophen, 109, 274

Hyperactivity
  in ADHD, 2
  in major depressive disorder with mixed features, 105

Hyperarousal, and fear as symptom of anxiety, 113.
  See also Arousal

Hypersexuality
  in hypomanic episodes of bipolar II disorder, 58
  in manic episodes of bipolar and related disorder due to HIV infection, 63, 64

Hypersomnolence disorder, 234–236

Hypertension, and sexual dysfunction, 249

Hypochondriasis (DSM-IV diagnosis), 187, 188, 196–197.
  See also Illness anxiety disorder

Hypocretin deficiency, and DSM-5 diagnostic criteria for narcolepsy, 230, 236

Hypomanic episode. *See also* Manic episode
  as characteristic of bipolar disorders, 45
  cyclothymic disorder and, 62
  depressive symptoms of bipolar II disorder and, 55, 59

major depressive disorder with mixed features and, 104–105
other specified bipolar and related disorder and, 73
requirements for diagnosis of, 46

Hypoxemia, and anxiety, 165

ICD. *See International Classification of Diseases*

Identity. *See also* Self
  borderline personality disorder and, 329
  dissociative disorders and, 176, 179
  gender and, 252
  schizophreniform disorder and, 32

Illness anxiety disorder
  DSM-5 approach to diagnosis of, 187–188
  OCD and, 139–140
  panic disorder and, 119, 195–198
  psychological factors affecting other medical conditions and, 206
  separation anxiety disorder and, 117

Impairment, as requirement for diagnosis. *See* Distress

Impulsivity
  in ADHD, 2
  in disruptive, impulse-control, and conduct disorders, 257
  in major depressive disorder with mixed features, 105

Inattention. *See* Attention

Insight. *See also* "Absent insight/delusional beliefs" specifier
  antisocial personality disorder and, 325
  body dysmorphic disorder and, 142
  brief psychotic disorder and, 43
  conduct disorder and, 260
  hoarding disorder and, 145
  OCD and, 134, 137

Insomnia. *See also* Insomnia disorder
  in ADHD, 10
  cocaine use disorder and, 98
  grief and, 84
  major depressive disorder with mixed features and, 105
  other specified depressive disorder and, 109–111
  substance-induced depressive disorder and, 98

Insomnia disorder, 229, 231–233

Insomnia Severity Index (ISI), 232

Insurance, and documentation of diagnosis in clinical chart, 340

illness anxiety disorder and, 196, 197
and reactions to trauma, 154
schizoaffective disorder and, 36
Panic disorder. *See also* Panic attacks
alcohol use disorder and medication-
induced anxiety disorder, 130
illness anxiety disorder and, 195–198
neurodevelopmental disorders and, 10–14
panic attacks and diagnosis of, 113–114,
118–120
schizoaffective disorder and, 37
separation anxiety disorder and, 117
Paranoia
bipolar II disorder and, 55
cannabis-induced psychotic disorder
and, 39, 40
mild neurocognitive disorder and
psychotic disorder due to
Huntington's disease, 304–307
Paranoid personality disorder, 316–318,
322–324, 326
Paraphilic disorders.
See also Fetishistic disorder;
Pedophilic disorder; Sexual sadism
disorder
clinical cases of, 348–361
overview of, 345–348
suggested readings on, 348, 351, 354, 357,
361
Parenting style
separation anxiety disorder and, 117
social anxiety disorder in adolescents
and, 123
Parent-Rated Anxiety Scale for Autism
Spectrum Disorder (PRAS-ASD), 9
Parkinsonian symptoms, and major
neurocognitive disorder with Lewy
bodies, 302
Parkinson's disease, 99–102, 299, 303, 305
Paroxetine, 331
Partial hospitalization, and disruptive mood
dysregulation disorder, 78, 79
Party and play (PNP) subculture, and
substance abuse, 272, 273
Patient Health Questionnaire 9-item
depression scale (PHQ-9), 232–233
Patient history.
See also Developmental history;
Family history; *specific disorders*
diagnosis of bipolar and related disorders
and, 45–46, 47

disruptive, impulse-control, and conduct
disorders and, 258
Pedophilic disorder, 346, 347, 348, 354–357
Penile plethysmography, 355, 356
Perceptual disturbances, and substance-
related and addictive disorders, 265
Perfectionism, and obsessive-compulsive
personality disorder, 317, 343
Peripartum onset, of bipolar I disorder,
69–71
Peripheral neuropathy, and restless legs
syndrome, 241
Persecutory delusions, and delusional
disorder, 34
Persistent (chronic) motor or vocal tic
disorder, 19
Persistent complex bereavement disorder (in
DSM-5 chapter "Conditions for Further
Study"), 76, 85, 149, 171.
See also Prolonged grief disorder
Persistent depressive disorder, 92–94, 108,
111, 171, 328–329
and bipolar disorder, 52, 53
parallelism with cyclothymic disorder, 43
Personality changes
after military deployment, 159
after traumatic brain injury, 310
Personality disorders.
See also Antisocial personality disorder;
Avoidant personality disorder;
Borderline personality disorder;
Dependent personality disorder;
Histrionic personality disorder;
Narcissistic personality disorder;
Obsessive-compulsive personality
disorder; Paranoid personality
disorder; Personality traits; Schizoid
personality disorder; Schizotypal
personality disorder
Alternative DSM-5 Model for Personality
Disorders, 313–315, **315**, 329, 343
bipolar disorder and comorbidity with,
73
clinical cases of, 316–343
intermittent explosive disorder and, 263
"micropsychoses" and, 43
overview of, 313–315
suggested readings on, 315, 318, 321, 324,
327, 330, 332, 335, 338, 341, 343
Personality disorder not otherwise specified
(DSM-IV diagnosis), 315

Personality traits
   dimensional conceptualization of, 313–315
   Five Factor Model of, 314
   associated with anxiety disorders, 114, 119
   in persistent depressive disorder, 93–94
   problematic responses to medical care
      and, 206
Pervasive developmental disorder not
      otherwise specified (DSM-IV diagnosis),
      1, 8
Physical examination
   alcohol withdrawal and, 270
   bipolar I disorder and, 49
   hypersomnolence disorder and, 235
   major depressive disorder and, 87, 88
   obstructive sleep apnea hypopnea and, 237
   pica and, 212
   schizophreniform disorder and, 30
   steroid-induced bipolar and related
      disorder, 66–67
Pica, 210, 211–213
Pittsburgh Sleep Quality Inventory (PSQI),
   232
Police. See also Criminal behavior
   bipolar disorder case and, 48
   delirium case and, 292
   pedophilic disorder and, 354
   schizophrenia cases and, 24, 27
   violence against Black men by, 280, 282
Polysomnography, and sleep disorders, 102,
   230, 235, 236, 238, 239
Positive symptoms, of schizophrenia, 22, 26
Postpartum period
   bipolar I disorder and, 69–71
   major depressive disorder and, 81–83
   somatic symptom disorder and
      depression in, 193, 195
Posttransition, as specifier for gender
   dysphoria, 255
Posttraumatic amnesia, 308–311
Posttraumatic stress disorder (PTSD)
   adjustment disorder with anxiety and,
      282
   characterization of, 149
   comorbidity with schizophrenia, 31
   dissociative amnesia and, 177–179
   female sexual interest/arousal disorder
      and, 246
   opioid use disorder and, 275
   requirement for diagnosis of, 149–150
   schizophreniform disorder and, 30, 32

social anxiety disorder in adolescents
      and, 121–123
   somatic symptom disorder and, 189
   temper in older adult and, 158–161
Prednisone, 46, 128, 129
Pre-exposure prophylaxis (PrEP) regimen,
   and HIV, 272
Pregnancy
   bipolar I disorder with psychotic features
      and, 69–71
   major depressive disorder with
      peripartum onset and, 81
   pica and, 210
   restless legs syndrome and, 241
Premature (early) ejaculation, 244
Premenstrual depression, 193
Premenstrual dysphoric disorder (PMDD),
   77, 94–96
Premenstrual syndrome (PMS), 94, 95, 96
Prevalence
   of brief psychotic disorder, 44
   of generalized anxiety disorder, 127
   of obstructive sleep apnea hypopnea, 238
   of other specified dissociative disorder, 185
Primary care clinics, and somatic symptom
      disorder, 190, 191
Primary nocturnal enuresis, 228
Prodrome/prodromal phase
   of schizophrenia, 318
   of schizophreniform disorder, 31–32
Prolonged grief disorder (new DSM-5-TR
      diagnosis), 76, 85–86, 149, 150, 169–173
Propranolol, 248, 249
Provisional diagnosis
   of "atypical migraine variant," 193
   of generalized anxiety disorder, 351
   of major depressive disorder and
      prolonged grief disorder, 172
   of premenstrual dysphoric disorder, 96
   of schizophreniform disorder, 22, 32
Provisional tic disorder, 18–20
Pseudocyesis, 188, 189
Pseudodementia, 299
Psychogenic nonepileptic seizure, 189
Psychological factors affecting other medical
      conditions (PFAOMC), 166, 187–188,
      204–207
Psychosis. See also Psychotic depression;
      Psychotic disorder due to Huntington's
      disease; Schizophrenia spectrum and
      other psychotic disorders

cannabis-induced psychotic disorder
and, 39–41
major depressive disorder and, 88
pedophilic disorder and, 355–356
postpartum period and, 69–71
schizoaffective disorder and, 36–38
Psychosomatic, misuse of term, 241
Psychotherapy. *See also* Cognitive-
behavioral therapy; Couples therapy;
Supportive psychotherapy
bipolar II disorder and, 58
separation anxiety disorder and, 116
tobacco use disorder and, 361
"Psychotic depression," and restless legs
syndrome, 241
Psychotic Depression Assessment Scale
(PDAS), 87
Psychotic disorder due to Huntington's
disease, 304–307
PTSD Checklist for DSM-5, 30

Quality of life, and obstructive sleep apnea
hypopnea, 239
Quetiapine, 103, 259, 333

Rapid cycling, in bipolar mania, 53–54
Rapid eye movement (REM) sleep disorder,
99–102, 230, 302, 303
Reactive attachment disorder (RAD), 150, 152
Reality testing
in bipolar II disorder, 55
in borderline personality disorder, 329
Reference, delusions of
body dysmorphic disorder and, 142
delusional disorder and, 34
schizophreniform disorder and, 31
Religion
anorexia nervosa and, 217
bipolar I disorder and delusions related
to, 69
bipolar and related disorder due to HIV
infection and, 63–65
schizophreniform disorder and, 29–32
Repetitive behaviors
autism spectrum disorder and, 8, 9
body dysmorphic disorder and, 133, 142
OCD and, 137
Respiratory distress, and psychological
factors affecting other medical
conditions, 204–207
Restless legs syndrome, 230, 240–242

Restricting subtype, of anorexia nervosa, 219
Risperidone, 39, 355
Rumination disorder, 210

Sadness. *See also* Depression
cyclothymic disorder and, 60–62
depressive symptoms and, 75
dissociative amnesia and, 177–179
grief and, 84
major depressive disorder with
peripartum onset and, 81–83
schizoaffective disorder and, 36–38
Sadomasochism, and sexual sadism
disorder, 348–351
Safety, and bipolar I disorder, 49.
See also Self-harm; Suicide
Schizoaffective disorder
bipolar I disorder and, 49, 50
delusional disorder and, 35
depression and psychosis, 36–38
pedophilic disorder and, 356
schizophrenia and, 29
Schizoid personality disorder, 319–321
Schizophrenia
antisocial personality disorder and, 326
behavioral symptoms of, 27–29
catatonia and, 21–22, 67
diagnostic criteria for, 22
emotional disturbance and, 24–26
obsessive-compulsive personality
disorder and, 314
overdiagnosis of in African Americans,
50
paranoid personality disorder and
obsessive-compulsive personality
disorder, 318
as prototypical psychotic disorder, 21
PTSD and, 31
schizotypal personality disorder and
paranoid personality disorder, 323
Schizophrenia spectrum and other
psychotic disorders.
See also Brief psychotic disorder;
Delusional disorder; Psychosis;
Schizoaffective disorder;Schizophrenia;
Schizophreniform disorder
clinical cases of, 24–44
overview of, 21–23
schizotypal personality disorder and, 317
suggested readings on, 23, 26, 29, 32–33,
35, 38, 41, 44

rapid eye movement sleep behavior disorder and, 99–102

specific learning disorder and generalized anxiety disorder, 15

Sleep-wake disorders.
See also Hypersomnolence disorder; Insomnia; Insomnia disorder; Narcolepsy; Obstructive sleep apnea hypopnea; Restless legs syndrome
clinical cases of, 231–242
overview of, 229–230
suggested readings on, 230, 233, 236, 239, 242

Snoring, and obstructive sleep apnea hypopnea, 238

Social anxiety disorder, 16, 117, 143, 234–236, 336–338

Social phobia. *See* Social anxiety disorder

Social (pragmatic) communication disorder, 2, 9

Social interactions.
See also Interpersonal relationships
autism spectrum disorder and, 8
avoidant personality disorder and social anxiety disorder, 336–337
cyclothymic disorder and, 61
grief and withdrawal from, 84
major neurocognitive disorder and withdrawal from, 294–297
schizoid personality disorder and isolation, 319–321
schizotypal personality disorder and withdrawal from, 323

Social media, 280, 328

Somatic symptom disorder, 119, 190–192, 192–195, 206, 276

Somatic symptom and related disorders.
See also Factitious disorder; Functional neurological symptom disorder; Illness anxiety disorder; Psychological factors affecting other medical conditions; Somatic symptom disorder
clinical cases of, 190–207
histrionic personality disorder and, 332
overview of, 187–189
suggested readings on, 189, 192, 195, 198, 201, 204, 207

Specific learning disorder, 2, 10–17

Specific phobia, 124–125

Specifiers. *See also* Severity
for ADHD, 2

for adjustment disorder, 150
for autism spectrum disorder, 9
for anxiety disorders, 113–114, 117, 119
for bipolar and related disorders, 50, 67, 71, 76, 105
for conduct disorder, 258, 260, 261
for depressive disorder due to another medical condition, 101–102
for depressive disorders, 76, 82, 90, 93
dissociative fugue as, 176
for gender dysphoria, 255
for major neurocognitive disorder, 310
for obsessive-compulsive and related disorders, 133–134, 137, 139, 140, 142, 145
panic attacks as, 113–114, 117, 119
for schizophrenia, 28
for sexual sadism disorder, 351
for somatic symptom and related disorders, 188, 191, 200
for specific learning disorder, 2
for specific phobia, 125
for substance-related and addictive disorders, 265, 271

Speech patterns. *See also* Mutism
disorganized, as criterion for schizophrenia, 22, 25
in hypomanic or manic episodes, 45, 50, 52, 55, 57–58, 63, 69–70
in depression, 52, 81–82, 107, 110

Speech sound disorder, 2, 9

Startle response, and acute stress disorder, 158

Stereotype, of gay subculture, 273

Stereotypy, and steroid-induced bipolar and related disorder, 67

Steroids, and body dysmorphic disorder, 143. *See also* Prednisone

Steroid-induced bipolar and related disorder, 66–68

"Steroid psychosis," 46

Stigma
documentation of diagnosis in clinical chart and, 340
mental health care in African American culture and, 90

Stimulant-induced mania, 64

Stimulant use disorder, 272

Stress. *See also* Acute stress disorder; Trauma- and stressor-related disorders
adjustment disorder with anxiety and, 280–282

suicidal behavior disorder, 168–169

Supportive psychotherapy
  for OCD and major depressive disorder,
    135
  for persistent depressive disorder and,
    93

Symmetry preoccupation, and body
  dysmorphic disorder, 143

Symptoms.
  See also Behavior; Diagnosis; Duration;
    Emotional features; Negative
    symptoms; Positive symptoms;
    specific disorders
  of acute stress disorder, 155–156
  of alcohol withdrawal, 270
  of bipolar disorders, 45
  of borderline personality disorder, 328
  cannabis-induced psychosis and rapid
    resolution of, 40
  depression as, 75
  of factitious disorder, 204
  of major depressive disorder, 88
  PTSD and categories of, 160
  schizophrenia and requirements for
    diagnosis, 21, 25, 28
  of substance abuse, 266
  of trauma- and stressor-related disorders,
    150

System for Assessment and Group
  Evaluation (SAGE), 309

Telehealth system, and obsessive-
  compulsive disorder, 139

Temper tantrums
  affective dysregulation in children and,
    76
  autism spectrum disorder and, 7–9
  differential diagnosis of age-incongruent,
    79
  enuresis and, 226–228
  PTSD and, 158–161

Theft. *See also* Criminal behavior
  antisocial personality disorder and, 325
  conduct disorder and, 259
  opioid use disorder and, 277, 278

Therapeutic alliance.
  See also Countertransference
  avoidant personality disorder and social
    anxiety disorder, 336–338
  narcissistic personality disorder and,
    333

"Three windows approach" (Bancroft) to
  assessment of sexual dysfunctions, 247

Tics, as specifier for obsessive-compulsive
  disorder, 139, 140

Tic disorders, 2–3, 137.
  See also Provisional tic disorder

Tobacco use disorder, 274–276, 358–361

Tourette's disorder, 3, 19

Toxicology screen
  bipolar and related disorder due to HIV
    infection and, 65
  cyclothymic disorder and, 62

Trail Making Test, 100, 129, 131

Transgender, nonbinary, agender, and other
  individuals. *See also* Lesbian, gay,
    bisexual, transgender, queer, and
    gender minority individuals
  gender dysphoria and, 252, 254–255
  sexual dysfunctions in, 244

Transvestism, and fetishistic disorder, 353

Trauma.
  See also Posttraumatic stress disorder
  adjustment disorder with anxiety and,
    280
  evaluation of in adolescents, 123
  normative stress reaction compared to
    acute stress disorder, 154–156
  psychotic disorders and, 31
  rates of schizophrenia and, 22

Traumatic brain injury
  acute stress disorder and, 156
  cognitive decline and, 288
  mild neurocognitive disorder due to,
    308–311

Trauma- and stressor-related disorders.
  See also Acute stress disorder;
    Adjustment disorder; Disinhibited
    social engagement disorder;
    Posttraumatic stress disorder;
    Prolonged grief disorder
  clinical cases of, 151–173
  overview of, 149–150
  suggested readings on, 150–151, 153, 156,
    158, 161, 163–164, 166, 169, 173

Trichotillomania, 134, 146–148

Tricyclic antidepressants, 249, 293, 294

"Trigger points," and intermittent explosive
  disorder, 263

"Tri-morbidity," of somatic symptom
  disorder, depressive disorders, and
  substance use disorders, 191

Clinical Case Index

This index is a guide to the Clinical Cases of specific disorders. Disorders are listed under Diagnostic Categories, which are printed in **boldface** type. More detailed information on specific topics can be found in the **Subject Index.**

387